Practical Manual of Vitreoretinal Surgery

Ahmed B. Sallam • Ferenc Kuhn
Giampaolo Gini • Ron A. Adelman
Editors

Practical Manual of Vitreoretinal Surgery

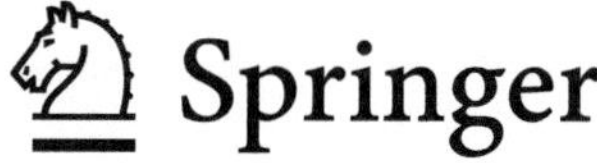

Editors
Ahmed B. Sallam
Jones Eye Institute
University of Arkansas for Medical Science
Little Rock, AR, USA

Giampaolo Gini
Department of Ophthalmology
University Hospitals Sussex NHS
Foundation Trust
Worthing, West Sussex, UK

Ferenc Kuhn
Helen Keller Foundation for Research and
Education
Birmingham, AL, USA

Department of Ophthalmology
University of Pécs Medical School
Pécs, Hungary

Department of Ophthalmology
University of Halle
Halle, Germany

Ron A. Adelman
Department of Ophthalmology
Mayo Clinic
Jacksonville, FL, USA

Ophthalmology and Visual Science
Yale University School of Medicine
New Haven, CT, USA

ISBN 978-3-031-47829-1   ISBN 978-3-031-47827-7   (eBook)
https://doi.org/10.1007/978-3-031-47827-7

This Springer imprint is published by the registered company Springer Nature Switzerland AG
The registered company address is: Gewerbestrasse 11, 6330 Cham, Switzerland

If disposing of this product, please recycle the paper.

Foreword

The topic of this book needs no introduction. Vitreous surgery has been at the forefront of ophthalmic procedures for more than 50 years. Retinal diseases are an important cause of ocular morbidity and visual impairment globally. Population-based studies have reported the prevalence of retinal disorders ranging from 5.35% to 21.02% at age 40 years and above. In developed countries, retinal diseases are the most common cause of irreversible blindness. Nevertheless, advances in surgical repair of retinal detachments, and macular diseases, including small-incision surgery, use of perfluorocarbon liquids, and silicone oil and gas tamponade, have made treatment very effective and visual recovery possible in many cases. Despite these advances, retinal diseases continue to be a leading public health issue that will grow in importance as the population increases and life expectancy is extended worldwide. Not to mention the prevalence of trauma in young males worldwide that frequently affects the retina and requires vitreoretinal surgery.

Many contributed to the development of vitreoretinal surgery, and the history of vitreoretinal surgery is beyond the scope of this "Foreword." However, I cannot avoid mentioning Robert Machemer, better known as the "Father of Modern Vitreoretinal surgery," who devised VISC (vitrectomy, infusion, suction, cutter) with Jean Marie Parel at Bascom Palmer in Miami, USA. After experimenting and succeeding in removing the egg albumin through the motorized instrument via 17-gauge ports, in order to improve the visibility, he later added a fiber optic light pipe for endoillumination. In 1970, he obtained good results in cases of vitreous hemorrhage and poor results in a case of proliferative vitreoretinopathy. Significant advances have taken place during the last 50+ years.

For these reasons, the appearance of this *Practical Manual of Vitreoretinal Surgery* edited by Drs. Ahmed Sallam, Ferenc Kuhn, Giampaolo Gini, and Ron Adelman to help ophthalmologists learn the newest techniques on vitreoretinal surgery is a wonderful gift to us all and our patients. The book has been beautifully illustrated and divided into 34 masterful chapters including important topics such as applied anatomy and physiology, preoperative evaluation of vitreoretinal surgery patients, vitreoretinal anesthesia, pars plana vitrectomy set up, vitreous substitutes, vitreous hemorrhage and opacities, retinal breaks and pneumatic retinopexy, pars plana vitrectomy for primary retinal detachment, scleral buckle surgery, giant retinal tear detachment, proliferative vitreoretinopathy detachment, retinoschisis, epiretinal membrane and vitreomacular traction, surgical management of lamellar macular hole, surgical management of macular holes, optic pit maculopathy, myopic traction maculopathy, diabetic delamination surgery, sickle cell retinopathy surgery, subretinal and suprachoroidal hemorrhage, uveoscleral effusion, choroidal patch graft, vitreoretinal surgery and pressure-dependent optic neuropathy, vitreoretinal surgery for anterior segment complications, vitreoretinal surgery in uveitis, vitreoretinal surgery in endophthalmitis, vitreoretinal surgery in trauma, vitreoretinal surgery in pediatrics, vitreoretinal surgery for ocular tumors, three-dimensional retina surgery, vitrectomy in the presence of corneal opacity, and cataract surgery and vitreoretinal surgery. With 177 color images, 123 videos, and 61 authors from 21 countries, this *Practical Manual of Vitreoretinal Surgery* is a must read for anyone interested in Vitreoretinal Surgery and helping our patients.

Contributors to this book are both educators and practitioners. There was no way for them to have developed these techniques and expertise except by performing them themselves. Their accumulated knowledge is the result of tremendous clinical and academic effort, and their expertise flows to the reader with the hope that individual lives will benefit. In bringing their work to press, Drs. Ahmed Sallam, Ferenc Kuhn, Giampaolo Gini, and Ron Adelman have done a great service to patients living with vitreoretinal diseases and to the doctors caring for them. Those who will read and study this *Practical Manual of Vitreoretinal Surgery* have already demonstrated that they care for their patients and that they want to learn. We now just need to move forward together to give our patients the gift of sight.

Retina Division, Department of Ophthalmology,   J. Fernando Arevalo
Johns Hopkins Bayview Medical Center
Wilmer Eye Institute,
The Johns Hopkins University School of Medicine,
Baltimore, MD, USA

Preface

We are pleased to present our book on retina surgery—*Practical Manual of Vitreoretinal Surgery.*

The purpose of this book is to impart clinical and surgical skills to retina surgeons and provide invaluable insights and recommendations from experienced practitioners in the field. Our aim is to deliver the fundamentals of retina surgery in a clear and practical manner, emphasizing efficient and straightforward approaches. By simplifying surgical procedures, we hope to instill confidence in new surgeons, minimize the risk of errors, and enhance the proficiency of experienced surgeons. One of our main focuses is to provide the easiest and "no faff about ways" for doing surgery. Throughout our journey, we have discovered that the saying "less is more" holds true for vitreoretinal surgery, and in many cases, it is indeed the best approach!

In these 34 chapters, we have endeavored to cover all aspects of retina surgery, spanning preoperative care, surgical planning, intraoperative techniques, and postoperative management. We delved into the most frequently encountered conditions, such as primary retinal detachment and macular hole, as well as the most complex surgery, including advanced diabetic surgery and pediatric retinal surgery. Each chapter presents a step-by-step methodology for various techniques, accompanied by valuable pearls of wisdom and clinical scenarios to help guide clinical decisions. Additionally, we provide insights into the latest technologies and advancements in retina surgery, including surgical endoscopy and 3D surgery.

We hope this book serves as a convenient guide and indispensable resource for new retina surgeons as they learn the basics of the field, as well as an aid for experienced surgeons who are looking for new tips and tricks to refine their surgical skills and make their surgery both "smoother" and "slicker!" We hope that it will serve as a helpful companion to all readers throughout their journey in retina surgery.

We have asked the most experienced and knowledgeable retina surgeons from all over the world to write the book chapters, but we also paid attention to editing the book to avoid the inclusion of contradicting statements. We would like to express our greatest appreciation to each author who contributed to this book. Their effort, time, and dedication made it possible for this book to reach publication, and we owe them a great debt of gratitude. We are privileged to have had the opportunity to collaborate with these distinguished scholars and outstanding teachers.

Our heartfelt thanks extend to the professional team at Springer for their invaluable assistance and guidance in bringing this book to fruition.

Surgical techniques continually evolve as various surgeons adapt and refine them over time. In this book, the editors and contributors share the techniques that have proven effective in their hands. Due to space constraints and the frequently unclear origins of many technical modifications in surgical techniques, which are traditionally passed from one surgeon to another, this book is lightly referenced. We acknowledge our teachers, innovators, and thought leaders for teaching us vitreoretinal surgery and sharing their knowledge. Without them, this book would not have been possible.

We are truly excited about the prospect of sharing our knowledge and experience with the readers, and we hope that, like us, you will continue to enjoy the fascinating world of retina surgery.

Sincerely,

Little Rock, AR, USA

Ahmed B. Sallam

Little Rock, AR, USA   Ahmed B. Sallam
Birmingham, AL, USA   Ferenc Kuhn
Worthing, West Sussex, UK   Giampaolo Gini
New Haven, CT, USA   Ron A. Adelman

Preface

Books, like people, have different destinies. Many eventually end up making a beautiful display of themselves in a book case only to be used as an occasional reference. This book is certainly not one of them. It is a practical compendium born from the experience of thousands of hours spent in the operating theater by some of the best surgeons in the world. The book covers all major vitreoretinal scenarios. Each chapter aims to give simple guidelines to address even the more complex issues. This is done in an easy-to-read, straight-to-the-point format, which is meant to prevent the surgeon from getting into trouble or getting him/her out of it as best and as quickly as possible. We as Editors believe this book should be a faithful, everyday companion to have in the doctor's debriefing room. Something to rely on as well as something which will stimulate further discussion. If one day we should venture into an operating theater and find a copy of the book with its pages wrinkled, dog-eared, and perhaps having a few coffee stains here and there, we will know we have been successful.

President of the European VitreoRetinal Society　　　　　　Giampaolo Gini

Acknowledgments

I have nurtured the idea of editing a manual on vitreoretinal surgery for a long time. While there exist numerous outstanding textbooks on the subject, to the best of my knowledge, there is currently no contemporary book that serves as a concise and handy manual that presents the information in a concise and practical manner, making it easily accessible for practitioners.

It was during one of the European Vitreoretinal Society Meetings 2 years ago that I had the opportunity to discuss the idea with my esteemed colleagues and dear friends, Drs. Ferenc Kuhn, Giampaolo Gini, and Ron Adelman. Their enthusiasm and eagerness to collaborate on this project were evident from the start. Bringing this project to fruition required extensive planning and a tremendous amount of teamwork.

I am indebted to all the contributing authors for generously sharing their knowledge, insights, and expertise, as well as for providing us with their invaluable videos and photographs.

Additionally, I would like to express my gratitude to the publisher, Springer, for their professional guidance throughout the entire process.

The assistance provided by my exceptional residents and fellows, particularly Drs. Riley Sanders and Zia Siddiqui, deserves special recognition. Their invaluable contributions in editing the videos and offering excellent suggestions for the writing played an instrumental role in shaping this manual.

Last but certainly not least, I want to extend my heartfelt thanks to my beloved wife, Sherin, and my children (and young friends), Abdel, Farida, and Amina. Their constant love, encouragement, and understanding have been the cornerstone of my journey. I am deeply grateful for their unwavering support, which allowed me the necessary time and space to dedicate myself to the creation of this book.

Ahmed B. Sallam

Contents

Applied Anatomy for the Vitreoretinal Surgeon

Abdelrahman M. Elhusseiny, Yousef Ahmed Fouad, Ahmed M. Alkaliby, and Ahmed M. Habib

This chapter discusses the surgical anatomy of the eye that is relevant to the vitreo-retinal surgeon.

1 Important Definitions and Numbers

- Average anteroposterior diameter of the eye: 24 mm.
- Average horizontal diameter of the eye: 24 mm.
- Average vertical diameter of the eye: 23 mm.
- Average volume of the adult eye: 7 ml.
- Average volume of the vitreous cavity: 5 ml.

Supplementary Information The online version contains supplementary material available at https://doi.org/10.1007/978-3-031-47827-7_1.

A. M. Elhusseiny
Ophthalmology, University of Arkansas for Medical Sciences, Little Rock, AR, USA
e-mail: ElhusseinyAbdelrahma@uams.edu

Y. A. Fouad
Ophthalmology, Ain Shams University Hospitals, Cairo, Egypt

A. M. Alkaliby
Ophthalmology, Cincinnati Eye Institute (CEI) Vision Partners, Maumee, OH, USA

A. M. Habib (✉)
Ophthalmology, Vitreoretinal Surgery, Ain Shams University, Al Mashreq Eye Center, Cairo, Egypt
e-mail: Ahmed.mohamedh@med.asu.edu.eg

A. B. Sallam et al. (eds.), *Practical Manual of Vitreoretinal Surgery*, https://doi.org/10.1007/978-3-031-47827-7_1

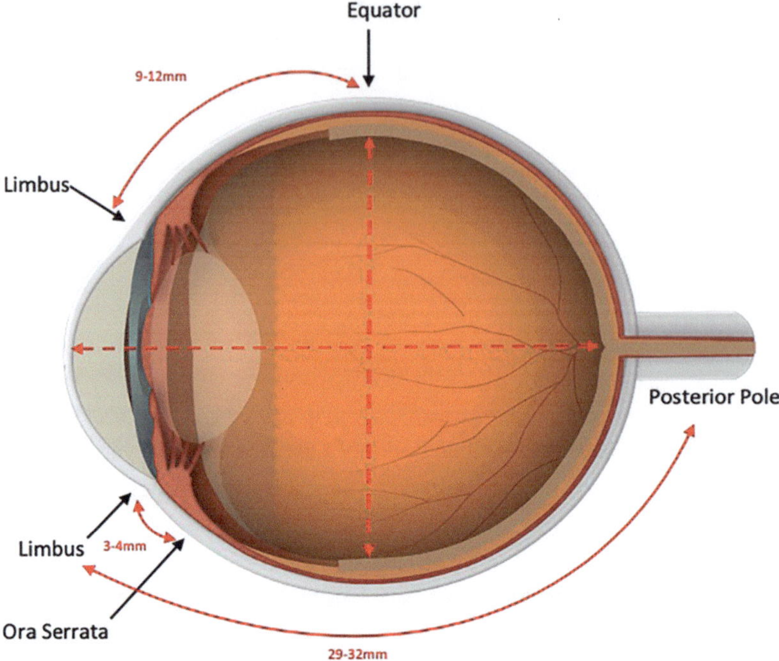

Fig. 1 Schematic representation of the distance from the corneal limbus to important surgical landmarks

- Surgical equator:
  - It is an important surgical landmark, particularly for scleral buckle surgery.
  - From outside, it is the part where the globe has the greatest circumference, located about 9–12 mm from the limbus (Fig. 1) and 2–4 mm anterior to the exit of the vortex veins.
  - From inside, it corresponds to the ampulla of the vortex veins and just anterior to the second bifurcation of the retinal blood vessels.

2 Vitreous

2.1 Biochemistry

- Water constitutes 98% of the vitreous, while proteins, extracellular matrix, and other substances represent the remaining 2%.
- The main collagen in the vitreous is collagen type II, which constitutes 75% of the total collagen in the vitreous. Collagen type II fibers are linked together by

collagen type IX. Staining patterns of other collagen fibers, including types I, III, IV, and XVIII, were previously confirmed in human retinas [1, 2].

- Hyaluronan is a polyanion that is entangled within the collagen fibers and is mainly responsible for maintaining vitreous transparency. It affects the diffusion of intravitreal drugs and plays a role in regulating the phagocytic activity of hyalocytes.
- Fibrillin is a non-collagenous structural protein, the mutation of which leads to vitreous liquefaction and subsequent higher incidence of retinal detachment (RD) in patients with Marfan syndrome.
- High concentrations of ascorbic acid in the vitreous are responsible for its antioxidant reducing the exposure of the crystalline lens to reactive oxygen species and maintaining the lens transparency.
- Significance

  - Removal of the vitreous in pars plana vitrectomy increases the risk of cataract formation.
  - This may also explain why diabetic retinopathy may exert a protective effect against the development of post-vitrectomy cataract formation; there is substantially lower oxygen tension in the vitreous cavity of diabetic eyes compared to non-diabetics.

- The vitreous holds on to chemicals such as vascular endothelial growth factor (VEGF) and transmits oxygen less readily than the aqueous.

- Significance:

  - Vitrectomy helps with improved oxygenation of the retina.
  - However, it facilitates the transport of VEGF down to its concentration gradient from the posterior segment to the anterior segment reducing the risk of retinal neovascularization but increasing the risk of rubeosis and neovascular glaucoma.
  - Silicone oil and the presence of the crystalline lens may act as a barrier to VEGF transport to the anterior segment, reducing the risk of neovascularization.

2.2 Gross Anatomy

- The vitreous volume is about 5 mL in normal eyes and up to 10 mL in high myopic eyes [1].

  Significance

  - Knowing the normal volume of the vitreous cavity, any discrepancies in the volume of tamponade injected or removed from the eye should raise suspicion during surgery. For example, removing a small volume of silicone in a recurrent case of retinal detachment should alert the surgeon that there could be some silicone under the retina not yet extracted. In another case, too little silicone injected in a retinal detachment repair with choroidal detachment could give the surgeon an idea of the magnitude of silicone underfill after the choroidal detachment is resolved.

- The vitreous can be divided anatomically into the vitreous body, vitreous base, and vitreous cortex (hyaloid surface).
- Anteriorly, it is bound by the posterior surface of the crystalline lens and the zonules. The lens is a biconvex structure that is more curved posteriorly, leading to the indention of the anterior vitreous called the patellar fossa.
- The radius of the anterior lens surface ranges from 10 to 14 mm compared to the radius of the posterior lens surface, which ranges from 6 to 7.5 mm. The retrolental space separating the lens from the anterior vitreous is called Berger's space.
  Significance

  - During pars plana vitrectomy, surgeons need to be cautious not to injure the posterior lens surface, which is more curved, while crossing the midline to the opposite quadrants.

- The anterior vitreous face is attached to the posterior part of the lens in an annular fashion called the hyaloideocapsular ligament of Weiger, which is about 1–2 mm wide and 8 mm in diameter.
- It is of note that the ciliary body, lens, and retina continue to develop in the first 6 years of life.

  Significance

  - When planning pars plana surgery in newborns, the small size and anterior position of the ciliary body and the relatively large size of the crystalline lens necessitate anterior placement of sclerotomies. Chap. 29 "Vitreoretinal Surgery in Pediatrics."

2.3 Vitreous Body (Core)

- Forming the main bulk, fibers are more densely packed in infants than adults.

  During eye movements, forces are transmitted from the eye wall to the vitreous body. Being highly viscoelastic, the vitreous movement lags behind the rotational forces of the eye wall "slack and lag," which markedly reduces the forces transmitted to vitreous attachments. Disruption of the hyaloid membrane results in an altered shape of the vitreous body which in turn causes abnormal stress on the retina. The inferonasal location of the optic nerve reduces the strain on the vitreous attachments inferiorly and nasally.

Significance

- The point of maximum strain is on the superotemporal retina, which may explain why it is the most common site of retinal tears.

• With age, liquefaction and spaces form within the vitreous gel. By the age of 40 years, 20% of vitreous is liquified, while at 80 years, 50% is liquified. Vitreous liquefaction is present more in myopic eyes and after recurrent episodes of vitreous hemorrhage.

Significance

- Vitreous hemorrhage absorbs faster in liquified vitreous (and vitrectomized eyes).
- During a vitrectomy, liquified vitreous may give a false impression of posterior vitreous detachment (PVD).
- The interface between liquified and gel vitreous has been studied in multiple mechanical models and has been shown to exert the most traction on the retina, causing retinal tears.
- A more formed vitreous with no PVD as seein in young patients favors the decision of a scleral buckle for the repair of a retinal detachment over pars plana vitrectomy (PPV). Detaching the posterior hyaloid during PPV in these cases is very challenging with risks of causing retinal tears.

2.4 Vitreous Base

• It straddles the ora serrata and extends 2 mm anterior and 2–3 mm posterior to the ora serrata (Fig. 2, Video 1). It also has the highest concentration of collagen and calcium among vitreous parts and contains fibroblasts. It is firmly attached to the retina, so it is anatomically impossible to induce a PVD of the vitreous base [3]. The vitreous base posterior boundary is where the vitreous gel exerts the most traction on the retina in cases with PVD [4].

Significance

- Since it is impossible to perform PVD of the vitreous base, shaving (trimming/cutting short the vitreous by the vitrector very close to the retina) is the only way to remove most of it.
- The posterior boundary of the vitreous base is a frequent site for retinal tears. Traction and subsequent retinal breaks increase with an increased angle between the vitreous and retina in cases with PVD. This increases further with the irregular posterior boundary of the vitreous base.
- Part of the vitreous base covers the pars plana, so shaving it during vitrectomy is not necessary.

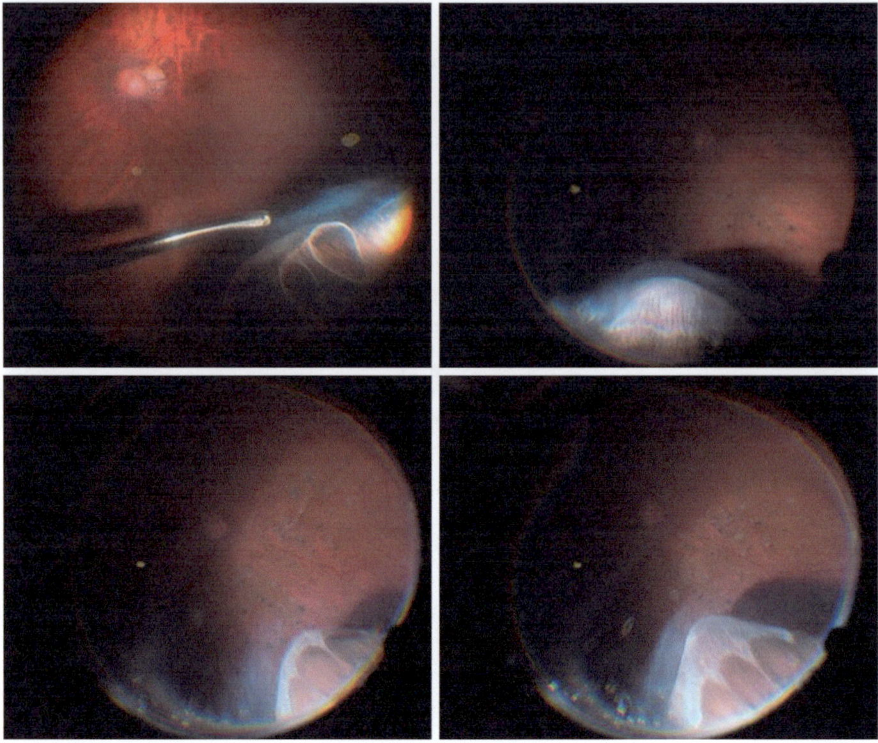

Fig. 2 Different morphological forms of the normal ora serrata. Top left, oral bays; top right, flat serrations; and bottom right and left, oral folds. Note the shaved vitreous base over the pars plicata and peripheral retina after pars plana vitrectomy with scleral indentation

- Posterior insertion of the vitreous base is an uncommon condition where the vitreous base is inserted more posteriorly down to the mid-periphery/ equator [3]. This is more common in high myopic eyes. In these cases, it will not be possible to propagate the PVD further anteriorly. It is also possible that these eyes may have an abnormal vitreoretinal interface with a high risk of iatrogenic retinal tears with PVD induction [5].

2.5 *Vitreous Cortex*

- It is a condensation of the vitreous and rich in hyaluronic acid for a single firm layer. Anteriorly, it separates the crystalline lens, and posteriorly, it separates the retina from the vitreous gel. Posterior vitreous detachment—a key step in vitrectomy surgery—is not done unless the posterior cortical vitreous is completely detached from the retina up to the vitreous base. Liquified vitreous does not mean that a PVD is present.

Significance

- High suspicion of still attached posterior cortical vitreous is advised, especially in myopic eyes and tractional retinal detachment.
- PVD is induced during vitrectomy by exerting sustained active suction by the vitreous cutter near the disc margin and then moving along the retina surface.
- Inducing anterior vitreous detachment is not necessary in every case but may be useful in removing hemorrhage stuck behind the lens. However, caution should be taken not to injure the posterior lens capsule.

2.6 Sites of Strong Vitreous Attachment

1. Vitreous base (most adherent).
2. Around the optic disc.
3. The fovea.
4. Along the vessels.
5. Areas of lattice degeneration.
   Significance
   - These are the areas to pull on with caution during PVD induction so as not to inflict injury or retinal tears.
   - Mid-peripheral areas of abnormally strong attachment of the vitreous could be mistaken for posterior displacement of the vitreous base, especially in myopic eyes.

2.7 Vitreous Cisterns

- Certain liquid spaces, known as vitreous cisterns, exist within the vitreous gel, including the pre-macular bursa, the space of Mertigioni over the optic nerve, and the retrolental space (Fig. 3).

Significance

- Vitreous hemorrhage can be trapped in the retrolental space, which can be challenging to remove in phakic patients during surgery without touching the lens. Also, vitreous hemorrhage can trap in the pre-macular bursa, causing a pre-macular hemorrhage.
- Pre-macular bursa could be used to start the dissection in diabetic delamination using the 'in-out technique,' ensuring a clean entry between the hyaloid/membranes and the retina.
- The 'wolf's jaw" configuration of diabetic fibrovascular proliferation along the temporal vascular arcades can be explained by neovessels' growth along the bursal wall.

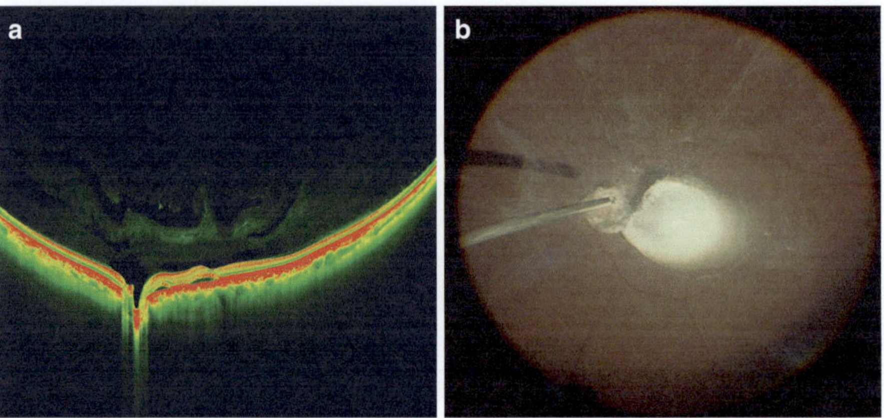

Fig. 3 A high-resolution OCT scan of the vitreous in a patient with central serous chorioretinopathy (note the 2 areas of subretinal fluid at the macula) and attached posterior hyaloid, depicting different vitreous cisterns, notably the pre-macular bursa and the adjacent space of Mertigiano over the optic nerve. (**a**). Staining of the 2 mentioned vitreous cisterns in another patient with triamcinolone acetonide during surgery for epiretinal membrane in the absence of posterior vitreous separation (**b**) (Courtesy of Adil El Maftouhi MD, Switzerland)

3   Retina and Optic Nerve

3.1   Gross Anatomy

- For description purposes, the retina extends from the optic disc to the ora serrata. The circumference from the temporal to the nasal retina is approximately 43 mm.
- The retina starts 5.5 mm (ciliary body size, 2.5 mm pars plicata and 3 mm pars plana) from the limbus nasally and 7 mm (ciliary body size, 2.5 mm pars plicata and 4.5 mm pars plana) temporally.

Significance

- Given that the vitreous base extends 2 mm into the pars plana, it is safest to place PPV sclerotomies at 3.5–4 mm from the limbus.

3.2   The Optic Disc

- It is a circular structure where axons of the ganglion cells converge and exit the globe into the optic nerve. Also, it is where major vessels (i.e., central retinal artery and vein) emerge.

Significance

- Damage to the disc results in augmented damage to the nerve fibers carrying visual impulses resulting in an augmented visual defect. Hence, cautery, laser photocoagulation, or excessive mechanical pressure on the disc should be avoided. Also, care is needed while draining fluid over the disc.

- – Damage to areas near the disc has a greater impact on vision than areas farther away.
- The optic disc is approximately 1500 μm in diameter.

  Significance

  - – This can be used as a measuring unit for other areas, e.g., macular holes, submacular hemorrhage, or areas of capillary obliteration.

3.3 The Macula

- *The anatomical macula* or the area centralis is a 6 mm circle with a diameter equal to the length between the superior and inferior temporal arcades.
- *The clinical macula* is a 1.5 mm circle at the center of the area centralis.
- *The clinical fovea* or the anatomical foveola is a 350 μm circle that is 3.4 mm temporal to the disc margin and 0.8 mm inferior to the center of the disc.

  Significance

  - – The position of the fovea in relation to the disc is to be considered in cases of 360° retinectomy to avoid retina rotation.
- The pressure in retinal arteries is approximately half than that of the systemic blood arteries.

  Significance

  - – If the intraocular pressure is set during surgery at a higher number than half the diastolic pressure, disc pulsations will denote compromised disc perfusion. Some vitrectomy machines are equipped for measuring disc perfusion utilizing this concept.
- The thickness of the retina ranges from 2 to 4 mm in the posterior pole to 1–2 mm near the ora serrata.

  Significance

  - – Breaks in the posterior pole can be left unlasered as the thickness of the retina supports it against detachment.
  - – Peeling of epiretinal membranes (ERMs) is best to be done from the posterior to the anterior.
- The macula supplies a large number of ganglion cell fibers into the papillomacular bundle, and the fibers serve the temporal periphery curve around it.

  Significance

  - – It is best to avoid starting/pinching the internal limiting membrane (ILM) peel nasal to the fovea.

3.4 The Ora Serrata [6]

- It is the anterior-most region of the retina, after which pars plana starts.
- It is about 2 mm wide and located 5 mm anterior to the equator and approximately 5.5 mm from the limbus.
- It represents the transition between the ciliary epithelium and the multilayered photosensitive neurosensory retina.
- At the ora serrata, variations in morphology are present. Ora bays are extensions of the pars plana into the retina. They can be enclosed by extensions of the retina to form ora islands or "enclosed ora bays." Ora folds are thickened retinal tissue extending into the pars plana. If they are not thickened, they are called "dentate processes" (Fig. 2).

Significance

- – Vitreoretinal surgeons should be familiar with ora serrata morphology to avoid confusing the different variations with breaks or retina folds prompting surgical action.

3.5 Microscopic Anatomy

- The retina is composed of ten layers: the retinal pigment epithelium, photoreceptor layer (composed of outer and inner segments), external limiting membrane (formed by the junctions between the photoreceptors and Muller cells' stomata), outer nuclear layer (nuclei of photoreceptors), outer plexiform layer (synapses between photoreceptors and bipolar cells), inner nuclear layer (nuclei of bipolar cells), inner plexiform layer (synapses between bipolar cells and ganglion cells), ganglion cell layer, nerve fiber layer, and ILM (Fig. 4).

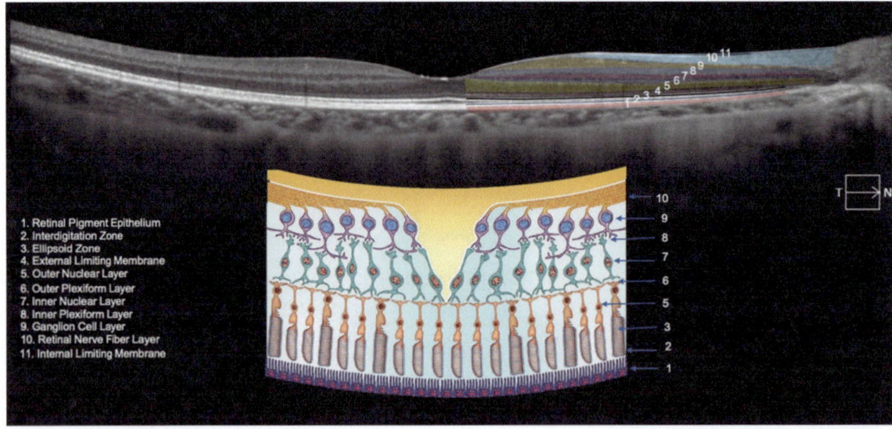

Fig. 4 Retinal microstructure as seen on optical coherence tomography (top) and corresponding diagram of the different retinal layers (bottom, photo by Ilusmedical, Shutterstock.com)

- Muller cells are an important glial cell type. They span nearly the whole retinal thickness. Their stomata form the external limiting membrane (ELM) with those of the photoreceptors. They send processes among photoreceptor discs and others up to the retinal surface, where they form footplates that coalesce together to form the ILM.
- Muller cells provide mechanical support for retinal layers acting. They also provide biochemical support aiding in transporting nutrients and washing out waste products. They form a sheath around the superficial vascular plexus.
- They are entangled with retinal cells forming the core of the so-called functional retinal columns, the smallest unit of "forward information processing." Each column contains a cone, several rods, inner nuclear layer neurons, and ganglion cells. Columns have more neurons in the fovea than the periphery.
- Two types of Muller cells exist. The first type is the foveal cone Muller cells which are present at the foveal center. They extend from the ELM to ILM, where their processes form an inverted cone at the foveal center, which forms the naval appearance of the fovea and is continuous with the rest of the ILM. The second type is the parafoveal Muller cells which assume a Z-shaped configuration. They are present in the parafoveal region and form the Henle layer and cone axons [7].

Significance

- One of the theories of epiretinal membrane formation is that incomplete PVD induces increased traction on Muller cells at the remaining points of attachment. This causes a fibrosis reaction along Muller cells leading to ERM and microscopic intraretinal fibrosis formation.
- Foveal cone Muller cells are vertically arranged in the central 100μm region of the fovea (central bouquet) as they connect with the cone photoreceptors. This makes this area most susceptible to traction from ERM leading to outer retinal changes such as upward displacement of cone receptors, foveal detachment, and subretinal pigment epithelium deposits [8].

- The ILM is a rigid membrane providing nearly half the retinal mechanical strength. It can pull on the retina and cause distortion and even schisis (as in myopic foveoschisis). Hence, the rationale for ILM removal in cases of macular distortion where removal of the ILM decreases the retinal strength and increases its elasticity, thus relieving traction and aiding in retinal relaxation.
- On the other hand, removal of the ILM can cause damage, hypertrophy, and even glial apoptosis of the Muller cells. This can cause macular holes (due to loss of focal cone Muller cells), loss of foveal contour (due to damage or hypertrophy/fibrosis of the parafoveal Muller cells), and macular cystic spaces or edema due to damage of the blood-retinal barrier [9].
- However, if the parafoveal Muller cells are not damaged, they contribute significantly to the centripetal force exerted by the circle of cells around macular holes with formation of temporary glial tissue, leading to their closure [9].
- Lastly, the fact that the cone Muller cells form the central foveal depression and, at the same time, are connected to the ILM led to the recommendation of leaving the ILM just above the fovea (fovea-sparing ILM removal) by some authors.

- The ILM thickness ranges from 1.4 µm at the macular center down to 0.4 µm at the macular periphery.
  Significance

  – ILM removal near the macular center is easier than the macular periphery.

- The macular area has multiple layers of ganglion cells (three to four layers) and has the highest concentration of cones responsible for color vision and high-definition vision. The convergence ratio of cones to bipolar cells is 1:1 (that means that for every cone, there is a bipolar cell synapsing with it).
- As we go toward the periphery, the concentration of cones decreases, while the concentration of rods increases (highest concentration in the mid-periphery and nasal retina). The convergence ratio increases up to 1:20 (20 rods converge to synapse with 1 bipolar cell), aiding the retinal periphery's function to detect motion rather than detailed vision.

  Significance

  – Breaks in the posterior pole translate into bigger, more noticeable field defects than those in the peripheral retina.

4   Extraocular Muscles

- All four recti muscles originate from the annulus of Zinn at the orbital apex and insert into the sclera at variable distances from the limbus. The medial, inferior, lateral, and superior recti muscles are inserted 5.5, 6.5, 6.9, and 7.7 mm from the nasal limbus, respectively.
- The spiral of Tillaux is an imaginary line connecting the insertions of the recti muscle (Fig. 5). It is an important anatomical landmark, especially during scleral

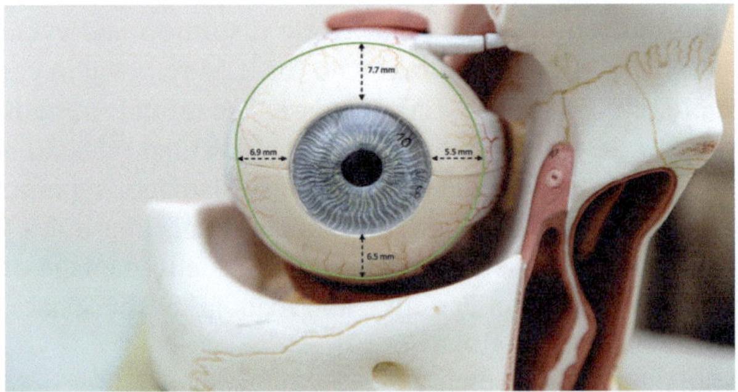

Fig. 5 All four recti muscles originate from the annulus of Zinn at the orbital apex and insert into the sclera at variable distances from the limbus. The medial rectus muscle is inserted 5.5 mm from the nasal limbus, the lateral rectus muscle is inserted 6.9 mm from the limbus, and the superior rectus muscle is inserted 7.7 mm from the limbus, while the inferior rectus muscle is inserted 6.5 mm from the limbus. The spiral of Tillaux (green circle) is an imaginary line connecting the insertions of the recti muscle

buckle surgery for retinal dialysis, as it roughly corresponds to the ora serrata location from the outside.

- The superior oblique muscle originates superomedial to the optic foramen. The muscle then runs forward and passes through the trochlea before changing its direction to be inserted in the supertemporal aspect of the globe.

Significance

- On hooking the superior rectus muscle, avoid sweeping the hook posteriorly to prevent inadvertent hooking or disinsertion of the superior oblique muscle. It is best to hook the superior rectus muscle from the temporal side. Hooking the rectus muscle from the nasal side may injure the trochlea.

5   Sclera

- The scleral thickness differs at different locations: at the limbus (0.8 mm), rectus muscle insertion (0.3 mm), equator (0.6 mm), and peripapillary (1 mm). This explains why scleral rupture tends to happen more commonly around the recti muscle insertion with blunt trauma. Also, this is important to note during scleral incisions for subretinal fluid drainage and when placing scleral sutures. Figure 6 shows the important structure at the posterior aspect of the sclera.

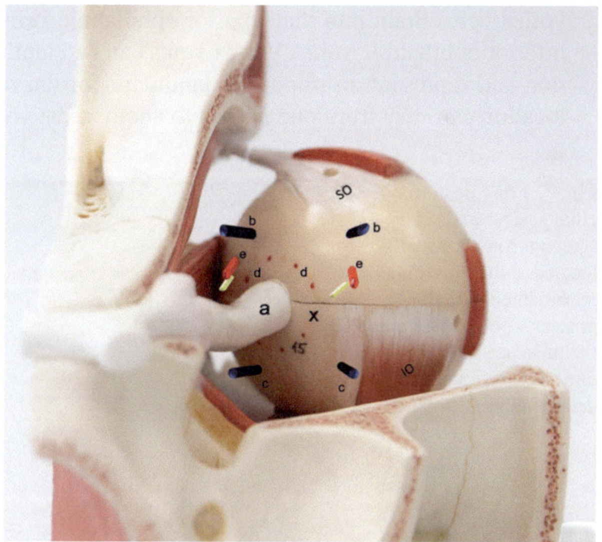

Fig. 6 The anatomy of the posterior aspect of the globe and the related important structures. IO, inferior oblique; SO, superior oblique; a, optic nerve; b, superior vortex veins; c, inferior vortex veins; d, short posterior ciliary vessels and nerves; e, long posterior ciliary vessels and nerves; x, fovea

6 Blood and Nerve Supply of the Globe [10]

- The globe is supplied by the ophthalmic artery through its branches. These include the central retinal artery and short posterior ciliary arteries supplying the retina and the short ciliary arteries supplying the anterior part of the eye, including the anterior ciliary arteries and the long posterior ciliary arteries. The anterior ciliary arteries travel along the recti muscle (one along each muscle border of the superior, medial, and inferior recti and one only along the lateral rectus).

  Significance

  – These arteries can serve as a good anatomical landmark to the recti muscles and explain why a tight encirclement buckle can lead to anterior segment ischemia.

- The long posterior ciliary arteries (usually 2) pierce the sclera near the posterior pole (approximately 4 mm around the optic nerve on each side) and then travel anteriorly between the sclera and choroid at the 3 and 9 o'clock positions (Fig. 7) to join the anterior ciliary arteries in forming the major arterial circle of the iris. The major arterial circle of the iris gives off branches to the iris and ciliary body.
- Venous drainage of the eye is mainly through the central retinal vein and the vortex veins (Fig. 8). Most of the venous drainage from the anterior segment is directed posteriorly into the choroid and then into the vortex veins. There are four to eight veins that represent the venous drainage system for the ocular choroid. Most people have at least one vortex vein for each retinal quadrant. Some vortex veins drain into the superior ophthalmic vein, while others drain into the inferior ophthalmic veins. Vortex veins can be identified during fundus examination and represent an important landmark for the retinal equator. Though their location can vary from one person to another, the vortex veins tend to be present

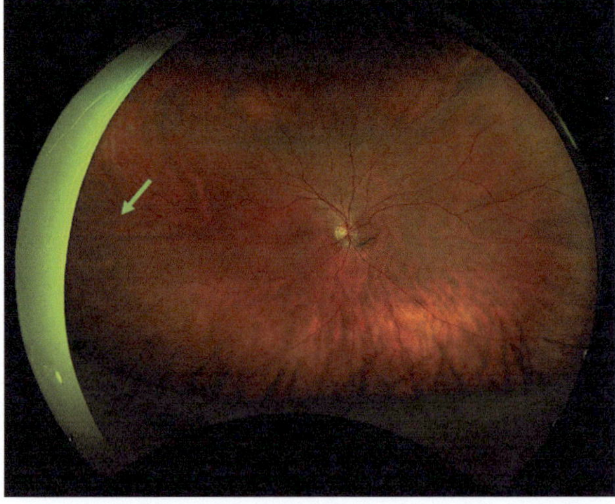

Fig. 7 Long posterior ciliary nerve and artery (green arrow) is usually located at the horizontal meridian outside the posterior pole. Also, note the presence of Weiss ring due to posterior vitreous detachment

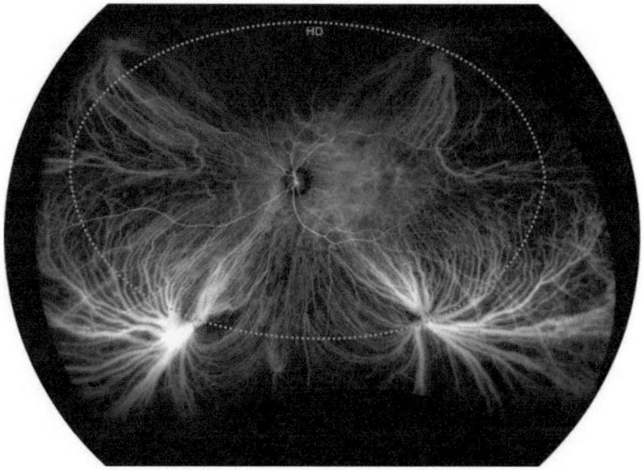

Fig. 8 Location and structure of the vortex veins highlighted by indocyanine green angiography. The ampulla of the vortex veins is an important landmark of the equator of the eye (green dotted line)

more toward the vertical meridian at the 1, 5, 7, and 11 o'clock positions. Drainage of subretinal fluid during scleral buckle surgery is therefore ideally performed above or below the horizontal muscles to avoid injury of the choroidal vasculature.

- The long posterior ciliary nerve arises from the nasociliary branch of the ophthalmic nerve. It passes along the horizontal meridian of the eye between the sclera and choroid together with the artery.
- The short ciliary nerves are branches of the ciliary ganglion located in the orbit and carry parasympathetic fibers. They penetrate the sclera around the optic nerve and continue their course in the suprachoroidal space to innervate the iris sphincter and the ciliary muscle. Their location is variable.

Significance

- Heavy retinal laser during surgery can cause neurotrophic keratopathy, cycloplegia, or paralysis of the iris sphincter. One needs to be cautious not to place heavy laser spots at the horizontal meridian.

References

1. Wolf E. The anatomy of the eye and orbit. 4th ed. London: Lewis; 1954. p. 226, 231.
2. Salzmann M. The anatomy and histology of the human eyeball. Brown EVL, trans., vol. 7. Chicago, IL: University of Chicago Press; 1912. p. 8.
3. Schepens CL. Clinical Aspects of Pathologic Changes in the Vitreous Body*. American Journal of Ophthalmology. 1954;38(1):8–21.
4. Foos RY, Allen RA. (1967) Retinal Tears and Lesser Lesions of the Peripheral Retina in Autopsy Eyes American Journal of Ophthalmology. 1967;64(3):643/125-655/137.
5. Sohn EH, Strohbehn A, Stryjewski T, Brodowska K, Flamme-Wiese MJ, Mullins RF, Eliott D. POSTERIORLY INSERTED VITREOUS BASE Retina. 2020;40(5):943–50.

6. Whitnall SE. Anatomy of the human orbit. 4th ed. London: Frowde; 1932. p. 257, 279.
7. Reichenbach A, Bringmann A. Glia of the human retina Abstract Glia 2020;68(4):768-796. 10.1002/glia.v68.4. 2020.
8. Govetto A, Bhavsar KV, Virgili G, Gerber MJ, Freund KB, Curcio CA, et al. Tractional abnormalities of the central foveal bouquet in epiretinal membranes: clinical spectrum and pathophysiological perspectives. Am J Ophthalmol. 2017;184:167–80.
9. Bringmann A, Unterlauft JD, Barth T, Wiedemann R, Rehak M, Wiedemann P. Müller cells and astrocytes in tractional macular disorders Progress in Retinal and Eye Research. 2022. 86100977.
10. Siam ALH, El-Mamoun TA, Ali MH. A restudy of the surgical anatomy of the posterior aspect of the globe: an essential topography for exact macular buckling. Retina. 2011;31(7):1405–11.

Preoperative Evaluation of Vitreoretinal Surgery Patients

John R. Chancellor, Ron A. Adelman, and Mohammad Z. Siddiqui

1 Introduction

- Becoming a proficient vitreoretinal surgeon begins with the ability to accurately evaluate and identify many subtle factors in the preoperative clinic that will enable a successful surgical outcome. This examination will guide your choice of anesthesia, surgical technique, tamponade, and expectations to discuss with the patient.
- The preoperative clinical examination can greatly impact the success or failure of vitreoretinal surgery. It is also the opportunity for the surgeon to discuss outcomes with the patient to mitigate any postoperative surprises. Patients should be given realistic expectations for anatomic success and vision improvement. Recovery and rehabilitation time may differ significantly depending on the surgical technique and tamponade required. Planning for this and discussing it before surgery enhance the patient's trust and confidence in the surgeon throughout the perioperative period.

J. R. Chancellor (✉)
Vitreoretinal Diseases & Surgery, Baylor College of Medicine, Houston, TX, USA
e-mail: John.Chancellor@bcm.edu

R. A. Adelman
Department of Ophthalmology, Mayo Clinic, Jacksonville, FL, USA

Ophthalmology and Visual Science, Yale University School of Medicine,
New Haven, CT, USA
e-mail: ron.adelman@yale.edu

M. Z. Siddiqui
Jones Eye Institute, University of Arkansas for Medical Sciences, Little Rock, AR, USA

© The Author(s), under exclusive license to Springer Nature
Switzerland AG 2024
A. B. Sallam et al. (eds.), *Practical Manual of Vitreoretinal Surgery*,
https://doi.org/10.1007/978-3-031-47827-7_2

2   The Patient

- All patients have different levels of comfort and tolerability with ocular procedures. This can be determined early into the exam with their ability to fixate on the examiner's light or hold a gaze position during scleral depression.
- If the patient has a poor ability to tolerate a clinic exam and high levels of anxiety, the surgeon would likely do a disservice to themselves and the patient by attempting to perform a case under local anesthesia.
- Even a relatively straightforward surgery or procedure could be dangerous or difficult if the patient becomes anxious or moves too much during surgery. It is important to remember that trying to force surgery under difficult patient circumstances does not make one a better surgeon or lead to better outcomes.
- Suppose the patient must frequently travel for work or has an important flight planned. In that case, they may prefer the option of silicone oil tamponade and a second surgery over intraocular gas that would force the cancellation of flights.

3   Visual Acuity

- Preoperative visual acuity plays a unique role in retina surgery as there are many circumstances to consider based on the pathology. A patient with counting fingers vision from a vitreous hemorrhage is not the same as a patient with a similar vision from a retinal detachment.
- Epiretinal membrane (ERM)/vitreomacular traction: the surgeon should carefully determine the visual impact of the membrane compared to other ocular factors. The retina surgeon should evaluate for corneal pathology, lens or intraocular lens opacity, and media changes. Classical teaching recommends waiting until the patient is 20/40 or worse before considering surgery, but significant metamorphopsia with good vision may give this cohort of patients the most significant subjective improvement after surgery [1]. It is also important to explain that vision improvement is not immediate after most macular surgery and it takes about 3 months on average to feel a difference [2].
- Diabetic surgery: surgery for chronic complex diabetic traction is often unpredictable regarding final visual acuity outcomes. The decision to perform surgery on a diabetic eye will depend on several factors, including the visual acuity of the fellow eye. A slowly progressing tractional retinal detachment with good vision may best be observed, given the risk of retinal tears or persistent postoperative vitreous cavity hemorrhage in such cases.
- Macular hole and rhegmatogenous retinal detachment: a patient with decreased vision from damage to the fovea from a detached macula or macular hole must be counseled appropriately. They often expect their acute vision loss to be cured and returned to baseline after surgery. Educating the patient about the level of

their current vision (e.g., showing a patient the best line they can read) at the preoperative clinic can help patients appreciate any postoperative improvement, even if only minimal. Counseling about the level of vision expected is essential. For example, in most cases of macula-off retinal detachment, vision does not return to baseline, and distortion is present.

- One last note about visual acuity is the difference between VA line gains and absolute postoperative vision. Patients with poor preoperative vision can have more line gains after retinal procedures or surgery compared to patients with better preoperative vision due to a ceiling effect. However, what matters the most for the patient is the absolute postoperative vision. For example, reaching a 20/40 vision which is the vision needed for driving from a baseline 20/60 is more impactful than gaining several more lines with change of vision from CF to 20/100 [3].

4 Intraocular Pressure

- High intraocular pressure: patients with significant elevation in intraocular pressure, for example, due to coexisting uveitis or, in some cases, retinal detachment (Schwartz-Matsuo syndrome), may require optimization before surgery. If the pressure is acutely elevated, the cornea may decompensate in the time between the clinic visit and surgery if not properly controlled. Additionally, the cornea may decompensate early into surgery, making the retina's view more difficult.
- Low intraocular pressure: placing trocars in a hypotonus eye can be difficult and dangerous. Taking note of the patient's hypotony and planning can allow for alterations in trocar insertion, for example, using an anterior chamber maintainer or injecting pars plana BSS to firm up the eye. In long-term retinal detachment and uveitis, hypotony is a poor prognostic sign for vision, indicating ciliary body damage. Finally, hypotony in a silicone-filled eye is a contraindication for SO removal [4].

5 Cornea

- As discussed above, it is important to evaluate the health of the cornea in the clinic to determine how well it will tolerate vitreoretinal surgery.
- Patients should be asked about and evaluated for previous refractive surgery, especially LASIK, as these patients should not have their epithelium removed as it may disrupt the entire flap permanently. Also, special arrangement needs to be made for IOL calculations if combined cataract PPV surgery is contemplated.
- Patients with corneal decompensation from trauma, endothelial dystrophy, ocular hypertension, or other factors would benefit from optimization before any non-emergent retina surgery. Even urgent surgery may have a better outcome if delayed for a few days if the corneal view can be improved before retina surgery.

6 Iris and Pupil Size

- Patient dilation and pupil size should be noted in preparation for retina surgery, just as a surgeon would prepare for cataract surgery.
- A small pupil may limit the view of the peripheral retina, and iris hooks or rings may be necessary to perform an adequate vitrectomy.
- Additionally, posterior synechiae may require lysis with or without cataract surgery before vitrectomy to provide an adequate view.
- Intracameral epinephrine/lignocaine works well if the pupil is large at the beginning of the surgery and comes down with anterior segment manipulations.
- Always look for iris rubeosis in diabetic patients and patients presenting with vitreous hemorrhage for unknown reason (retinal vein occlusion or diabetic retinopathy might be the cause). Manipulation of the anterior chamber in these patients may result in intracameral hemorrhage that will significantly lengthen the surgical time and require tamponade and removal for optimal view.

7 Lens Status

- Preoperative evaluation is the lens status of the patient and may dramatically impact surgical planning. Alterations in surgical technique will be discussed later in this book, but below are some basic considerations.
- Phakic patients: older patients with a clear lens must be counseled appropriately on the formation of cataract or may benefit from sequential or combined cataract extraction and vitrectomy.
- The type of surgery and type of cataract must also be considered. Significant cortical spoking may cause difficulty in peripheral view for retinal detachment surgery or panretinal photocoagulation but will have less impact on posterior pole surgery. Conversely, a small posterior subcapsular cataract will have a minimal impact on retinal detachment surgery or peripheral laser but may have a dramatic impact on internal limiting membrane peel or diabetic membrane removal.
- Pseudophakic patients: the surgeon should note the type of intraocular lens material and the status of the posterior capsule. Posterior capsule opacity may limit detailed retinal work, while an open posterior capsule can cause lens condensation under air or gas. The presence of a sulcus three-piece lens may suggest zonular instability that can allow air or gas to migrate into the anterior chamber. Multifocal lenses can cause distortion that hinders the view of the surgeon during macular work.
- Aphakic patients: the surgical view in unicameral eyes can become very difficult once the surgeon transitions to air. Additionally, if silicone oil is required, it is at further risk of migration into the anterior chamber. Depending on the urgency and the complexity of the surgery (e.g., ERM or retinal detachment surgery), it may benefit the patient to have secondary lens placement at or after the time of vitrectomy.

8 Vitreous Status

- The most basic evaluation of the vitreous is determined by taking the patient history and examining to determine if the patient has been previously vitrectomized. If the vitreous body is still present, then there are several important considerations.
- If vitreous hemorrhage or opacity prevents a view of the retina, B-scan ultrasound will provide useful information about the presence or absence of retinal detachment, posterior vitreous detachment, and vitreous traction.
- If possible, the surgeon should document the presence or absence of a posterior vitreous detachment (PVD). If one can determine in clinic if there is a PVD or, conversely, very adherent hyaloid with membranes, it will help the surgeon estimate a case duration and complexity. For example, it is good to know that PVD is usually absent in young patients with RRD due to atrophic retinal holes or dialysis, in macular holes, and in diabetic TRD cases. PVD is usually present in most ERM cases (without vitreomacular traction) and in retinal detachment due to horseshoe retinal tears.
- Optical coherence tomography (OCT), B-scan ultrasound, and close examination for a Weiss ring or posterior vitreous face can all be helpful for determining if there is the presence of a PVD. However, this can only be truly established once the patient is in the operating room and the surgeon has confirmed the full separation of the hyaloid!

9 Retinal Exam

- Given a clear view and cooperative patient, it is imperative to document all retinal pathology and perform a thorough scleral depressed exam when appropriate, for example, in retinal detachment cases and patients presenting with acute vitreous floaters.
- Optic nerve: often overlooked during routine retinal exams, it is important to consider if there is advanced cupping or pallor of the optic nerve before surgery. Perhaps the decrease in vision is due to the optic nerve pathology and not the ERM that is present? Always ask yourself whether the pathology fully explains the patient's symptoms. Sometimes, it may be best to defer retina surgery entirely in the setting of irreversible optic nerve pathology due to the risk of poor visual outcomes or limitations of visual improvement. Discussion with a glaucoma or neuro-ophthalmology specialist may be indicated to determine visual potential. Assessing the patient for a relative afferent pupillary defect at a subsequent clinic visit prior to dilation and surgical approval may be indicated.
- Macula: care should focus on the retinal layers' health and the retinal pigment epithelium. OCT is an important adjuvant for macular disorders and their classification, for example, macular holes and ERM [5]. If there is significant disorganization of retinal layers from ischemia or loss of the ellipsoid

zone/interdigitation zone from chronic pathology, then postoperative visual potential may be limited. This can guide the surgeon in setting expectations with the patient and may also help determine if surgery should even be performed.

- Retinal vessels: areas of ischemia can be determined with preoperative fluorescein angiography and/or indocyanine green (ICG). This can be used to perform targeted laser during surgery for branch artery or vein occlusions. In neovascular disease, angiography and clinical exam can be used to determine sites of neovascularization at risk for epicenter formation and adhesion. These areas may require more careful surgical dissection during vitreous removal. Peripheral ischemia with large areas of neovascularization can be at higher risk of resultant tractional retinal detachments (Fig. 1).
- Peripheral retina: an examination of the peripheral retina is of particular importance for retinal detachments, retinoschisis, and other peripheral retinal pathology.

  - Examination with indentation is an essential skill that the starting surgeon must master.
  - It is important to note subtle signs; for example, retinal folds with limited mobility during indentation can suggest the presence of proliferative vitreoretinopathy, even in primary detachments, and may significantly alter the surgical duration and tamponade options. This entity needs to be differentiated from retinal edema or hydration folds in primary RRD [6] that still allow the retinal to move freely during the examination (Fig. 2).
  - OCT of the periphery can be important, for example, in differentiating RD from retinoschisis (Fig. 3).
  - Figure 4 shows a case of peripheral exudative hemorrhagic chorioretinopathy (PEHCR) [5] that was referred for suspected retinal detachment and hemorrhagic PVD. ICG was helpful in making the diagnosis.

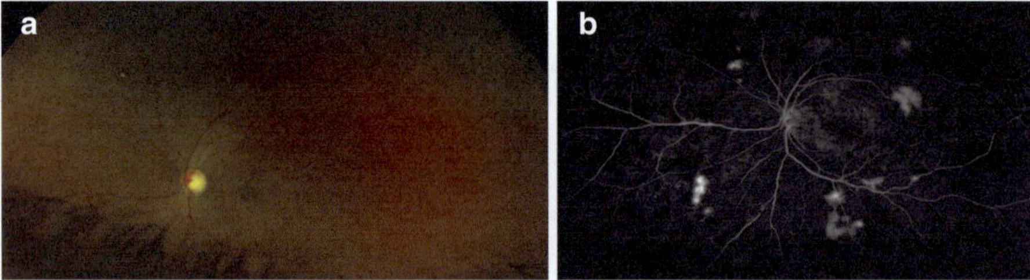

Fig. 1 (**a**) Fundus photograph depicting areas of peripheral ischemia with neovascularization in a patient with proliferative diabetic retinopathy. (**b**) Late-phase fluorescein angiography showing areas of neovascularization with leakage and also areas of peripheral ischemia with capillary dropout

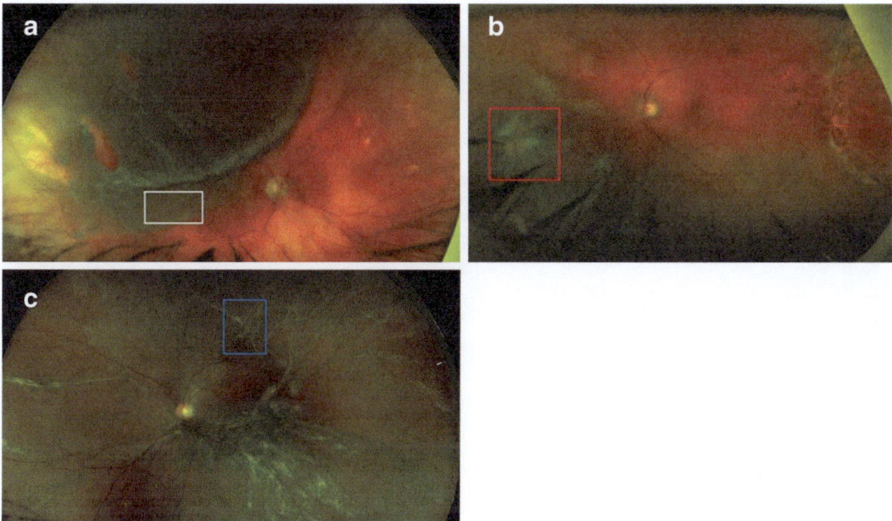

Fig. 2 (**a**) Fundus photographs of a patient with rhegmatogenous retinal detachment (RRD) and multiple retinal tears. Notice the retinal hydration folds of the RRD and the small undulating and repeating nature (white rectangle). (**b**) Fundus photograph of a patient with a history of retinal detachment repaired with pars plana vitrectomy and scleral buckle. The patient developed proliferative vitreoretinopathy (PVR) with a tractional retinal detachment. Notice the linear and more vertically oriented bands (in contrast to the retinal hydration folds) depicting the PVR (red rectangle). (**c**) Fundus photograph depicting tractional membranes and fibrotic bands (blue rectangle)

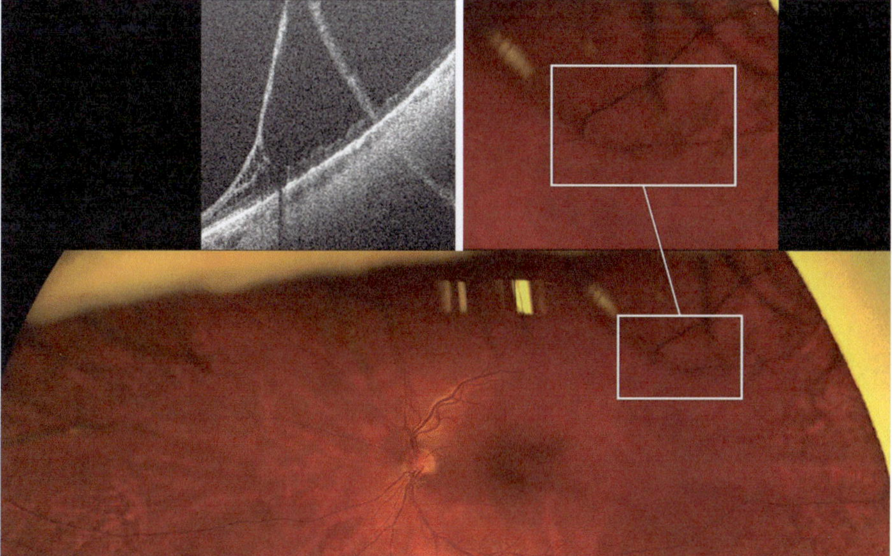

Fig. 3 Fundus photograph showing area of elevation in superotemporal periphery. Optical coherence tomography scanning over this area confirms an area of peripheral retinoschisis

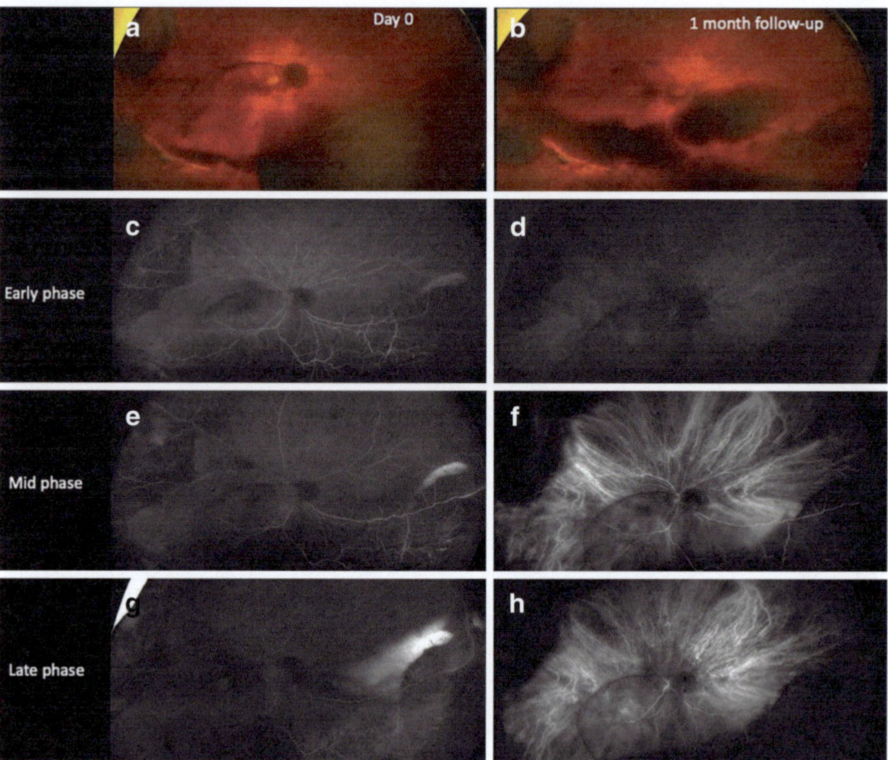

Fig. 4 Patient with peripheral exudative hemorrhagic chorioretinopathy (PEHCR). (**a**) Widefield fundus image showing areas of subretinal and sub-pigment epithelium hemorrhage and area of exudative mass in temporal and inferonasal periphery on initial presentation. (**b**) Widefield fundus photo of the same patient with PEHCR showing resolving areas of hemorrhage at 1-month follow-up. (**c**, **e**, **g**) Fluorescein angiography of the same patient with PEHCR showing classic findings of blockage of choroidal fluorescence related to hemorrhage in the early phase and areas of diffuse peripheral hyper- and hypoautofluorescence in areas of retinal pigment epithelium loss or hyperplasia in the mid and late phases. (**d**, **f**, **h**) Indocyanine green angiography (ICG) of the same patient showing areas of irregular choroidal vascular networks in all phases corresponding to the areas of hemorrhagic lesions seen on the fundus photos and more prominent blockage of the choroidal fluorescence at the subretinal level seen better in the mid and late phases

References

1. Wang LC, Lo WJ, Huang YY, Chou YB, Li AF, Chen SJ, Chou TY, Lin TC. Correlations between clinical and histopathologic characteristics in idiopathic epiretinal membrane ophthalmology 2022;129(12):1421–8.
2. J. Corbin, Norton Mohamed K, Soliman Yit C, Yang Shree, Kurup Ahmed B., Sallam (2022) Visual outcomes of primary versus secondary epiretinal membrane following vitrec-

tomy and cataract surgery Graefe's Archive for Clinical and Experimental Ophthalmology 2022;260(3):817–25.
3. Ross A, Donachie P, Sallam A, et al. Which visual acuity measurements define high-quality care for patients with neovascular age-related macular degeneration treated with ranibizumab? Eye. 2013;27:56–64.
4. Schubert HD. Postsurgical hypotony: relationship to fistulization inflammation chorioretinal lesions and the vitreous Survey of Ophthalmology. 1996;41(2)97–125.
5. Safir M, Zloto O, Fabian ID, Moroz I, Gaton DD, Vishnevskia-Dai V. Peripheral exudative hemorrhagic chorioretinopathy with and without treatment-clinical and multimodal imaging characteristics and prognosis. PLoS One. 2022;17(9):e0275163.
6. Dalvin LA, Spaide RF, Yannuzzi LA, Freund KB, Pulido JS. Hydration folds in rhegmatogenous retinal detachment. Retin Cases Brief Rep. 2020;14(4):355–9.

Vitreoretinal Anesthesia

Joseph W. Fong, Mohammad Z. Siddiqui, and Ahmed B. Sallam

1   Introduction

- Historically, vitreoretinal surgery has been performed under general anesthesia due to the prolonged duration of the surgery, the intensity of the surgical stimulus, and the need for a motionless surgical field.
  Over the past decades, vitreoretinal surgery has been increasingly performed with local anesthesia [1, 2].
- Several factors must be considered when selecting anesthesia for vitreoretinal surgery, including the age of the patient, the general health of the patient, the length and complexity of the surgery, the surgeon's preference and level of experience, and the patient's previous experiences with ophthalmic surgery [1].

Supplementary Information The online version contains supplementary material available at https://doi.org/10.1007/978-3-031-47827-7_3.

J. W. Fong
Hamilton Eye Institute, University of Tennessee Health Science Center, Memphis, TN, USA
e-mail: jfong2@uthsc.edu

M. Z. Siddiqui · A. B. Sallam (✉)
Jones Eye Institute, University of Arkansas for Medical Sciences, Little Rock, AR, USA

A. B. Sallam et al. (eds.), *Practical Manual of Vitreoretinal Surgery*,
https://doi.org/10.1007/978-3-031-47827-7_3

2   Anesthesia Techniques

2.1   General Anesthesia

– It is more suitable for prolonged, complex vitreoretinal procedures; individuals who have difficulties remaining quiescent, such as children; patients with developmental delay; patients with movement disorders; and those with certain psychiatric issues, such as profound claustrophobia, and also in complex diabetic and proliferative vitreoretinopathy cases that are expected to last for a long time.
– Drawbacks of general anesthesia include its systemic risks in elderly and morbid patients, prolonged recovery and the potential for an abrupt intraocular pressure spike upon emergence and extubation [1]. There are also increased costs and operation room utilization time as compared to local anesthesia [3].

2.2   Retrobulbar Block/Peribulbar Blocks

– It is mandatory to have intravenous access and cardiovascular monitoring before any sharp needle anesthesia.
– A **retrobulbar or intraconal block** is performed by inserting the needle tip *inside* the muscle cone and injecting a low volume (4–5 mL) of local anesthetic (Fig. 1, Video 1). Retrobulbar blocks are highly effective and induce rapid onset of analgesia and akinesia.

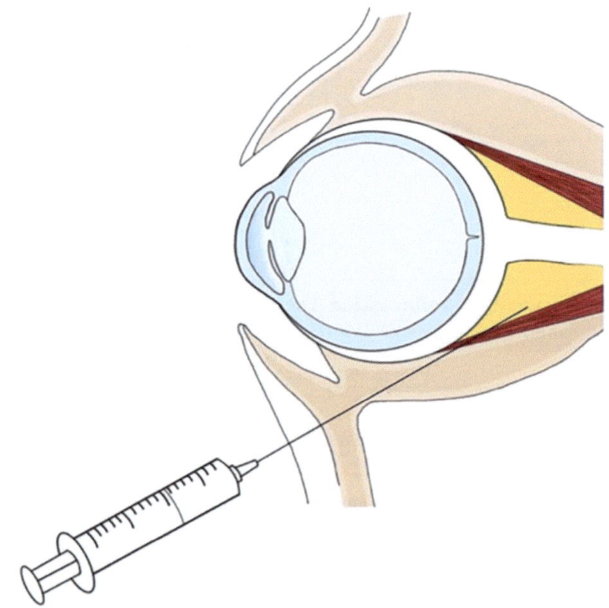

Fig. 1 A retrobulbar or intraconal block is performed by inserting the needle through the intermuscular septum and injecting a low volume of local anesthetic (4–5 mL) into the muscle cone. Note the upward redirection of the needle once it is in the retro-equatorial extraconal space that is necessary to properly insert the needle into the intraconal space

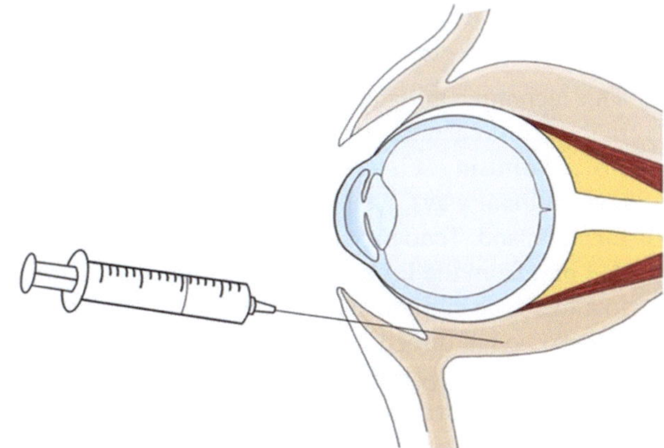

Fig. 2 A peribulbar block is performed by inserting the needle into the extraconal space and injecting a slightly larger volume of anesthetic (5–10 mL). Note the posterior trajectory of the needle, remaining safely in the extraconal space

- Similarly, a **peribulbar block** is performed by injecting a slightly larger volume of local anesthetic (5–10 mL) *outside* of the muscle cone (Fig. 2, Video 1). Inward diffusion of the anesthetic similarly renders the globe insensate and akinetic, although with more gradual onset compared to retrobulbar blocks.
- Complications associated with sharp needle blocks (more with a retrobulbar block but still can happen with peribulbar) include retrobulbar hemorrhage, precipitation of the oculocardiac reflex, postoperative diplopia from inadvertent injury to the extraocular muscles, penetration of the globe with possible intraocular injection of local anesthetics, optic nerve trauma, central retinal artery occlusion, and intravascular injection of local anesthetics [4].
- The surgeon must consider the increased risk of globe perforation during retrobulbar injection in patients with high or very short axial length or previous scleral buckle placement.

2.3 Subconjunctival Anesthesia

- Subconjunctival anesthesia is used infrequently in intraocular surgeries, especially in vitreoretinal surgery.
- A recent prospective randomized clinical trial by Fan et al. showed that subconjunctival anesthesia for selected patients undergoing 23- or 25-gauge (g) pars plana vitrectomy resulted in satisfactory analgesia without increased complication rates from lack of akinesia [5].
- We advise only using this technique for simple vitrectomy cases if it is ever to be used.

2.4 Sub-Tenon's Block

- This technique mitigates the risk of complications related to using sharp needles in the orbit (cannula-based block).
- Instead of using scissors to dissect the conjunctiva [6] to sub-Tenon's space (the conventional way), we use an 18-gauge needle to initiate a puncture in the conjunctiva and Tenon's capsule in the inferonasal conjunctiva, approximately 3–4 mm from the limbus. A 20-g intravenous cannula (angiocatheter) is secured to a luer lock syringe and navigated along the plane of sub-Tenon's space in the posteromedial direction along the contour of the globe with a slow injection of local anesthetic [7] (Fig. 3, Video 2).
- There are few drawbacks to sub-Tenon's block. If the angiocatheter is not maximally inserted, the block can sometimes result in significant chemosis that can hinder visualization and access to trocars during surgery. This may require conjunctival cutdown to relieve the chemosis. Additionally, the degree of akinesia achieved with sub-Tenon's block alone is often inadequate for delicate vitreoretinal steps like internal limiting membrane peeling, as the eye is usually left with a slight but troublesome "shimmering" movement.

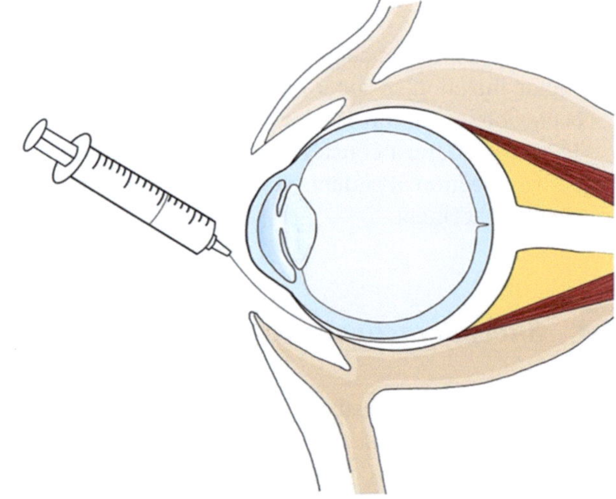

Fig. 3 A modified sub-Tenon's block is performed by creating a small puncture in the inferonasal conjunctiva with an 18-gauge needle, followed by the insertion of a 20-gauge intravenous cannula secured to a luer lock syringe. The cannula is then slowly and maximally advanced along the curvature of the globe within sub-Tenon's space

3 Sedation with Local Anesthesia

- **Sedation** using propofol, morphine-class analgesics, and benzodiazepines can be an option if the patient is anxious [8].
- However, it is not a substitute for analgesic, and heavy sedation could be counterproductive as it increases the risk of disinhibition and poor patient cooperation.

4 What Do We Do?

- We generally use a combined peribulbar block (5 mL) with a sub-Tenon's block (5 mL) for most cases. We opt for general anesthesia in select cases where patients are young and very anxious or complicated cases that are expected to last more than 1.5 h.
- For local anesthesia, we inject a 50% mix of 2% lignocaine + 0.5% bupivacaine. 0.75% ropivacaine alone is a good single anesthetic alternative. For peribulbar blocks, we add 0.5 mL hyaluronidase for every 5 mL of anesthetic.
- Our use of sedation with local anesthesia is low (approximately 20% of cases with local anesthesia). In many cases, patients are anxious because they do not understand what is coming. It is important to think of local anesthesia as both local and vocal—you must talk to your patient and reassure them. This makes a lot of difference!

5 Potential Problems During Vitreoretinal Anesthesia

1. Oculocardiac reflex during scleral buckle surgery

   - The oculocardiac reflex (OCR) is a well-known phenomenon where the heart rate decreases by greater than 20% from the manipulation of extraocular muscles, globe, or conjunctiva [9]. The connection between the ophthalmic branch of the trigeminal nerve and the vagus nerve mediates the reflex. In vitreoretinal surgery, the OCR is especially important during scleral buckle surgery. Local anesthesia delivered via ophthalmic block (i.e., retrobulbar, peribulbar, sub-Tenon's anesthesia) prevents the OCR. Scleral buckle surgery is more commonly done under general anesthesia, so in these cases, using local anesthesia along with general anesthesia can prevent the OCR. If the OCR is encountered, it is typically easily managed by the anesthesiologist. Although very rare, serious cardiac arrhythmias leading to cardiac arrest can occur, making OCR an important consideration. If significant bradycardia is encountered, the anesthesiologist may treat it with certain medications (i.e., atropine).

2. Intraocular perforation with sharp needle anesthesia

   - It is discussed in chap. 25 "Posterior Segment Complications of Cataract Surgery: When the Anterior Segment Meets the Posterior".

3. Valsalva-induced suprachoroidal hemorrhage during pars plana vitrectomy under general anesthesia

   - Valsalva-induced suprachoroidal hemorrhage is a serious complication that can occur during vitreoretinal surgery [10]. It generally happens toward the conclusion of a case where general anesthesia becomes light. If a painful stimulus like scleral indentation for retinal periphery check is done while a patient is under light sedation, there is a risk the patient would feel pain and react. If this happens, the patient may cough or "buck," which can result in suprachoroidal hemorrhage. To minimize this risk, it is important to notify the anesthesiologist to maintain deep sedation till the end of the case. Additionally, using local anesthesia during general anesthesia can provide additional analgesia and decrease pain with scleral indentation. We routinely place a sub-Tenon's block in all general anesthesia cases from the outset.

4. Venous air embolism

   - Ocular venous air embolism (OVAE) is a rare complication during vitreoretinal surgery that can be fatal. OVAE can occur during pars plana vitrectomy by an improperly positioned infusion line, leading to the entry of pressurized air into the suprachoroidal space and tearing of the vortex veins [11]. This could also happen in cases where a large area of the choroid is exposed to air infusion as in ocular trauma, choroidal tumor excisions and large choroidal biopsies. Air may then be transmitted from the suprachoroidal space into the systemic venous circulation and ultimately to the right ventricular outflow tract, causing impaired gas exchange in the lungs. Intraoperatively, OVAE is discovered based upon anesthesia monitoring, specifically by a sudden drop in end-tidal carbon dioxide level (Fig. 4), followed by signs of cardiovascular collapse during vitrectomy and air infusion. To decrease the risk of OVAE, the surgeon must ensure that the infusion line is always in the vitreous cavity, especially with air exchange.

Key Points
- The majority of retinal surgery can be performed under local anesthesia, which is safer, quicker, and more cost-effective than GA.
- Sedation is not a substitute for adequate local anesthesia/analgesia.
- Local anesthesia is both local and vocal.
- The use of supplemental sub-Tenon's anesthesia with general anesthesia prevents OCR and decreases intraoperative and postoperative pain sensation.

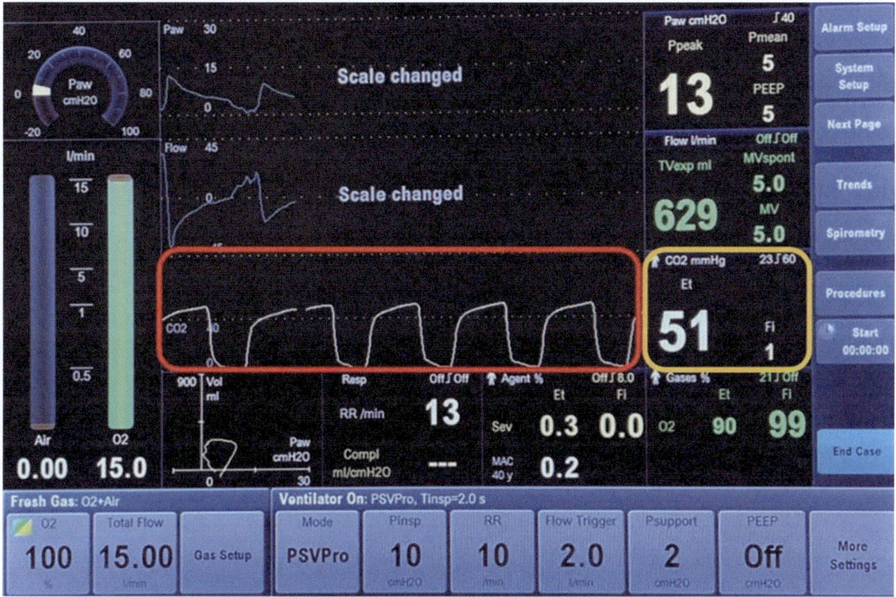

Fig. 4 Intraoperative hemodynamic monitoring with normal capnography waveform (red box) and end-tidal carbon dioxide reading (orange box)

References

1. Sallam AAB, Donachie PHJ, Williamson TH, Sparrow JM, Johnston RL. The Royal College of Ophthalmologists' National Ophthalmology Database Study of vitreoretinal surgery: report 5, anaesthetic techniques. Br J Ophthalmol. 2016;100:246–52.
2. Yannuzzi NA, Sridhar J, Flynn HW Jr, Gayer S, Berrocal AM, Patel NA, Townsend J, Smiddy WE, Albini T. Current Trends in Vitreoretinal Anesthesia. Ophthalmol Retina. 2019;3(9):804–805.
3. Siddiqui MZ, Chauhan MZ, Stewart AF, Sallam AB. Analysis of Operational Efficiency and Cost Differences between Local and General Anesthesia for Vitreoretinal Surgery. Healthcare (Basel). 2022;10(10):1918.
4. Bir R, Tanvi S, Victoria K, Chhavi L, Wonkyung S, Sukhman C, Partap SK, Agarwal SA. Ocular complications of perioperative anesthesia: a review graefe's archive for clinical and experimental ophthalmology. 2021;259(8):2069–83.
5. Malik A, Foster RE, Correa Z, Peterson M, Miller D, Riemann C. Anatomical and visual results of transconjunctival sutureless vitrectomy using subconjunctival anesthesia performed on select patients taking anticoagulant and antiplatelet agents. Retina. 2012;32:905–11.
6. Lai MM, Lai JC, Lee WH, Huang JJ, Patel S, Ying HS, Melia M, Haller JA, Handa JT. Comparison of retrobulbar and sub-Tenon's capsule injection of local anesthetic in vitreoretinal surgery. Ophthalmology. 2005;112(4):574–9.
7. Mather CM. Comparison of i.v. cannula and Stevens' cannula for sub-Tenon's block. Br J Anaesth. 2007;99(3):421–4.

8. Morley HR, Karagiannis A, Schultz DJ, Walker JC, Newland HS. Sedation for vitreoretinal surgery: a comparison of anaesthetist-administered midazolam and patient-controlled sedation with propofol. Anaesth Intensive Care. 2000;28(1):37–42.
9. Dunville L, Sood G, Kramer J. Oculocardiac reflex. Treasure Island, FL: StatPearls Publishing; 2022.
10. Pollack AL, Richard McDonald H, Ai E, Johnson RN, Dugel PU, Folk J, Gilbert Grand M, Michael Lambert H, Schwartz S, Miller RD. Massive suprachoroidal hemorrhage during pars plana vitrectomy associated with valsalva maneuver. Am J Ophthalmol. 2001;132:383–7.
11. Morris RE, Boyd GL, Sapp MR, Oltmanns MH, Kuhn F, Albin MS. Ocular venous air embolism (OVAE): a review. J Vitreoretin Dis. 2019;3(2):99.

Pars Plana Vitrectomy: The Basics

**Mostafa Hanout, Rachid Tahiri Joutei Hassani,
and Athanasios Nikolakopoulos**

This chapter discusses basic concepts in vitrectomy that apply to every vitrectomy surgery, including the basic setup, tips for maintaining excellent visualization during surgery, and basic surgical steps.

1   Getting Started

- The vitreoretinal surgeon is the lead person who is most responsible for all details related to the surgery. This mandates a thorough preoperative ophthalmic and physical examination of the patient, which is essential for proper surgical planning. Inadequate evaluation or planning can significantly impact the flow of surgery and the surgical outcome.
- The goal of the evaluation is to determine:

    - Retinal pathology and the level of its complexity and the appropriate intervention.

Supplementary Information The online version contains supplementary material available at https://doi.org/10.1007/978-3-031-47827-7_4.

M. Hanout (✉)
Ophthalmology, Apex Eye Institute, Corner Brook, NF, Canada

Department of Ophthalmology and Vision Sciences, Dalhousie University, Halifax, Canada

R. T. J. Hassani
Ambulatory Surgery Department, Avranches Granville, Granville, France

A. Nikolakopoulos
Thessorasi Retina Clinic and Drama Ophthalmology Day Center, Thessaloniki, Greece

- Lens status: phakic, pseudophakic, or aphakic and presence of cataract or posterior capsular opacity.
- Type of anesthesia required.
- Prominent facial features that may dictate a specific head position during surgery.
- Physical conditions that may be associated with increased risk or require special consideration during surgery or may interfere with the patient's ability to position after surgery, for example, anticoagulant use.
- Any medications or special surgical instrumentations that must be prepared ahead of time.

- The patient should also be counseled thoroughly regarding the surgical plan, expected prognosis, and important risks and complications. It is always advisable to "under-sell" and "over-deliver" to increase patient satisfaction. It is important and helpful to the patient to have trained staff to explain what to expect during the whole process after assessment until admission to the surgical suite.

2 Basic Setup in the Operating Room

The operating room (OR) setup should be personalized to the surgeon to improve the workflow. These are several essential points to achieve this goal:

- It is very effective to have a fixed arrangement of the OR with floor markings to indicate the position of the surgical microscope, the vitrectomy machine, and the surgical table. It is also the surgeon's responsibility to orchestrate the positions of the surgical assistant and scrub nurse (Fig. 1).
- A list of the surgeon's preferences can be placed in a visible place (hanged on the task board), including glove size, the number of pumps on the surgical table to

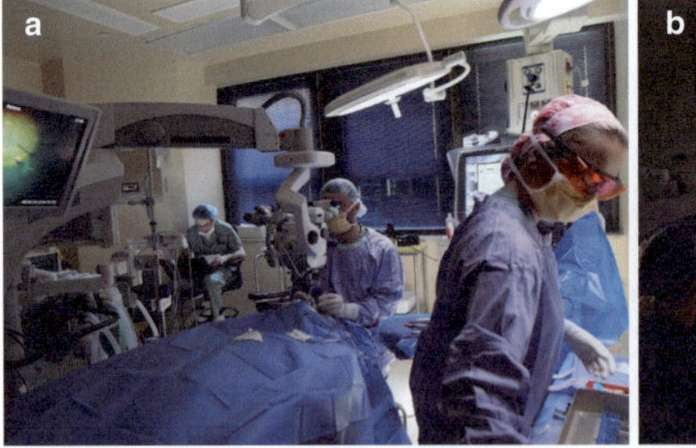
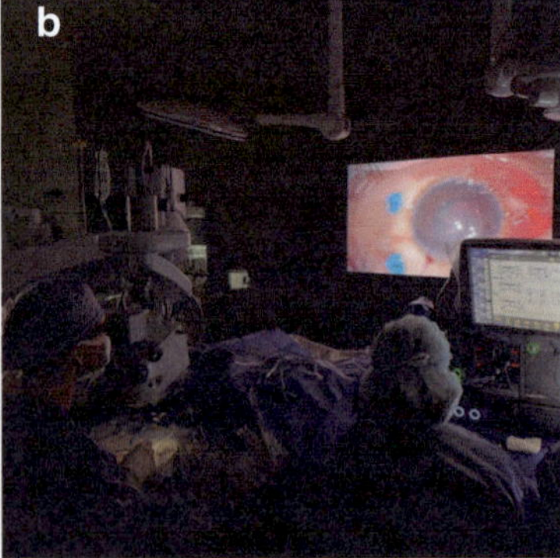

Fig. 1 An example of the operating room setup when operating with the microscope (**a**) and with 3D surgery platforms (**b**)

achieve the desired height, a photograph of the preferred arrangement of the surgical tray, the concentration of intraocular or subconjunctival drugs, etc.

- Surgical briefing before each surgery is important to confirm the patient's identity and operative eye and to list any particular drugs or instruments needed, e.g., special forceps or subretinal cannula.
- The vitrectomy machine and the surgical microscope are the most essential equipment that will be used throughout every vitrectomy surgery. It is imperative for surgeons to fully master the control of both pieces of equipment so that they operate them seamlessly and subconsciously.
- The arrangement of foot pedals is based on the surgeon's preference and should be fixed. Learning all potential functions of all buttons and kicks of the vitrectomy foot pedal, e.g., intraocular pressure (IOP) control, proportional reflux, activating or deactivating cutting, and switching between different modes, could be very critical during surgery. Similarly, learning potential functions of the microscope pedal, e.g., video recording and screenshot functions, may come in handy (Fig. 2).
- Each surgeon should have their personalized settings saved on the surgical microscope and the vitrectomy machine under their name to be easily activated by a single click of a button.
- The surgeon should be well versed in how to set up the vitrectomy machine and troubleshoot simple errors. This is especially important in less common procedures, e.g., obtaining dry vitreous samples. There may be a time when you have a nurse or technician that is not fully experienced with the machine!

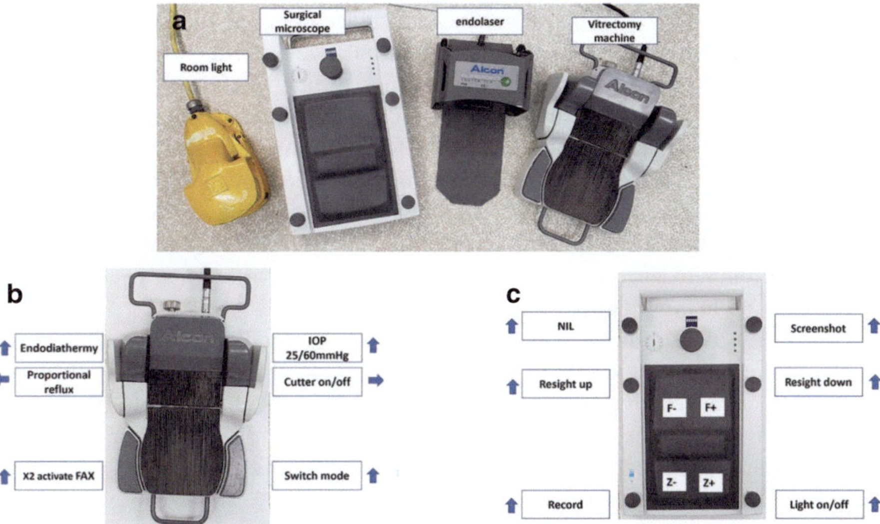

Fig. 2 Foot pedal arrangement (**a**) and different functions assigned to vitrectomy machine (**b**) and microscope foot pedals (**c**)

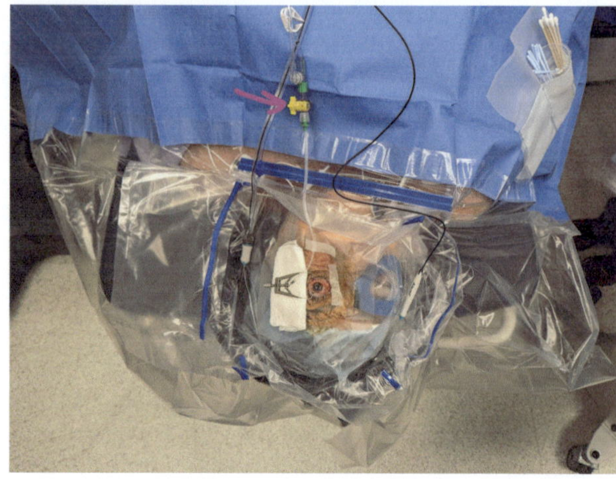

Fig. 3 Draping for vitreoretinal surgery. Note the tape covering the exposed skin over the medial canthus after the drape is cut to limit fogging of the non-contact lens from condensation. Also note the three-way stopcock to facilitate air-gas exchange (arrow), the ring surrounding the head for surgeon's wrist support, and the protective shield over the non-operated eye

- Standard aseptic technique is essential, including draping, prepping the eye with 5% povidone-iodine, proper draping to displace the eyelashes away from the surgical field, and using an eyelid speculum. Tape (Steri-Strip) can be used as an adjuvant to the draping to cover any exposed skin (Fig. 3).

3 Fluid Dynamics for Safe and Efficient Vitreous Removal

- Historically, surgery with 20-gauge (g) instruments used to be the standard in the past. The widest array of instruments can be placed through these larger sclerotomies. Sclerotomies needed suturing, and turbulence of fluid currents at the ports existed. Today, smaller-gauge instrumentation through self-sealing trocars is the standard because of its advantage of faster recovery and more precision including the ability to perform some actions of forceps, scissors, or backflush needles.
- Understanding the fluidics of vitreous removal and its impact on the vitreous gel and nearby tissues (e.g., mobile detached retina) at the cutter port will allow surgeons to tailor the parameters of the vitrectomy machine to enhance the safety and efficiency of vitreous removal. The ideal fluidics will aim at faster vitreous removal while minimizing retinal traction.
- Efficient vitreous removal was previously misunderstood as having a higher flow rate of the vitreous and was highest in larger-gauge probes (i.e., 20-g). With the modern advances in cutter technology, our understanding of efficiency was revised to the volume of vitreous removed vs. volume of infusion per minute.
- The VR surgeon needs to understand the various factors contributing to efficient vitreous removal and how each impacts the process.
  - **Size of vitrectomy probe and flow rate:** While larger-gauge probes have higher flow rate, small-gauge transconjunctival probes are favored due to

faster patient recovery and better outcomes. The flow rate in small-gauge probes can be increased by increasing the inner lumen size. This will lead to thinner walls which are addressed by using more stiff materials to minimize bending. Faster flow is driven by a higher vacuum level. However, a higher vacuum increases the risk of retinal traction and iatrogenic breaks.

- **Cutter design:** Sharp guillotine cutters are the most widely adapted design in most of the currently available vitrectomy platforms. Pneumatic cutters are favored over electric cutters given their lighter weight that enhances dexterity. Recently, the return spring has been eliminated and replaced with dual pneumatic action in the newer probe designs for better and more consistent control. Single-action and dual-action designs are available. The former cuts the vitreous only with the close stroke, whereas the latter cuts the vitreous in both the close and open strokes due to its dual blade (Fig. 4).

- **Cutting rate, duty cycle, and the sphere of influence:** Duty cycle is the percentage of open port time during a complete cut cycle. With single-action cutters, the port is closed at least 50% of the time. At low cut rates, the vitreous "bites" are relatively larger and are usually not completely detached from the main vitreous block. This often leads to aspiration of the main vitreous

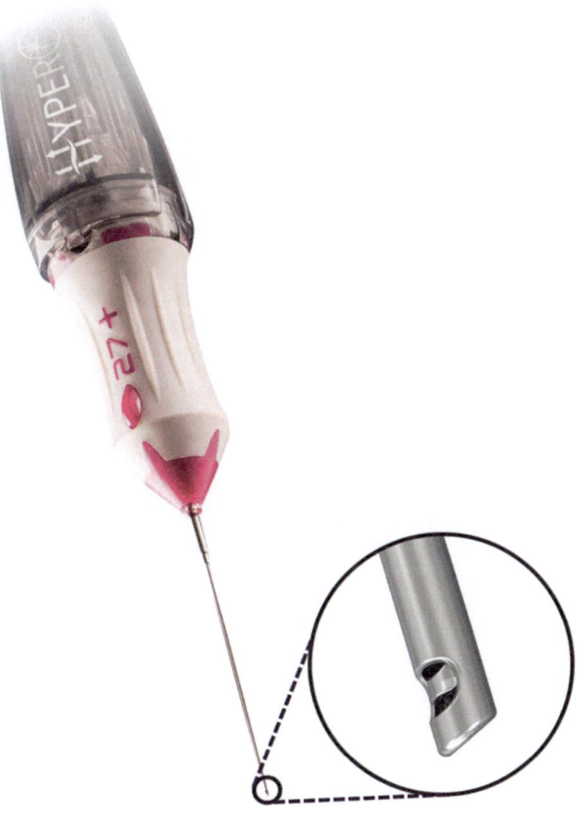

Fig. 4 Dual-blade high-speed 27-gauge cutter. Note the proximity of the cutter opening to the tip and the beveled design

block with consequent surging and pulsatile traction on the retina when the port opens. Vitreoretinal traction is worse if the surgeon moves the cutter away from the retina. The area around the cutter port influenced by the fluid dynamics is referred to as the sphere of influence, which is greater at low cut rates and increased cutter diameter with increased risk of vitreoretinal traction. Higher cut rates reduce the size of vitreous "bites" which reduces traction and reduces the sphere of influence allowing safer vitreous removal while working near a detached retina or during shaving of the vitreous base. However, higher cut rates in single-action cutters also reduce the duty cycle, hence reducing the flow and efficiency of vitreous removal. The introduction of dual-blade cutters, such as HYPERVIT (Alcon Vision LLC, Fort Worth, TX) that produces 20,000 cpm, remarkably improved vitreous fragmentation into much smaller "bites" while maintaining a nearly 100% duty cycle with a continuously open port. This allowed *faster and smoother* vitreous removal even with smaller-gauge probes and lower vacuum levels while reducing the sphere of influence and risk of traction. David Steele et al. demonstrated over 44–47% and 26–32% increase in vitreous flow in 25+ and 27+ HYPERVIT dual-action cutters (20,000 cpm), respectively, vs. corresponding gauge in ULTRAVIT single-action cutters (10,000 cpm) [1].

- In summary:
  - Dual-action cutters with high cut rates can help faster and safer vitreous removal. Lowering the vacuum level and increasing the cutting rate are advisable while working near a detached retina or shaving the vitreous base to minimize the sphere of influence and reduce the risk of traction.
  - The beveled tip design makes the port opening closer to the retina, facilitating steps such as drainage of subretinal fluid and epiretinal membrane dissection.
  - 23-g systems offer the most efficient cutter probes for core vitrectomy and allow for the utilization of larger forceps and scissors when bimanual surgery is required. At this size, the instruments are the sturdiest compared to 25- and 27-g, but there is a slightly higher need for sclerotomy suturing.
  - The finer size of the 27-g instruments makes the sphere of influence small, and thus, the cutting is very precise [1]. But at this size, the instruments are the least sturdy, and the most available illumination probes are focal and not wide-field. Core vitrectomy is also the least efficient with the 27-g.
  - 25-g is an ideal size and offers advantages of both 23- and 27-g in terms of small size, good sturdiness, and bright wide-field illumination. 25-g vitrectomy probes are reasonably efficient in removing the vitreous, and the ports allow an intermediate array of instruments.

4   Illumination

Advances in illumination include brighter wide-field illumination probes and chandelier lights. We prefer wide-field illumination probes and seldom use focal light pipes. In selected cases where bimanual surgery is needed, we use chandelier lights, as in some cases of diabetic delamination and proliferative vitreoretinopathy (PVR) surgery. With 3D surgery, the surgeon uses [2] much less illumination than when operating with the conventional microscope due to the ability to increase the camera gain.

5   Tips for Excellent Visualization During Vitrectomy

To perform a vitrectomy, we need to see through a specific set of media that must be clear to provide an excellent surgical view (Video 1).

- The eyepiece of the surgical microscope should be clean and the interpupillary distance (IPD) set. The refractive dial should be neutralized to +0.00 D or adjusted to the surgeon's refraction as per preference.
- **Non-contact wide-angle viewing system:** Clarity of the non-contact lens, such as RESIGHT® 500/700 fundus viewing system from Zeiss or BIOM® 5 from Oculus Surgical, Inc., should be maintained throughout the surgery. Effective draping is vital to prevent fogging of the non-contact lens from condensation. Sometimes, cutting the upper part of the face mask to make it shorter can expose a larger area of the patient's bare skin, thus improving the adhesiveness of the drape. This can help redirect the steam from the patient's breath to minimize lens condensation. Using available anti-fogging agents is also helpful [3]. Bringing the lens too close to the corneal surface can cause fogging or lens-corneal touch. On the other hand, raising the lens too high will significantly decrease the area seen of the retina. Therefore, it is important to keep the lens at a "sweet" distance from the corneal surface that does not cause fogging while maintaining an adequate field of the retina.
- **Cornea:** Lubricating the corneal surface is critical to maintaining surgical view during vitrectomy. Using dispersive viscoelastic material immediately after inserting the eyelid speculum can maintain adequate corneal lubrication throughout the procedure. Alternatively, balanced salt solution (BSS) can be used frequently on the cornea during the procedure. In complex diabetic vitrectomies, prolonged use of high IOP for hemostasis can lead to corneal epithelial edema. If mild, reducing the IOP, if appropriate, and massaging the corneal epithelium using a sterile cotton swab or a cannula may resolve epithelial edema and restore the view. However, debridement of the corneal epithelium may occasionally be needed.

- **Anterior chamber (AC):** Any media opacity in the AC needs to be dealt with before approaching the posterior segment. This includes hyphema, air bubbles, fibrin, prolapsed silicone oil droplets, etc. Two paracenteses are created, one for irrigation using an AC maintainer or the posterior segment infusion cannula while using the vitrectomy probe through the other port to aspirate and remove the undesired material. Unless the patient is aphakic, it is best to avoid placing the infusion in the posterior segment during this step, as doing so usually results in AC shallowing.
- **Crystalline and intraocular lens:**

  - Cataracts of enough density to preclude adequate visualization of the posterior segment must be removed with or without intraocular (IOL) insertion, as indicated. Therefore, preparing IOL measurements before vitrectomy surgery in any phakic patient is important.
  - If the crystalline lens is clear or there is a mild cataract that does not preclude the surgical view, we do not endorse removing the lens simultaneously in the same procedure. This is mainly to make surgery short and to avoid intraoperative complications such as narrowing of the pupil and postoperative complications such as posterior synechia, significant postoperative inflammation, or IOL optic incarceration. Every effort should be made to avoid damaging the lens, which most commonly occurs due to posterior lens capsule touch with surgical instruments.
  - There are several essential tips to avoid lens touch during vitrectomy in phakic patients. Firstly, sclerotomies should be created 4 mm posterior to the limbus, which should be measured carefully. Secondly, there are certain limits to the range of movement of straight surgical instruments inside the vitreous cavity that should be respected as follows:

    Working inferiorly near the 6 o'clock position, the vitrector should not cross a virtual line that passes across the fovea (Fig. 5).
    Working in the mid-vitreous cavity, the instruments should not cross beyond the equator.
    Working superiorly, the vitrector in one hand can reach the other superior sclerotomy.
    To reach outside the above-described ranges, hands should be switched to avoid lens touch (Fig. 5).
    It is advisable to move the instruments instead of rotating the globe to reduce the risk of lens touch.
    There is more lens clearance with curved instruments such as curved endolaser probes; thus, crossing to the other side is safe (Fig. 6).

  - Posterior capsular opacity in pseudophakic patients can be managed by surgical posterior capsulotomy using the vitrectomy cutter.
  - Fogging of the IOL may happen when the vitreous cavity is filled with air and the posterior capsule is opened. This can be managed by placing a small amount of dispersive viscoelastic material at the back of the intraocular lens within the area of the capsular defect.

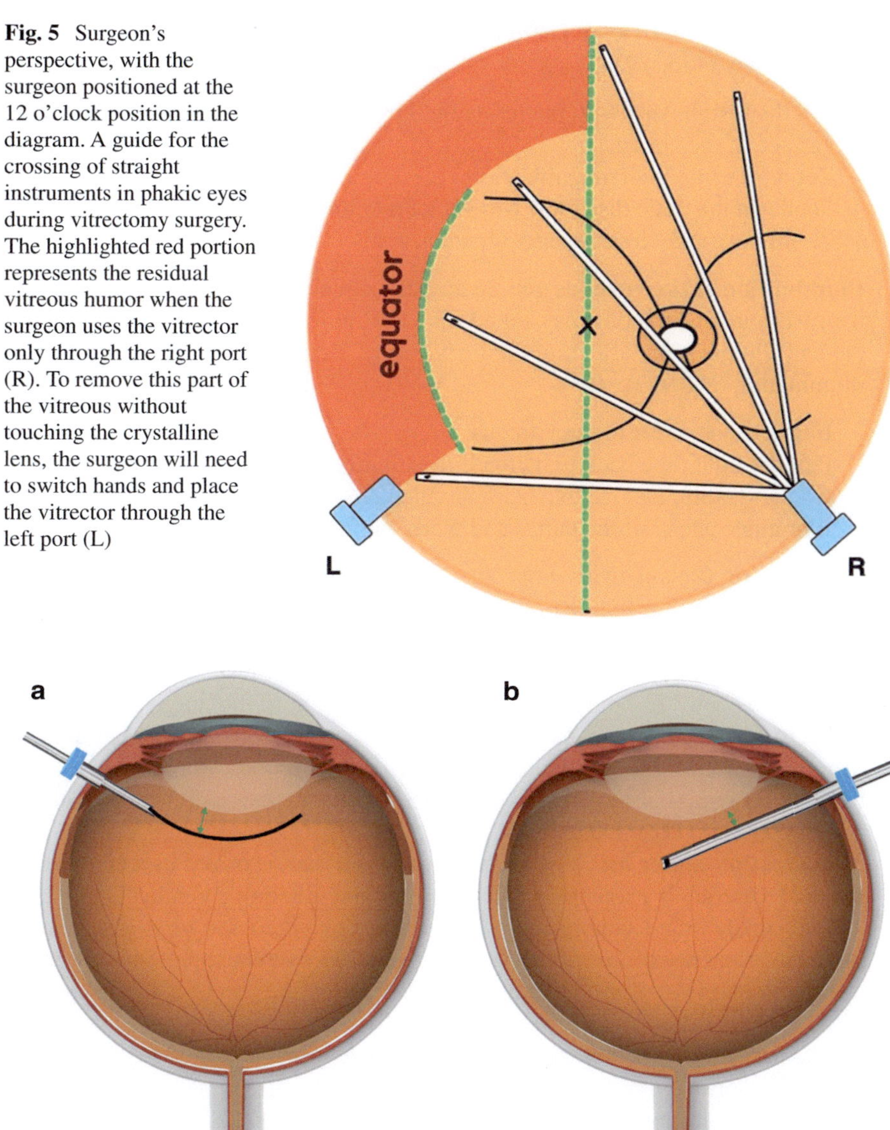

Fig. 5 Surgeon's perspective, with the surgeon positioned at the 12 o'clock position in the diagram. A guide for the crossing of straight instruments in phakic eyes during vitrectomy surgery. The highlighted red portion represents the residual vitreous humor when the surgeon uses the vitrector only through the right port (R). To remove this part of the vitreous without touching the crystalline lens, the surgeon will need to switch hands and place the vitrector through the left port (L)

Fig. 6 Distance between the back of the crystalline lens and vitrectomy instruments when crossing the midline (green arrow). There is more clearance between the curved instruments such as the curved laser probe and the lens (**a**) than with straight instruments (**b**)

- **Adjusting surgical view:** There are four steps to establish an excellent initial surgical view (Video 2):

  - Fill the resight lens with the retina field by bringing it adequately close to the surface of the cornea.
  - Zoom in using high magnification.
  - Focus on the optic disc until you get a crisp image.
  - Zoom out to the desired magnification.

- **Illumination of the vitreous gel:** Seeing the vitreous is key to removing it effectively. Beginner surgeons may spend time aspirating BSS if they incorrectly use the end illumination, affecting their efficiency. Here are some tips for effective illumination (Video 3):

  - Illuminate anterior to the vitreous.
  - Pull the light pipe back to increase the illuminated area, reduce phototoxicity risk, and eliminate overexposure in video recording.
  - Illuminate ahead of the cutter and work within the "light cone."

- **Centralizing the surgical view:** This is an essential step for visualization that takes time to master but can be taught to the novice VR fellow using surgical simulation. When the surgeon reaches the peripheral part of the vitreous, the viewing lens and the eye become no longer aligned. This results in a shifted, non-centralized view. To compensate for this decentration, the surgeon frequently learns to X-Y the microscope during the surgery. It is good to remember that, for example, to remove the superotemporal peripheral vitreous, the surgeon tilts the eye up and temporal as much as possible and moves the microscope (with the viewing system) up and temporal.

- **Visualization under air:** Visualization under air can be tricky, especially if the residual vitreous is present peripherally near the infusion cannula. This breaks air into many small bubbles as it flows into the vitreous cavity, significantly obscuring the view for a few precious moments. To overcome this issue, perform a core vitrectomy to thoroughly clear the vitreous at the port of the infusion cannula. This will allow a more constant influx of air during the fluid-air exchange (FAX) with minimal bubbling and will minimize visual disturbances during this step. Also, refocus the microscope as the presence of air makes the eye very myopic. Decreasing the magnification and a very slight X-Y movement also improve the view (Video 4). We do not advocate performing vitrectomy under air. Although air stabilizes a detached retina, it pushes the remaining vitreous toward the retina, which may increase the risk of hitting the retina during vitreous removal. Finally, one needs to be wary of high velocity of BSS fluid current if the surgeon switches from air back to BSS, which may cause retinal damage. This can be prevented by placing the light pipe between the infusion cannula and the retina at the beginning of the exchange (Video 5).

- **The use of vitreous stains and dyes:** Use of diluted triamcinolone or trypan blue to highlight the vitreous cortex could be particularly important in specific pathologies such as myopic traction maculopathy (MTM) and diabetic traction detachment, where vitreoschisis is almost universal. Please see further discussion on tissue stains in Chap. 13 "Surgical Management of Epiretinal Membranes and Vitreomacular Traction".

6 Basic Steps of Vitrectomy Surgery

Basic surgical steps that are performed in every vitrectomy surgery should be mastered by the surgeon so that they become second nature. Below is a brief overview of the most fundamental steps in basic vitrectomy.

- **Creating pars plana sclerotomies and setting up the infusion:** sharp trocars are used to facilitate the passage of the cannulas, typically creating three pars plana sclerotomies 3.5 or 4 mm posterior to the limbus depending on the lens status. In phakic patients, a 4 mm distance will help reduce the risk of iatrogenic lens injury, whereas 3.5 mm is safe in pseudophakic or aphakic eyes. If bimanual maneuvers are planned, a fourth sclerotomy may be needed to insert a chandelier light. After removing the trocars, the cannulas will remain in position, allowing easy insertion and retrieval of micro-instruments. Unlike non-valved cannulas, they avoid the inconvenience of needing plugs and provide more stable fluidics, especially if perfluorocarbon liquids (PFCL) are to be used. However, the downside of valved cannulas is inserting soft-tip cannulas could be trickier. This could be easily overcome by cutting the soft tip shorter or inserting it under direct visualization through the surgical microscope.

  It is ideal for creating beveled self-sealing sclerotomies to achieve sutureless surgery. The key steps to achieve this include:

  - Conjunctival displacement gently using a Q-tip or forceps to misalign the conjunctival and scleral incisions.
  - It is safer to measure the desired distance from the limbus (3.5 or 4 mm) using the marks at the heel of the trocar.
  - Insert the trocars in an angled fashion 30–45° radial to the limbus with the flat aspect (not the sharp aspect) facing the sclera, and then penetrate in the same orientation or toward the center of the vitreous (Video 6).
  - Creating sclerotomies can be tricky in soft eyes, such as in a previously vitrectomized eye. To overcome this situation, BSS could be injected to pressurize the globe using a 30-g needle. Alternatively, adequate counter-pressure could be applied by holding the globe firmly using suitable toothed forceps. Once the first sclerotomy is created, the infusion line can be inserted, and the IOP can be raised to facilitate subsequent sclerotomies.
  - In case a 20-g sclerotomy is needed for a fragmatome or intraocular magnet, it is usually made parallel to the limbus, and a localized peritomy is needed.
  - The superior sclerotomies should be located at 10 and 2 o'clock meridians or between 9–10 and 2–3 o'clock meridians. Placing the sclerotomies directly at

3 and 9 o'clock or more superior to 10–2 o'clock will compromise intraoperative access and make the surgery more difficult.

- The infusion line should be inserted in the inferotemporal sclerotomy with the infusion line clamped. The silver shining of the infusion cannula should be visualized through the pupil (sometimes, you need to shine the light pipe through the pupil with room lights out) before the infusion is opened to avoid misdirection of the infusion to the subretinal or suprachoroidal space (Video 7).
- Caution should be used in cases with preexisting choroidal detachment or dense vitreous hemorrhage with impossible visualization of the cannula. In the former cases, a 6-mm-long cannula can be helpful, and infusion may not necessarily be inserted inferotemporally but instead in the quadrant with no choroidal detachment or where choroidal detachment is most shallow.
- In cases of dense VH, the light pipe can be inserted through the trocar to confirm passage into the vitreous cavity before inserting the infusion line.

- **Detaching the posterior hyaloid**: inducing a posterior vitreous detachment (PVD) is a fundamental step in almost every vitrectomy surgery except on uncommon occasions such as core vitrectomy for some endophthalmitis cases and vitrectomy in some pediatric eyes, where detaching the posterior hyaloid could be unnecessary, too risky, or even impossible! Although many surgeons can detach the posterior hyaloid in most cases without using any stain, staining the posterior hyaloid with triamcinolone is helpful and is especially advisable when vitreoschisis is expected, such as in high myopic cases or in cases of diabetic vitreoretinal traction to ensure complete dissection of all epicenters.

  Detaching the posterior hyaloid is usually performed using the vitrectomy cutter alone with maximum suction and cutter-off mode. Aspiration may be started over the optic disc edge until occlusion occurs, and then the hyaloid is elevated straight up. You can move tangentially to grasp the hyaloid better before elevating up, but this needs to be for a very small distance so as not to induce traction on the opposite retinal quadrant (Video 8). Some surgeons would prefer to turn the port of the cutter down and hover over the nasal peripapillary area until they engage the hyaloid and start elevating it. In some challenging cases with anomalous sticky hyaloid, a macular pick can be useful to initiate elevation, which could then be completed by the vitrectomy cutter [4] (Video 9). If inducing PVD proves very difficult, a partial internal limiting membrane (ILM) peel can be performed. This will create an opening in the posterior hyaloid, facilitating the induction of a PVD,
- **Core vitrectomy:** it is a good practice to clear the vitreous thoroughly at the ports at the beginning of surgery to clear the infusion port and to eliminate traction while inserting or retrieving instruments. Core vitrectomy, however, can only be completed after detaching the posterior hyaloid, where the vitreous skirt can be trimmed to the periphery in a circumferential pattern.
- **Vitreous base shaving:** except for anterior PVR cases, we do not routinely endorse shaving of the vitreous base. It does not improve the surgery outcome

and it may be associated with increased risks such as creation of iatrogenic retinal tears and injury to the crystalline lens and the zonules. In primary retinal detachment, we still make sure we remove traction around retinal breaks.

- **Anterior hyaloid removal:** some surgeons prefer to start surgery by cutting and removing the retrolental anterior vitreous directly visualized through the surgical microscope. We do this in pseudophakic eyes. Because of the associated risk of hitting the crystalline lens in phakic eyes, we feel that this step is not needed unless the anterior hyaloid is dusted with blood or opacified and is interfering with visualization during pars plana vitrectomy (PPV).
- **Internal search of the peripheral retina:** in *all* cases, before flattening the retinal periphery with tamponade or directly before the closure of the eye on BSS, the surgeon has to search the peripheral retina for tears. Although the incidence of retinal breaks with trocar at the entry sites is very low compared to the previous 20-g vitrectomy without trocars (<1% vs. >10%, respectively) [5], it is best to look for a tear and deal with it using laser or cryopexy than having an avoidable postoperative retinal detachment after an ERM or macular hole case (Video 10). There is less access in the nasal quadrant, making an internal search more difficult. Tips for making this step easier include dropping the infusion pressure down to 15 mmHg and indenting the nasal quadrants after the eye becomes softer to improve peripheral visualization (Video 11). In general, it is best to do the indentation gently as it could be painful, particularly if anesthesia (local or general) is wearing off at the end of surgery. If the eye is filled with PFCL, non-gentle indentation and sudden release of indentation can also lead to PFCL sloshing, resulting in temporary interference with visualization and, more importantly, migration of PFCL bubbles through a preexisting peripheral retinal tear into the subretinal space.
- **Closing sclerotomies:** it is critical to avoid the leak of gas or fluid resulting in postoperative hypotony, tamponade underfilling, or choroidal detachment. If silicone oil is used, leakage of oil into the subconjunctival space can cause a significant inflammatory reaction that is difficult to resolve, even with conjunctival excision. Properly fashioning the sclerotomy incision in a beveled design is key to making it self-sealing. Fluid-air exchange can indicate if the incision is leaking, as bubbling can be seen. Needling the sclerotomy bed with a 30G needle has been shown to assist with sclerotomy closure and minimize the need for suturing (Video 12) [6]. It is advisable, however, to have a low threshold to suture a leaking sclerotomy using 8–0 Vicryl. We routinely suture all sclerotomies in silicone-filled eyes.

7 Tamponade and Vitreous Substitutes

At the conclusion of vitrectomy, different substances can be used to fill the vitreous cavity to substitute the vitreous gel, including air, gas, or liquid substitutes. Less often, the eye can be left fluid-filled.

8 Complications of PPV

PPV may be associated with potential complications such as lens or retinal touch. Other complications may be more linked to the treated retinal condition such as retinal redetachment or vitreous cavity hemorrhage. In general, complications will be discussed under the relevant chapters. One subject we would like to touch on here is iatrogenic retinal touch by instruments such as the vitrector or the light pipe and the common scenarios to be aware of, particularly when surgeons are in their early learning phase.

- Early on, it is best to have all instruments out of the eye when performing steps such as checking the machine parameters or as the assistant wets the cornea and the viewing system is lifted off the eye so as to avoid hitting the retina (Video 13). Later on, you will learn how to 'lock' your hands in the anterior vitreous cavity during these steps, away from the crystalline lens and the retina (Video 14).
- Be wary of the curvature of the back of the eye as you are moving instruments from the posterior pole to the periphery particularly during laser. Also if you are introducing instruments in the eye under high magnification, for example introducing a forceps to peel the ILM.
- Injecting substances inside the vitreous cavity while maintaining the position of the light pipe can be challenging in the initial stages with a single-handed approach, risking the potential slippage of the cannula. The presence of an assistant can prove beneficial in such situations (Video 15).
- Iatrogenic retinal tears can occur as a result of vitreoretinal traction during surgery. Current rates, when compared to the previous 20-gauge surgery, are relatively low, given the utilization of trocars and modern high-cut vitreoretinal machines. It is noteworthy that the risk of this complication tends to be lower when a PVD is already present, as seen in epiretinal membranes, compared to cases where PVD induction is required, such as in macular holes [7].

Key Points
- Personalized protocols in the OR, including vitrectomy machine settings, the position of the foot pedals, and the arrangement of surgical instruments, help make the surgery day seamless and efficient.
- Visualization is key in vitrectomy surgery.
- Dual-action cutters with high cut rates can help faster and safer vitreous removal.
- Fundamental steps of vitrectomy should be mastered by the surgeon and become second nature. This includes optimum placing of sclerotomies, X-Y of the microscope to maintain a centralized wide-field view of the retina, and detaching the posterior hyaloid.
- The ability to maintain a centralized wide-field view during surgery is an important skill to learn early on.

References

1. Steel DH, Charles M, Zhu Y, Tambat S, Irannejad AM, Charles S. Fluidic performance of a dual-action vitrectomy probe compared with a single-action probe. Retina. 2022;42(11):2150–8.
2. Agranat JS, Miller JB, Douglas VP, Douglas KAA, Marmalidou A, Cunningham MA, Houston SK III. The scope of three-dimensional digital visualization systems in vitreoretinal surgery. Clin Ophthalmol. 2019;13:2093–6.
3. Kreps EO, Lemm JM, Ruagh EA, Ramkissoon YD. Fogging of Non-Contact Viewing Lenses During Vitreoretinal Surgery. Retina. 2016;36(12):2428–9.
4. Ellabban AA, Barry R, Sallam AAB. Surgical induction of posterior vitreous detachment using combined sharp dissection and active aspiration. Acta Ophthalmologica. 2016;94(6).
5. Ramkissoon YD, Aslam SA, Shah SP, Wong SC, Sullivan PM. Risk of iatrogenic peripheral retinal breaks in 20-G pars plana vitrectomy. Ophthalmology. 2010;117(9):1825–30.
6. Felfeli T, Altomare F, Mandelcorn ED. Sutureless closure of 23- and 25-gauge leaking sclerotomies with the scleral needling technique. Retina. 2020;40(5):838–44.
7. Fajgenbaum MAP, Neffendorf JE, Wong RS, Laidlaw DAH, Williamson TH. Intraoperative and postoperative complications in phacovitrectomy for epiretinal membrane and macular hole. Retina. 2018;38(9):1865–72.

Vitreous Substitutes

Alex U. Pisig, Robert Gizicki, and Mostafa Hanout

This chapter outlines the important properties, indications, and safety profile of the different vitreous substitutes/tamponades currently used.

1 Physical Properties of Tamponades

1. Specific Gravity (SG): The relative density of a material to that of water. Air or gas has a very low specific gravity at 0.001 g/mL, so it floats in the vitreous cavity. Silicone oil (SO) also floats but less than air as its specific gravity is only slightly lower than water (0.97). Perfluorocarbon liquid (PFCL) is heavier than water and thus sinks in it.
2. Buoyancy: The upward force, or buoyant force, that acts on an object in water. The "pressing" force for silicone oil is relatively small (0.03 g), as the specific gravity is close to that of water. The force is greatest with air or gas (0.999 g).

Supplementary Information The online version contains supplementary material available at https://doi.org/10.1007/978-3-031-47827-7_5.

A. U. Pisig
Retina and Vitreous Diseases, Asian Eye Institute, Makati City, Philippines

R. Gizicki (✉)
Ophthalmology, Surrey Memorial Hospital, University of British Columbia,
Surrey, BC, Canada
e-mail: rgizicki@retinabc.ca

M. Hanout
Ophthalmology, Apex Eye Institute, Corner Brook, NF, Canada

A. B. Sallam et al. (eds.), *Practical Manual of Vitreoretinal Surgery*,
https://doi.org/10.1007/978-3-031-47827-7_5

Table 1 Main physical properties of different vitreous tamponades

	Air/gas	PFCL	SO	Water
Specific gravity (g/mL)	0.001	1.7–2	0.97	1
Viscosity (mPas)	0.018	24–48	1000–5000	1
Interfacial tension against water (mN/m)	72	50	40	NA
Refractive index	1	1.3	1.4	1.33

3. Interfacial Tension: The force of attraction between the molecules at the interface of immiscible fluids. For example, the air-liquid interface substance with a high interfacial tension will have a greater tendency to stay as one large bubble without breaking into small bubbles. This force is highest at the air-aqueous interface (72 mN/m) followed by PFCL (50 mN/m). This has implications in PVR surgery in checking whether the retina has been sufficiently relaxed after membrane peel or retinectomy. Surgeons should judge retinal relaxation based on retinal flattening under PFCL and not under air since the high surface tension of air can flatten the retina even if some stiffness exists. However, retinal attachment is unlikely to be maintained with SO (lower interfacial tension at 40 mN/m) postoperatively in this situation.
4. Viscosity: The resistance of a substance to deformation under shear stress. The higher the viscosity, the higher the surface tension, and the lower the tendency for breaking into small droplets (Table 1).

1.1 Ideal Vitreous Substitute

A successful vitreous humor substitute should maintain the physical and biochemical properties of the original vitreous [1]. The vitreous gel is damaged in various vitreoretinal disorders and needs to be replaced, hence the need for substitutes. The ideal substitute should:

- Be easy to inject.
- Be long lasting with a good tamponade effect.
- Maintain physiologic intraocular pressure (IOP).
- Have a high surface tension and sufficient buoyancy to serve its intended purpose of providing tamponade to the retinal tear by resisting transretinal tear fluid flow.
- Be inert, slowly biodegradable, and transparent so that it does not opacify postoperatively.
- Avoid cellular proliferation.

1.2 Classification

There are several ways to classify vitreous substitutes, the most common of which is to organize them based on their molecular status—whether they are in gas or liquid form.

2   Intraocular Air/Gases

Unlike air, which immediately enters the dissolution phase after injection, pure expansile gases undergo three phases of expansion, equilibration, and dissolution before being completely resorbed by the eye. These gases' lower water solubility than nitrogen makes them expand when injected into the eye.

Phases of Gas Resorption:

1. Expansion happens when physiologic gases', mainly nitrogen's, diffusion rate into the bubble is higher than the rate of gas dissolving into the surrounding tissue fluid compartment.
2. Equilibration phase begins when the partial pressure of nitrogen in the bubble equals that in the surrounding fluid compartment.
3. Dissolution phase begins when gases dissolve into the fluid compartment and the gas gradually decreases in size. This phase is the longest of all three phases.

The duration of these phases differs for different gases and depends on their solubility. Tamponade is often effective only during the initial 25% of its life span since it requires at least 50% of its initial size to provide an effective tamponade. Fish eggs or bubbles smaller than 50% are ineffective even though they can remain in the eye for a long time. Additionally, evidence shows that there is greater diffusion into the uveal tissues than into the lens, presumably because the lens is less metabolically active and lacks blood flow. The life span of gases may be more than twice as long in phakic non-vitrectomized eyes than in aphakic vitrectomized eyes.

The following features are the basis of their value in vitreoretinal surgery:

- Buoyancy, which applies upward pressure to flatten the detached retina.
- Surface tension, which closes retinal breaks and prevents the bubble from passing into the subretinal space.
- Low solubility in water, which varies depending on the molecular structure of a given gas.

The first two properties provide internal tamponade. However, the high buoyancy of gas compared to water can result in displacement of the retina in rhegmatogenous retinal detachment (RRD) by displacing subretinal fluid posteriorly. The third factor maintains the retinal tamponade for a desired period, depending on specific surgical objectives and goals.

It is unclear whether air/gas tamponade works by sealing the break or just by reducing the turbulence of the fluid currents going in and out through the break and if this is enough to give the retinal pigment epithelium (RPE) adequate time to pump fluid to dry the retina. If the latter is true, then a big gas fill to have contact with the retinal tear may not be needed, and postoperative head positioning may not be that critical in RRD surgery [2].

2.1 Air (Non-expansile Gas)

Filtered room air is readily accessible and cheap or, rather, free. It is colorless and inert and diffuses easily in the blood circulation, reducing its tamponade effects quickly in a few days. Complete resorption of an air-filled eye can be expected in approximately 5–7 days postoperatively.

2.2 SF$_6$, C$_2$F$_6$, and C$_3$F$_8$ (Expansile Gases)

The most used expansile gases in practice in North America are sulfur hexafluoride (SF$_6$) and perfluoropropane (C$_3$F$_8$). Other forms of perfluorocarbon gases (such as C$_2$F$_6$) may be available elsewhere in the world. Expansile gases provide longer and more effective tamponade than air. These are inert, inflammable gases with no odor or color. For perfluorocarbons, water solubility varies according to the carbon chain length. The longer the carbon chain, the lower the solubility in water; hence, the longer the intraocular longevity of the gas. Table 2 summarizes the important features of different intraocular gases.

2.3 SF$_6$, C$_2$F$_6$, and C$_3$F$_8$ (Expansile Gases): Clinical Applications

Common indications for intraocular gas injection include:

- Pneumatic retinopexy.
- RRD surgery with pars plana vitrectomy or scleral buckle.
- Macular hole surgery.
- Displacement of subretinal hemorrhage.

Table 2 Intraocular gas properties and indications of use

	Air	SF$_6$	C$_2$F$_6$	C$_3$F$_8$
Expansion (times original size)	NA	2.0	3.3	4.0
Time to maximum expansion (hours)	NA	24–48	36–60	72–96
Non-expansile concentration	NA	18%	15–16%	14%
Longevity	5–7 days	1–2 weeks	4–5 weeks	6–8 weeks
Volume used in pneumatic retinopexy	1.2 mL	0.6 mL	0.4 mL	0.3 mL

2.4   SF₆, C₂F₆, and C₃F₈ (Expansile Gases): Techniques of Use

Air-gas exchange is done when the eye is filled with air.
Techniques for air-gas exchange:

1. Conventional technique: Before the removal of the trocars, gas of the proper concentration in a 50 mL syringe is delivered through a three-way stopcock in the infusion line. A 27-gauge (g) needle or a venting cannula is placed in one of the two remaining trocars to act as a vent. Once adequate gas exchange is achieved, the remaining trocars are removed (Video 1). At least, four times the eye volume of gas must be flushed through the eye to attain the final desired gas concentration. With the average vitreous volume being approximately 4.5 mL, a minimum of 35 mL of gas is flushed for optimal effect. In a highly myopic eye (>25 mm axial length), the vitreous cavity is larger and thus a larger amount of gas (up to 80 mL) may be needed for the flush [3].
2. After the removal of all trocars and confirming each sclerotomy is air-tight, gas in a syringe with a 27-g needle is delivered through the pars plana, while a second 27-g needle, on an empty syringe and with plunger removed, is also inserted through the pars plana and acts as a vent. In this technique, clear visualization of the injecting needle tip within the vitreous cavity is essential before any gas exchange is performed because inadequate placement may lead to suprachoroidal gas injection, intraocular hemorrhage, retinal or choroidal detachment, and insufficient gas fill postoperatively.
3. In an air-filled eye that is slightly on the hypotonus side, 1 mL of 100% gas is injected for SF_6. This will result in a gas concentration of about 25% at the end. For C_3F_8, 0.5 mL of 100% gas will result in a concentration of about 12%. An advantage of this technique is less use of intravitreal gas (1 mL vs. 50 mL) which has cost implications. However, the technique is more prone to dilution errors.

2.5   Gas Top-Up

Some degree of hypotony is usually accepted after air-gas exchange, and there is no need to top up the gas. Make sure that there is no leakage from sclerotomy that requires suturing. However, if the surgeon finds the IOP very low, gas top-up will be required. Video 2 shows a suggested technique for this step.

2.6   SF₆, C₂F₆, and C₃F₈ (Expansile Gases): Postoperative Care

Proper posturing of the head after intraocular gas injection ensures proper displacement of subretinal hemorrhage and opposition to retinal breaks and macular holes. The area of interest should be positioned at the uppermost part of the eye and be in direct contact with the bubble. Face-down posturing can also prevent gas bubble-induced pupil block glaucoma, IOL decentration resulting in pupil block glaucoma, and cataract development for phakic patients. Lying laterally on the opposite side of the break is also accepted (i.e., lying on the left for a right-side break) if face-down or prone posture is difficult.

2.7 SF_6, C_2F_6, and C_3F_8 (Expansile Gases): Complications

Complications of intraocular gas use include:

- Gas-induced cataracts (feathery posterior subcapsular cataracts).
- Elevated IOP, secondary to gas overfill or inappropriate/wrong gas dilution.
- Hypotony with leaking sclerotomies.
- Migration of gas into the subretinal space, which can affect proper retinal reattachment.
- Migration to the anterior chamber, especially in aphakic or pseudophakic eyes with a non-intact posterior capsule.

Avoiding lying supine and proper wound closure with optimal eye pressure control usually mitigate these complications.

In the event of elevated postoperative IOP in a gas-filled eye, it is critical to ascertain the nature of the issue. Urgent intervention will be needed, whether in the outpatient setting or the operating room. The specific intervention depends on the level of IOP elevation, visual status at presentation, and associated ocular pathology.

- If the IOP elevation is moderate (30–45 mmHg) and visual acuity measurable at HM or better, this indicates a patent central retinal artery. Aggressive medical treatment for IOP reduction is recommended with topical and systemic medication. Close monitoring of the IOP in the next few hours is recommended to confirm adequate IOP reduction.
- If the IOP elevation is severe (>45 mmHg) and visual acuity is LP, this indicates severe compromise of the retinal vascular perfusion and may lead to permanent severe vision loss if not treated with urgency. An urgent vitreous tap to remove excess gas is recommended using a 3 cc syringe and a 30G or 27G needle. The tap is carried out using active suction until the IOP is normalized on palpation or direct measurement. One needs to be careful to do gradual decompression of the eye to avoid the risk of suprachoroidal hemorrhage. Aggressive medical management of the IOP is then started. Following this, the IOP should be closely monitored. If the IOP rises again to a severe level within the next 2–3 h, this may indicate an elevated gas concentration within the eye. In this scenario, the patient should be brought urgently to the operating room to surgically evacuate the gas and complete the gas exchange with an appropriate concentration.

Gas bubble size changes at different altitudes and can cause a sudden increase in IOP and possible retinal arterial occlusion. It is therefore important to advise patients that air travel is strictly contraindicated, as is the passage through high mountain passes and rapid altitude gain. Some studies have suggested that air travel is safe if the intraocular gas bubble is 10% or less, but in general, air travel should only be permitted after the complete dissolution of the bubble. Should such travel be necessary, consideration should be given to using non-gas vitreous tamponades, such as silicone oil.

3   Liquid Vitreous Substitutes

These substitutes include agents that can act as temporary fillers of the vitreous cavity during surgical procedures.

3.1   *Perfluorocarbon Liquid (PFCL)*

Perfluorocarbon liquid (PFCL) is a synthetic fluorinated hydrocarbon containing carbon-fluorine bonds. These exist in liquid forms due to their long carbon chains (compounds with a carbon chain shorter than C5, e.g., C_3F_8, exist in a gaseous state).

3.2   *Perfluorocarbon Liquid (PFCL): Advantages*

PFCL use is popular because of the following:

- High density and specific gravity allow the flattening and unrolling of retinal folds. This is the basis of its usefulness in retinal surgery.
- Optical clarity, allowing surgical manipulations under PFCL.
- Different refractive indexes from saline allow a visible PFCL-fluid interface.
- No interference to laser wavelengths permitting endolaser under PFCL.
- Moderately high interfacial tension tends to hold it in a large confluent bubble and reduce the risk of PFCL migration into the subretinal space through the break.
- Low viscosity allows easy injection and aspiration even with small-gauge vitrectomies.
- PFCL is hydrophobic. Its immiscibility with water resists incursion by saline and blood and allows a clear operating field despite intraoperative bleeding.
- Its immiscibility with silicone oil (SO) allows PFCL-SO exchange, which is helpful in specific scenarios.

3.3   Perfluorocarbon Liquid (PFCL): Indications

Due to its versatility and ease of use, PFCL is utilized in different surgical scenarios where a temporary heavier-than-water tamponade is needed:

- Keeping the macula attached during RRD and PVR surgery.
- Giant retinal tears for unfolding the retina, and some authors use it for short-term postoperative tamponade (10 days).
- Vitreous base shaving, wherein the PFCL displaces the vitreous skirt anteriorly.
- Subretinal and suprachoroidal hemorrhage to displace the bleeding peripherally.
- Debatable: it may be that PFCL has a cushioning effect and protects the macula from an intraocular foreign body or lens fragments during fragmentation.

3.4   Perfluorocarbon Liquid (PFCL): Techniques of Injection

Below is the standard technique for injecting PFCL in the repair of an uncomplicated RRD:

- After standard core vitrectomy, removal of the posterior hyaloid face, peripheral trimming, and release of all traction, the surgeon begins filling the posterior pole with PFCL.
- Start the injection over the optic disc and proceed slowly to build up a bubble. Some surgeons prefer to start the injection over the nasal retina, outside the edge of the optic disc for fear that the PFCL jet penetrates through the disc.
- To prevent IOP elevation during injection, a dual-bore or fenestrated cannula (Video 3) may be used, or when a chandelier illumination is present, the injection can be done in one hand while fluid is being aspirated using a vitrector in the other. Injection speed should be gradual and sustained, keeping the tip of the cannula submerged within the PFCL bubble throughout the process. This will prevent turbulence within the PFCL and the possible formation of small bubbles, which may migrate through retinal breaks into the subretinal space.
- In the initial injection of PFCL, the eye should be tilted away from the retinal break to allow the PFCL to express as much fluid from the subretinal space through the retinal break. Injection of PFCL is stopped once the bubble level reaches the posterior edge of the retinal break.
- Note: another technique for injecting PFCL is to continue with the injection till the PFCL bubble crosses the retinal break and the peripheral retina is flat. This allows lasering the break under PFCL rather than under air for better visualization. This is mainly used in giant retinal break detachment. A disadvantage of this technique is that it may increase the chance of PFCL migration under the retina through the retinal break.

3.5   Perfluorocarbon Liquid (PFCL): Removal and PFCL-Air Exchange

- PFCL can be removed via active or passive aspiration with an extrusion needle through a PFCL-air exchange.
- Best to aspirate on top of the PFCL bubble high up in the anterior vitreous cavity till the air comes into the eye.
- Next, keep aspirating as more air comes into the eye till you reach the retinal tear.
- Spend some time aspirating from the break. Keep in the middle of the break away from any possible residual vitreous anteriorly (like what you do in the balanced salt solution (BSS)/air exchange).
- Opposite to what you do in BSS/air exchange where you tilt the eye, so the break and hence the subretinal fluid are dependent, do not do this in PFCL exchange. You want to keep the eye in the neutral position to avoid aspirating the PFCL supporting the retina posterior to the break before you remove all the subretinal fluid remaining at/anterior to the retinal tear.
- Keep aspirating at the tear until you see the retina stuck down to the RPE. At this point, your view of the PFCL bubble edge will be less, as there is not too much BSS in the eye. This is a great endpoint for aspiration from the tear.
- Now dip the aspiration tip in the PFCL and follow the bubble to the optic disc (Video 2).
- To avoid PFCL dispersion into droplets, try to take the heavy liquid in a smooth action and continuously observe the bubble as it gets smaller.
- Saline Rinse: Occasional at the end of the exchange, it can be challenging to visualize and remove the last droplets of PFCL. This can be solved by instilling a few drops of BSS over the optic nerve as a "rinse" and then completely removing the residual PFCL-water bubble. This will help ensure all/most PFCL have been removed (Video 4).

3.6   Perfluorocarbon Liquid (PFCL): Complications [4]

- PFCL has a good safety profile, but toxicity has been reported from extended intraocular use (>2 weeks); hence, complete removal toward the end of surgery is warranted.
- Chemical toxicity due to PFCL's high oxygen-carrying capacity and mechanical toxicity from the extended compression of the inferior retina are potential issues.
- Every effort should be made to remove PFCL that has accidentally gone under the retina as it can eventually migrate under the fovea with time and cause central scotomas and vision loss.

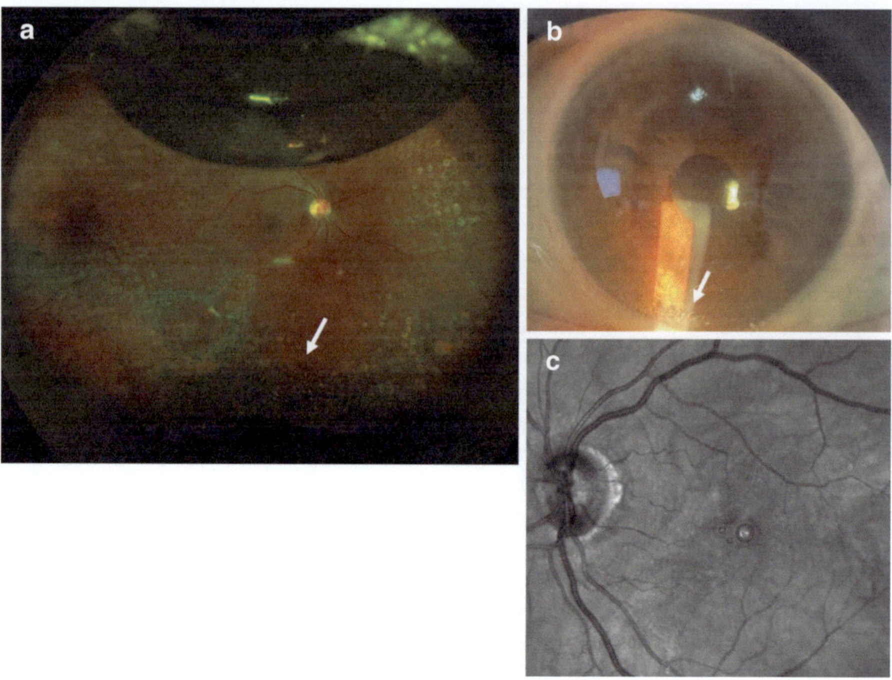

Fig. 1 Perfluorocarbon liquid complications with retained droplets (arrow) in the vitreous cavity (**a**) and anterior chamber (**b**). Subfoveal perfluorocarbon liquid bubble (**c**)

- PFCL in the anterior chamber may cause blockage of the visual axis, corneal endothelial loss, iritis, and elevated IOP (Fig. 1).
- Posterior segment complications include retained PFCL in the vitreous cavity (Video 5) and subretinal PFCL (Fig. 1).

Subfoveal PFCL

While peripheral stable subretinal PFCL bubbles can be left alone, PFCL under the macular area will result in RPE damage and central scotoma.

Below are our top tips for avoiding subfoveal PFCL:

1. Do not inject directly over the macula.
2. Inject slowly till a bubble forms and then keep injecting in the bubble as it builds up to avoid fish eggs.
3. Do not inject over traction areas until traction has been relieved.
4. Do not inject near retinal breaks, and it is best to always keep the edge of the bubble away from retinal breaks.
5. Avoid turbulence in the eye that may lead to PFCL bubble breakup "sloshing." Inject PFCL slowly, and be gentle when performing scleral indentation and when releasing the indent.

6. Do not double dip, i.e., do not re-aspirate over the retinal break after you moved over the optic nerve to aspirate the PFCL bubble with a backflush.
7. Finally, the best way to avoid the PFCL problem, in our view, is to minimize its use!

There are several ways to remove subfoveal PFCL, including direct aspiration with a fine-tipped cannula (38–41 g) [5] (Video 6) or dilution with subretinal BSS to push a PFCL bubble inferiorly.

Our Use of PFCL

In general, we try to avoid PFCL in routine cases and restrict its use to GRT and PVR RD. Although PFCL use in routine RRD may help simplify surgery, it is associated with several disadvantages, including extending the duration of surgery, increasing surgery cost, and all the aforementioned complications, the worst being subfoveal PFCL.

3.7 Silicone Oil

Repeating units of siloxane (silicone and oxygen molecule) are the primary compounds that make up silicone oils (SO). They are either lighter or heavier than water, depending on their viscosities. Most SO consist of polydimethylsiloxane (siloxane with two attached methyl side chains) and are known as PDMS. In contrast, the most common heavy SO are known as fluorosilicone oils, which are PDMS with methyl and trifluoropropyl side chains. Table 3 summarizes the properties of different types of silicone oils. As a reference, the unit value of water for specific gravity and viscosity is 1.0.

For all PDMS (which include 1000, 2000, and 5000 centistokes oil), specific gravity remains the same regardless of its chain length or molecular weight.

Table 3 Chemical properties of commonly used silicone oils

	Specific gravity (g/cm³ at 25 °C)	Viscosity (cSt at 25 °C)
Silicone oil (1000 cSt)	0.97	1000
Silicone oil (2000 cSt)	0.97	2000
Non-silicone oil (5000 cSt)	0.97	5000
Densiron 68	1.06	1349
Oxane HD	1.02	3300

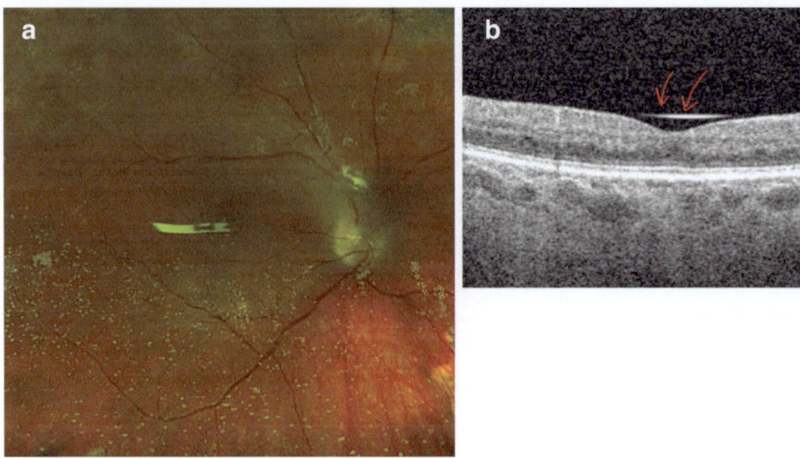

Fig. 2 An eye that is silicone filled after vitrectomy (**a**). Note the separation between the edge of the silicone oil bubble (red arrows) and the retinal surface. Preretinal aqueous film on the optical coherence tomography scan (**b**)

The second type of viscosity refers to extensional viscosity. This is a measure of the resistance of the SO to break up when a globule is drawn into a strand. When the strand breaks, satellite droplets tend to form. Higher-viscosity oils have less tendency to disperse and emulsify and hence are the preferred choice for longer or permanent intraocular tamponade.

It is virtually impossible to completely fill an eye with tamponade; therefore, there is always a retro-tamponade fluid space present. This space is more pronounced in SO-filled eyes as compared to gas-filled eyes (Fig. 2). Reports also show that a SO bubble virtually makes no contact with the retina until the eye is nearly 50% filled. Therefore, it is essential to achieve a greater fill, to have a good tamponade effect with SO. This is even more important if a buckle is also present as SO conforms to the shape of the eye less than gas.

3.8 Silicone Oil: Indications

Overall, silicone oil has inferior tamponade properties as compared to gas:

1. SO has significantly lower buoyancy and interfacial tension.
2. As the retina is hydrophilic, SO achieves less contact with the retina as compared to gas, particularly when SO underfill is present.
3. SO adapts less to the changes in the shape of the eye produced by a scleral buckle.
4. Presence of choroidal detachment or similar pathology with the RRD can result in significant SO underfill. With gas, a slightly expansile concentration can be used for, e.g., 30% SF_6 to compensate for gas underfill.
5. SO requires removal.

Hence, gas should be the tamponade of choice in primary RRD surgery.

The main advantage of SO is that it will remain longer and will not absorb. This makes it useful for PVR cases with retinectomies or unrelieved traction [6]. In the latter situation, SO will not counteract traction but will keep the retinal break sealed. Lastly, SO also has the advantage that it does not interfere with flying.

Conventional SO are mainly used for complex RRD with PVR that needs a prolonged tamponade duration. Some authors use SO in severe PDR-related tractional retinal detachment, but we do not favor this indication, as explained in the diabetic vitrectomy section. Heavier-than-water SO are designed for inferior tamponade purposes, especially when PVR is present with proven success [13], but they are still not available in the USA.

3.9 Silicone Oil: Techniques of Injection

A two-step procedure with an air-fluid exchange followed by an air-SO exchange or a direct exchange between PFCL and SO can be utilized for SO injection. The former technique is easier to do and has better IOP control but is associated with an increased risk of retinal slippage. Direct PFCL-SO exchange offers an improved visualization and mitigates the risk of retinal slippage in cases of GRTs or retinectomies; however, it is more difficult to master and has its associated risks.

The two-stage procedure involves the modification of techniques used for gas-fluid exchange:

- For aphakic patients, an inferior peripheral iridotomy for conventional SO and a superior peripheral iridotomy for heavy SO are performed to prevent pupillary block glaucoma. It is much easier to perform the PI with the vitreous cavity filled with BSS or PFCL (not air or SO) (Video 7).
- After complete vitrectomy and the release of all traction, the fluid-air exchange is performed, and any remaining subretinal fluid should be drained, and endophotocoagulation should be performed as necessary.
- Through one sclerotomy, a venting port or an extrusion cannula is placed. SO injection is then carried out through a second cannula using the automated viscous fluid injector controlled by the foot pedal.
- Before injection, it is important to verify that the tip of the injecting cannula is within the vitreous cavity to avoid injection in the subretinal or suprachoroidal space (Video 8).
- Aphakic eyes are filled with SO nearly to the level of the iris diaphragm. Phakic and pseudophakic eyes are filled to an amount reaching the posterior surface of the lens or IOL. IOP is monitored digitally during the process. An IOP of around 10–20 mmHg is desirable at the end of the surgery. Tonopen can also be used at the end of surgery to check IOP.
- Sclerotomies are closed by 7–0 or 8–0 Vicryl sutures to prevent subconjunctival oil migration and underfill of the vitreous cavity.

Direct PFCL-SO exchange can be done with a passive or active approach, based on how the PFCL is removed.

Passive Direct PFCL-SO Exchange

- This is the more conventional approach for direct PFCL-SO exchange (Video 9)
- SO is actively injected with the foot pedal, and PFCL is passively aspirated using a flute needle (Fig. 3a).
- Because passive aspiration of fluids is inherently slow, the inflow of SO during the exchange often exceeds the passive outflow of PFCL.
- As a result, the vitreous cavity can become over-pressurized, and IOP can rise at times. If the surgeon is not careful to stop the injection, significant elevation in IOP during surgery may lead to a dangerous situation resulting in corneal edema with impairment of the retinal view, SO migration into the anterior, or scleral rupture in extreme cases. Attention to details is very important in this step.
- The SO syringe is first connected to the viscous fluid injection kit. The infusion line is removed from the eye, and the oil injection syringe is connected to the infusion line. The pedal is pressed to prime the infusion line with SO, and the line is reconnected to the port. Oil is then injected by pressing the foot pedal while passively aspirating the PFCL simultaneously using a backflush. The other hand is holding the light pipe. As the oil enters the eye, it floats atop the saline and PFCL. The backflush cannula's tip is held first within the saline anterior to the break until the oil level has forced most of the saline out. Removing the saline first helps to ensure that saline does not go under the retina and cause re-detachment or retinal slippage. Once the saline is removed and the retinal tear edges are seen stuck down to the RPE, the backflush tip is moved posteriorly into the PFCL, and the PFCL bubble is followed to the optic nerve cup (Fig. 4). The infusion pressure of the oil forces all the PFCL out of the backflush. Silicone oil injection is usually maintained at relatively low pressure, typically 20–30 pounds per square inch (PSI), and may be modified as needed based on the IOP in the eye.

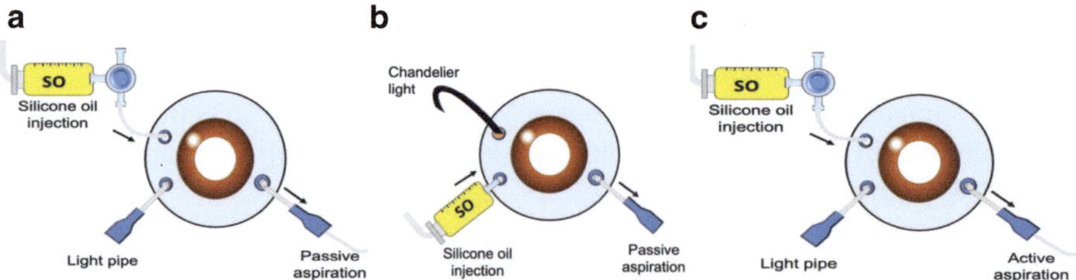

Fig. 3 Setup for passive perflurocarbon liquid (PFCL)-silicone oil (SO) exchange, the conventional way (**a**) and with the use of chandelier light (**b**). Setup for active automated PFCL-SO exchange (**c**)

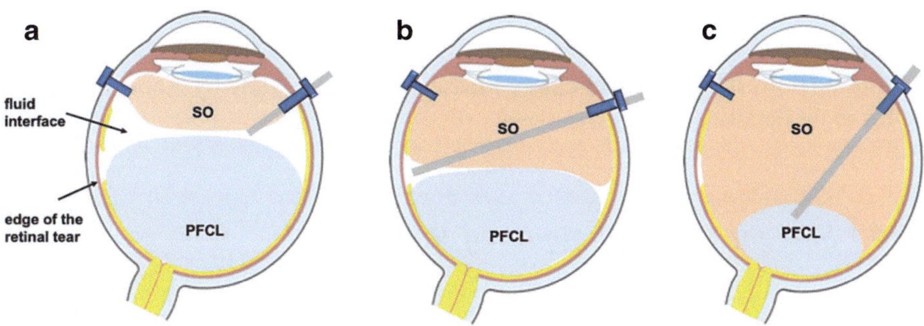

Fig. 4 Placement of the backflush for the removal of perflurocarbon liquid (PFCL) during PFCL-silicone (SO) exchange. The backflush is initially placed at the interface between the PFCL and SO (**a**) and then moved to the retinal break (**b**) as the SO advances in the eye and finally moved to the optic nerve (**c**). At all times, this cannula should not be immersed in the SO

- Notes
  - With 25-g vitrectomy, injection of the SO through the infusion cannula can be difficult. An alternative technique is to use a chandelier. The infusion cannula is completely removed from the eye in this setup and the chandelier placed in this port (Fig. 3b).
  - Indicators of high IOP are pallor of the disc and retinal arterial pulsations and, also, corneal haze with obscuration of the view. Slightly pressing the light pipe and the infusion cannula inward against the sclera provides tactile feedback on the IOP status.
  - To avoid IOP spikes, the surgeon must balance SO injection with PFCL aspiration. Injections should be eased off/stopped at the earliest signs of raised IOP. Also, the surgeon must always be careful *not* to allow SO to go into the backflush cannula, as it will block fluid egress and consequently raise the IOP. If SO blocks the cannula, it must be withdrawn and flushed out.
  - A modification for this passive exchange technique to decrease the risk of over-pressurization of the vitreous cavity is to use a larger-gauge backflush for PFCL removal (Video 9). For example, passive aspiration of the PFCL through a 23-gauge port while actively injecting the SO through a 25-g port increases the efficiency of PFCL by 1.5× [7].

Active Direct PFCL-SO Exchange

- The active extrusion technique allows for automated, precise control of both SO injection and PFCL removal using the foot pedal (Fig. 3c).
- As opposed to passive aspiration, active extrusion of PFCL allows for the removal of the PFCL at a rate that matches the silicone oil injection avoiding over-pressurization of the vitreous cavity.

- It is important to avoid hypotony with this technique as this may lead to retinal slippage.
- Video 10 illustrates the technique. Please refer to the study by Ahmad et al. [8] for more details.

3.10 Silicone Oil: Techniques of Removal

SO bubble is removed when it has served its purpose and when further retention may increase the risk of complications.

The Silicone Study Group allowed removal after a minimum of 8 weeks after surgery. However, removal within the first 4 months is generally acceptable.

Sometimes, it is best to leave SO and only consider removal if complications happen. This includes (1) PVR and persistent traction that was not possible to relieve during surgery and (2) chronic hypotony.

Techniques

- Infusion must first be secured at the pars plana to allow volume replacement with BSS as SO is being aspirated.
- The port through which SO is aspirated should be placed in the uppermost position because SO floats up.
- The aspiration of the SO should always be active. Active aspiration has to be achieved close to the eye with a minimum length provided by a short cannula. Plastic cannulas have a greater affinity to SO.
- When available, it is best to use specifically designed 23-g cannula and tubing system for SO removal to increase the efficiency of SO removal (Video 11).
- Alternately for heavy SO, a separate sclerotomy using a 20-g micro vitreoretinal (MVR) blade (a conjunctival peritomy) is created. A shortened 20-g venous catheter with just enough length to reach the posterior pole is used to aspirate the oil bubble that naturally sinks under BSS.
- Care is to be taken to observe the "vortex" developing within the oil and to make sure that the tip of the aspirating needle is always submerged within the SO bubble to avoid collapse of the eye.
- In cases where cataract surgery is performed simultaneously, a posterior capsulotomy/rhexis could be made for SO removal (Video 12). This is similar to the technique in aphakic eyes, wherein the aspirating needle is passed through a corneal incision instead of a sclerotomy. The technique is very efficient, particularly with the use of high viscosity SO, and avoids the need for creating a large sclerotomy to remove the SO (Video 13).
- We routinely have a pars plana vitrectomy (PPV) setup at the time of ROSO. In this case, we can inspect the retina after SO removal for retinal re-detachment or need for more laser treatment. We also routinely perform three cycles of air-fluid exchange to ensure a more complete removal of SO or retained PFCL bubbles (Videos 11–13). PPV is also required in the setting of heavy SO removal as the

last bubbles usually drops down towards the retina making removal difficult. Certain techniques have been described to remove the dropped heavy SO bubbles including injection of air in the bubbles to help them float up. [9].

3.11   Silicone Oil: Other Considerations

- SO retention sutures in aphakic eyes and iris loss can be employed to try to prevent SO migration to the anterior chamber. 10–0 Prolene sutures across the anterior chamber are placed to mimic the iris diaphragm and may act as a barrier between the SO and aqueous (Fig. 5).
- Silicone IOLs are prone to fogging during the fluid-air exchange, and SO droplets can remain stuck on the posterior lens surface during removal. IOL exchange is sometimes necessary to mitigate these risks. SO solvents are being used, but potential toxicity to intraocular tissues remains a concern.

3.12   Silicone Oil: Complications

- High IOP due to (a) SO overfill and (b) pupillary block glaucoma with inadequate peripheral iridotomies can both increase IOP. There can also be high IOP in (c) chronic hypotony where SO emulsifications can obstruct the trabecular meshwork. Overall, the rate of elevated IOP in the SO study was approximately 10%.
- SO in the anterior chamber can cause corneal decompensation (Fig. 6a).
- SO can migrate under the conjunctiva if the scleral ports are not well sutured or if there is overfill (Fig. 6b).
- SO use is associated with retinal toxicity that has been histologically proven.

Fig. 5 Silicone oil (SO) retention sutures in aphakic eyes with iris loss to prevent SO migration to the anterior chamber using 10–0 Prolene sutures across the posterior chamber. Sutures are placed 1.5–2 mm behind the limbus. (Courtesy of Mohamed Ahmed El-Masry, MD, Egypt)

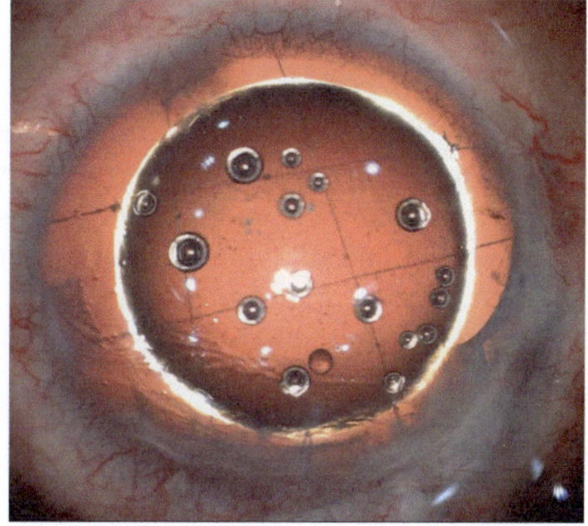

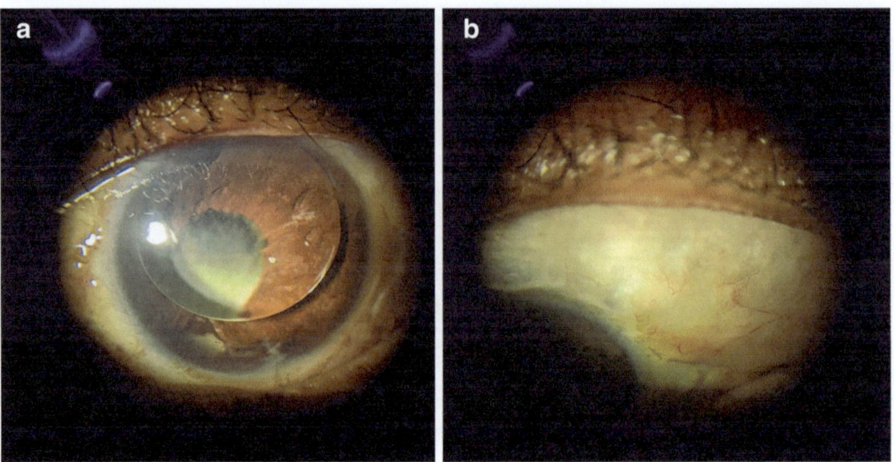

Fig. 6 Silicone oil complications with oil in the anterior chamber in an eye with hypotony (**a**) and under the conjunctiva (**b**)

- Chronic hypotony can also happen due to ciliary body alterations and SO under-fill. Insufficient SO tamponade can result in retinal re-attachment failure as it may not seal the retinal break.
- SO can stimulate epiretinal (retro-oil) membrane proliferation. This may be due to the concentration of inflammatory mediators and fibrogenic growth factors such as IL-6 and TGF-B in the retro-oil aqueous film. Retro-oil proliferations can be very marked in eyes with diabetic tractional retinal detachment.
- Heavier-than-water SO can result in significant inflammation, and it is advisable not to leave them in the eye for more than 8 weeks.
- Dispersion of SO and eventually emulsification happen when large bubbles break up into smaller droplets. This is time-dependent and can reach up to 10% after 3 months and 85% after 6 months. It has been thought that 5000 cSt emulsifies less than 1000 cSt due to higher viscosity. However, the viscosity of oil does not affect emulsification much as compared to intraocular inflammation and eye movement, which are the main drivers. It is also of note that 5000 cSt SO is more difficult to inject and remove as compared to 1000 cSt SO.
- RRD can occur after removal of SO (ROSO) in the range of 5–30% and is higher in eyes with persistent traction. Some advocate performing 360 degrees laser before ROSO to decrease this risk. If this is to be performed, we encourage waiting until after PVR settles down and laser is away from areas of traction and scar tissues. In one study, the risk of re-detachment was less when oil was kept for more than 12 months, but the vision was significantly better when SO was removed at 3 months [10].

- In general, it is best to avoid SO use in eyes with good visual potential. Vision in eyes operated with oil (after SO removal) is inferior to those where gas tamponade was used [11]. There are also reports of unexplained visual loss after ROSO. The reported incidence of this phenomenon ranges between 7% and 30% [12]. It has been attributed to several factors, including phototoxicity during ROSO or changes in the balance of ions and growth factors in the vitreous cavity.

Key Points
- Intraocular gas has superior tamponade properties over SO and should be used for primary RRD cases.
- SO provides longer-term tamponade and is of benefit in proliferative vitreoretinopathy (PVR) detachment.
- PFCL can provide many advantages during RRD surgery but is associated with significant potential complications. Use it only when you really need it!
- Direct PFCL-SO exchange in the context of GRT repair or with large relaxing retinectomy is associated with a significantly decreased risk of retinal slippage as compared to the two-stage air-PFCL/PFCL-SO exchange.
- As opposed to passive aspiration, direct PFCL-SO exchange using active aspiration allows for the removal of PFCL at a rate that matches SO injection. This helps prevent over-pressurization of the vitreous cavity during surgery.

References

1. Donati S, et al. Vitreous substitutes: the present and the future. Biomed Res Int. 2014;2014:351804, 12 pages.
2. Angunawela RI, Azarbadegan A, Aylward GW, Eames I. Intraocular fluid dynamics and retinal shear stress after vitrectomy and gas tamponade. Invest Ophthalmol Vis Sci. 2011;52(10):7046–51.
3. Shunmugam M, Shunmugam S, Williamson TH, Laidlaw DA. Air-gas exchange reevaluated: clinically important results of a computer simulation. Invest Ophthalmol Vis Sci. 2011;52(11):8262–5.
4. Scott IU, Murray TG, Flynn HW Jr, et al. Outcomes and complications associated with perfluoro-n-octane and perfluoroperhydrophenanthrene in complex retinal detachment repair. Ophthalmology. 2000;107:860–5.
5. Hanout M, Muni RH. Novel surgical technique to remove retained subfoveal perfluorocarbon liquid. Retin Cases Brief Rep. 2021;15(6):741–4.
6. The Silicone Study Group. Vitrectomy with silicone oil or sulfur hexafluoride gas in eyes with severe proliferative vitreoretinopathy: results of a randomized clinical trial. Silicone Study report 1. Arch Ophthalmol. 1992;110:770–9.
7. Elhusseiny AM, Sanders RN, Ellabban AA, Sallam AB. Hybrid 23/25 gauge direct perfluorocarbon liquid-silicone oil exchange. Retina. 2023;43(12):2123–5.
8. Ahmad KT, Sallam AB, Saad AA, Ellabban AA. Fully automated direct perfluorocarbon liquid-silicone oil exchange. Clin Ophthalmol. 2020;10(14):4355–8.

9. El-Khayat A, Sharma A, Mitra A. REMOVAL OF DROPPED HEAVY SILICONE OIL BUBBLE USING AIR. Retin Cases Brief Rep. 2023;17(2):152–153.
10. Huang D, Starr MR, Patel LG, Ammar MJ, Kaiser RS, Mehta S, Park CH, Khan MA, Gupta OP, Kuriyan AE, Yonekawa Y, Ho AC, Garg SJ, Cohen MN, Hsu J. Factors affecting retinal redetachment after silicone oil removal for rhegmatogenous retinal detachments. Retina. 2022;42(7):1248–53.
11. Funatsu R, Terasaki H, Koriyama C, Yamashita T, Shiihara H, Sakamoto T. Silicone oil versus gas tamponade for primary rhegmatogenous retinal detachment treated successfully with a propensity score analysis: Japan Retinal Detachment Registry. Br J Ophthalmol. 2022;106(8):1044–1050.
12. Roca JA, Wu L, Berrocal M, et al. Unexplained visual loss following silicone oil removal: results of the Pan American Collaborative Retina Study (PACORES) Group. Int J Retina Vitreous. 2017;3:26.
13. Tzoumas N, Yorston D, Laidlaw DAH, Williamson TH, Steel DH; British and Eire Association of Vitreoretinal Surgeons and European Society of Retina Specialists Retinal Detachment Outcomes Group. Improved Outcomes with Heavy Silicone Oil in Complex Primary Retinal Detachment: A Large Multicenter Matched Cohort Study Ophthalmology. 2023.
14. Kirchhof B, Tavakolian U, Paulmann H, Heimann K. Histopathological findings in eyes after silicone oil injection. Graefe's Archive for Clinical and Experimental Ophthalmology. 1986;224(1):34–7.

Vitreous Hemorrhage and Other Vitreous Opacities

Mohamed Kamel Soliman and Ahmed M. Habib

This chapter discusses the surgical management of vitreous opacities, mainly focusing on vitreous hemorrhage (VH).

1 Causes of Vitreous Opacities and Indications for Pars Plana Surgery

Table 1 summarizes the important causes of vitreous opacities. In practice, vitreous hemorrhage (VH) is the most important sight involving vitreous opacities encountered and may result from traumatic and non-traumatic causes.

- The most common etiology of non-traumatic vitreous hemorrhage is hemorrhagic posterior vitreous detachment (PVD) with/without retinal tears, prolifera-

Supplementary Information The online version contains supplementary material available at https://doi.org/10.1007/978-3-031-47827-7_6.

M. K. Soliman (✉)
Department of Ophthalmology and Visual Sciences, University Hospitals Eye Institute, Cleveland, OH, USA

Department of Ophthalmology, Assiut University Hospitals, Assiut, Egypt

A. M. Habib
Ophthalmology, Vitreoretinal Surgery, Ain Shams University, Al Mashreq Eye Center, Cairo, Egypt
e-mail: Ahmed.mohamedh@med.asu.edu.eg

A. B. Sallam et al. (eds.), *Practical Manual of Vitreoretinal Surgery*,
https://doi.org/10.1007/978-3-031-47827-7_6

Table 1 Causes of vitreous opacities

• Vitreous hemorrhage
– Trauma
– Vascular pathology: PDR, CRVO, macroaneurysm, neovascular AMD
– Intraocular tumor
• Asteroid hyalosis (Fig. 1)
• Vitreous syneresis and floaters
• Posterior uveitis and masquerade

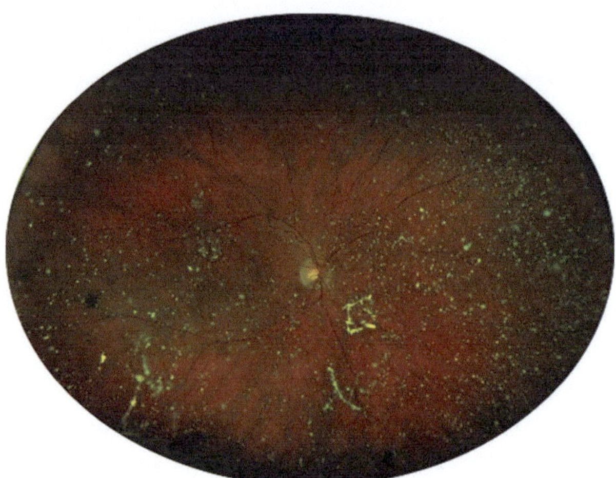

Fig. 1 Asteroid hyalosis. While many patients are not symptomatic, some patients with asteroid hyalosis may have floaters/ severe enough to affect their daily activities. Caution needs to be exercised during pars plana vitrectomy for asteroid hyalosis as posterior vitreous detachment is usually absent and strong vitreoretinal adhesion may be present

tive diabetic retinopathy (PDR), and then other vascular disorders, including central retinal vein occlusion (CRVO) and macroaneurysm. Pars plana vitrectomy (PPV) is required for significant VH affecting the vision or precluding retinal examination [1].

- In pediatric vitreous hemorrhage, consider shaken baby syndrome, X-linked retinoschisis, intermediate uveitis, retinopathy of prematurity, familial exudative vitreoertinopathy (FEVR), and systemic blood diseases such as leukemia [2].
- In addition to VH, vitreous opacities due to vitreous syneresis (floaters) may, in some cases, be treated with PPV. For this, we only advise surgery when floaters interfere with a patient's vision and affect their lifestyle. One needs to be cautious not to offer surgery to a patient with mild symptoms as PPV is a surgery that carries a small but still significant risk of severe loss of vision or blindness [3].
- Finally, other indications for PPV include posterior uveitis and uveitic masquerades such as lymphoma and amyloidosis. In these cases, PPV may be considered for diagnostic or therapeutic reasons, as discussed in the vitreoretinal surgery in the uveitis chapter, Chap. 26.

2 Preoperative Assessment

There are several points to consider when examining patients with VH.

- It is important to ask about the history of trauma and systemic conditions such as diabetes mellitus and sickle cell. If the patient recalls seeing flashes and floaters right before visual deterioration, this may point to hemorrhagic PVD. The duration of the VH is also important when planning the timing of PPV surgery. Ocular history, such as treatment with anti-VEGF or laser, can help identify the underlying causative pathology.
- The level of visual acuity in relation to the degree of VH is important—Acuity that is out of proportion with hemorrhage density raises the suspicion of existing central retinal pathology such as macular ischemia.
- The presence of neovascularization of the iris (NVI) with or without hyphema points to an ischemic retinal pathology such as PDR or CRVO as the cause of the hemorrhage. Raised intraocular pressure may be due to neovascular glaucoma (NVG) or ghost cell glaucoma.
- Assessment of lens clarity is important, and it is also important to note whether the cataract is dense enough to contribute to the poor fundus view. It is also helpful to note the relation of the hemorrhage to the back surface of the crystalline lens and whether there is a significant dusting of the anterior hyaloid with blood.
- When the fundus view permits, an examination of the retina can help point out the cause for VH, for example, retinal tears, PDR, or CRVO. A retinal break that causes significant bleeding is usually large or associated with a bridging vessel.
- In the context of acute symptomatic PVD, there is a 7–22% risk of retinal tear. This rate goes up to 80% if there is pigment in the vitreous or hemorrhage [4]. It is therefore essential to perform scleral indentation on these patients and to consider early surgery to clear the view and examine the retina.
- Retina examination of the fellow eye is crucial. For instance, the presence of PDR in the fellow eye of a diabetic patient with dense VH makes it more likely that the hemorrhage is caused by diabetic retinopathy. In contrast, the presence of only mild DR in the fellow eye favors the diagnosis of hemorrhagic PVD.
- Wide-field flourescein angiography can be considered in some cases with severe but non-total VH to help answer the question of whether the VH is due to PVD or vascular pathology.
- Ultrasound B-scan is also helpful in cases with no retinal view to assess the retinal status for retinal detachment (RD) and to exclude an intraocular mass. Table 2 provides some clues for differentiating PVD from RD on B-scan (Video 1).
- In general, we consider operating on most cases of fundus obscuring VH and those associated with NVI early to clear the vision and deal with any coexisting retinal pathology. This could range from a few days to 1 week. About 2/3 of cases of PVD associated with VH have at least one retinal break that will progress if untreated. In the presence of NVI, there is a high risk that the hemorrhage is associated with an active untreated vascular pathology that may result in permanent visual loss from NVG or tractional retinal detachment (TRD).

Table 2 Clues for differentiation between posterior vitreous detachment (PVD) and retinal detachment (RD) on B-scan

	PVD	RD
Attachment to the disc	May or may not be present	Nearly always present
Mobility on dynamic imaging	Freely mobile, show prominent "after movements"	Much less freely mobile, less prominent "after movements"
A-scan	Low but could be high in some parts of the posterior hyaloid which is thickened or layered with blood	Constantly high

- In cases of VH with stable previously treated vascular pathology such as PDR and previous panretinal photocoagulation (PRP), we usually wait for 1–2 months in anticipation that the hemorrhage may spontaneously clear.
- Preoperatively, we use intravitreal anti-vascular endothelial growth factor (VEGF) in patients with active vascular pathology, mainly diabetics with iris rubeosis or TRD, to decrease the risk and the severity of intraoperative and early postoperative hemorrhage. More discussion on this point is found in the diabetic delamination chapter, Chap. 18.

3 Considerations for PPV Surgery

- As standard in PPV, it is important to visualize the tip of the pars plana infusion cannula, inside the vitreous cavity, before opening the infusion.

  - If the VH is dense to preclude the visualization of the cannula, it can be placed at least temporarily in the anterior chamber, even in phakic patients. This will provide reasonable infusion to the posterior segment through the zonules until the anterior vitreous is cleared and the infusion is then moved to a pars plana trocar (Video 2).
  - Another option is to allow some air inside the infusion cannula. If the cannula is in the correct position in the vitreous cavity, opening the infusion momentarily would eject the air bubble in the vitreous cavity and be visible behind the lens. In addition, the light pipe can be turned on and introduced into the vitreous cavity through the infusion cannula. The lighted pipe can be easily visualized through dense VH. It is important to make sure that the light pipe is not dragging/pushing any pars plana or retinal tissues. Once this confirmed, this means that the infusion cannula is in the correct intravitreal location.

- During vitrectomy, if a hazy view persists, check the anterior chamber for dispersed blood as it may be the cause of the haze, solved by anterior chamber wash (Video 3).
- Be wary of the position of the instruments in relation to the crystalline lens. It is best to start in the central upper part of the vitreous cavity away from the lens until the view is cleared to avoid lens injury. This position is also favorable should a retinal detachment exist, as superior iatrogenic retinal breaks are more readily supported with vitreous substitutes than inferior breaks.

- In dense VH, caution is needed as the retina could be detached behind the VH, and sometimes layered VH may be challenging to differentiate from the retinal tissue. Clues for differentiating the vitreous from the retina include the absence of firm attachment of the vitreous to the disc and the absence of the retinal blood vessels. In cases where differentiation is not possible, you may create an opening in the layered vitreous/retina superiorly by cutting vertically through it and then introduce the light pipe through the hole to see what's underneath that layer. You may find retinal blood vessels indicating that you only cut through vitreous, or you may find bare RPE, which indicates this tissue was the retina (Video 4).
- Most cases of VH are associated with PVD. This makes surgery easy once the view is cleared to visualize the surgical instruments and the position of the retina is established. An exception is in patients with proliferative retinopathy, mainly diabetic and sickle cell retinopathy, where stronger connections exist between the posterior hyaloid and the retina at epicenters. The retina is thin at the epicenters and it can tear or bleeding from the vessels can happen. You cannot just pull as, for example, in macular hole surgery. The tactic is a bit of pull to get some separation of the vitreous from the retina, away from areas of traction, and then you cut deep at the epicenters to free up the hyaloid (Video 5).
- More discussion on the "pull and cut technique" for removing the posterior hyaloid in these cases is discussed in the diabetic delamination chapter.
- Caution must be exercised when removing the peripheral parts of the vitreous at the vitreous base. There are two benefits to removing these parts:

    - It decreases the risk of early postoperative vitreous cavity hemorrhage as a result of leaching from the remaining inferior peripheral hemorrhage.
    - It helps in improving the view for examining the retinal periphery.

    However, these benefits need to be weighed against the risk of retinal touch and lens injury in phakic eyes, particularly since the rate of intraoperative entry site retinal break with modern PPV is low.
- We do not routinely remove the internal limiting membrane unless a coexisting pathology exists with the VH, mainly a full thickness macular hole, or in the presence of sub-ILM hemorrhage (Video 6).
- Following the removal of the hemorrhage, any associated retinal pathology is dealt with as needed, for instance, applying PRP in PDR or air fluid exchange and laser in rhegmatogenous retinal detachment. In general, we do not use vitreous substitutes unless indicated for coexisting retinal pathology.

4 Dealing with Retrolenticular Anterior Hyaloid Hemorrhage

A significant dusting of the anterior hyaloid with hemorrhage can obscure the surgeon's view during PPV. This situation is difficult to manage in phakic eyes as the anterior hyaloid is firmly adherent to the posterior capsule of the crystalline lens. In young patients <45 years with a clear lens, we remove the anterior hyaloid hemorrhage under high magnification with the vitreous cutter using aspiration only first to pull the hyaloid away from the lens capsule and then cut. This can be repeated several times until an adequate view is obtained. Maintaining the cutter port to the side as much as possible rather than facing up toward the lens helps minimize the risk of opening the posterior capsule as the hyaloid is cut (Video 7). Another technique is to inject balanced salt solution in the anterior chamber with a 30-gauge needle. This is to hydrodissect the retrolental vitreous pushing it away from the lens and therefore more accessible to the vitreous cutter [5]. In older patients, we perform cataract surgery from the outset, simplifying the dissection of the anterior hyaloid.

5 Intraoperative and Postoperative Complications

Few complications are important to highlight in the context of PPV for VH, and these include:

1. Retinal touch

    This is likely to occur early in the course of PPV due to poor view from VH. It is therefore advised to work away from the retina and the crystalline lens at the beginning of surgery. Injury to the retina and lens can also happen during the trimming of the peripheral hemorrhage, as mentioned above.
2. Crystalline lens touch

    Like retinal touch, lens injury can happen early on when the view is poor or during the removal of peripheral hemorrhage at the vitreous base. Lens touch and breaching of the lens capsule during PPV are further discussed in the cataract chapter.

    - If only lens touch is present without breaching the posterior lens capsule and the view is not significantly compromised, we advise dealing with the lens at another time. In many cases, the cataract does not progress, and lens extraction later may not be complicated with dropped lens fragments, though this is not the case in about 10% of cases [6].
    - Breaching the lens capsule during surgery is different and can progress quickly post-surgery and result in intraocular inflammation. In this situation, we tend to remove the lens during the PPV surgery.

3. Postoperative vitreous cavity hemorrhage.

    This is not an uncommon complication, particularly in vascular causes of VH. The causes and management of this condition are discussed in the diabetic delamination chapter.

6 Case Scenario

A 70-year-old female presents with decreased vision in the right eye of several months' duration from Terson's syndrome. Right eye examination was consistent with HM vision, normal intraocular pressure, no NVI, nuclear 2+ cataract, and dense 4+ VH. B-scan showed no RD. Surgery showed dense VH. Initially, due to layered VH, it was challenging to be sure of the retinal status. The retina was found attached with no retinal tears (Video 8). The patient had vision of 20/25 post-surgery.

Key Points

- The most common causes of non-traumatic VH are hemorrhagic PVD with/without retinal tears and PDR.
- Always look for NVI in cases of VH. Its presence makes the diagnosis of an ischemic retinal pathology such as PDR or CRVO.
- B scan ultrasound is helpful to look for retinal tears and RD in cases of VH, but the senstivity is only about 30% and 60%, respectively.
- PPV for VH in diabetic eyes is usually not associated with PVD, and there are strong adhesions between the vitreous and the retina at epicenters.
- Dense-layered VH may be difficult to differentiate from the retinal tissue during the early stage of PPV.
- PPV for vitreous floaters should only be offered to patients with significant visually disabling symptoms after extensive discussion of the possible risks from surgery.

References

1. Pighin MS, Berrozpe C, Jürgens I. Outcome of acute nontraumatic vitreous hemorrhage in healthy patients. Retina. 2020;40(1):87–91.
2. Naik AU, Rishi E, Rishi PA. Pediatric vitreous hemorrhage. Narrative review. Indian J Ophthalmol. 2019;67(6):732–9.
3. Zeydanli EO, Parolini B, Ozdek S, Bopp S, Adelman RA, Kuhn F, Gini G, Sallam AB, Aksakal N, EVRS Floaters Study Group. Management of vitreous floaters: an international survey the European VitreoRetinal Society Floaters study report. Eye (Lond). 2020;34(5):825–34.
4. Boldrey EE. Risk of retinal tears in patients with vitreous. Floaters American Journal of Ophthalmology. 1983;96(6):783–7.
5. Surgical Detachment of the Anterior Hyaloid Membrane. From the Posterior Lens Capsule Journal of Vitreo Retinal Diseases. 2017;1(3):214–7.
6. Elhousseini Z, Lee E, Williamson TH. Incidence of lens touch during pars plana vitrectomy and outcomes from subsequent cataract surgery. Retina. 2016;36(4):825–9.

Retinopexy for Retinal Tears and Pneumatic Retinopexy for Primary Retinal Detachment

Mohamed Kamel Soliman and Ahmed B. Sallam

Primary rhegmatogenous retinal detachment (RRD) is a neurosensory detachment that develops due to retinal breaks. The annual incidence of primary RRD is about 10 per 100,000, and it is most common between 40 and 70 years. Primary RRD is a sight-threatening condition that requires emergent management. In this chapter, we discuss the management of retinal tears by laser or cryotherapy and the technique of retinal reattachment by pneumatic retinopexy.

1 Retinopexy

- Retinopexy is done by laser or cryotherapy, and it can be applied to precursors of RRD (retinal tears, holes, lattice degeneration, and traction tufts) to guard against progression to RRD.
- We typically apply the laser to symptomatic or traumatic breaks (horseshoe tears, operculated retinal tears, necrotic traumatic tears, and dialyses) as these are associated with a high risk of RRD. In those cases, we opt to perform the laser at the time of presentation and if not within 24 h.

Supplementary Information The online version contains supplementary material available at https://doi.org/10.1007/978-3-031-47827-7_7.

M. K. Soliman
Department of Ophthalmology and Visual Sciences, University Hospitals Eye Institute, Case Western Reserve University, Cleveland, OH, USA

Department of Ophthalmology, Assiut University Hospitals, Assiut, Egypt

A. B. Sallam (✉)
Jones Eye Institute, University of Arkansas for Medical Sciences, Little Rock, AR, USA

- Symptomatic retinal breaks are those associated with flashers and floaters secondary to a new-onset posterior vitreous detachment (PVD).
- The risk of retinal detachment with a symptomatic horseshoe tear is 1:2 and 1:6 if the tear becomes operculated [1]. New retinal breaks may arise in 5–15% after treatment, with the risk being higher in the first 6 weeks. Overall retinopexy cuts down the risk of RD to 5% [2].
- Laser retinopexy can be applied to the wall of retinal breaks associated with a cuff of subretinal fluid (SRF). There is no consensus about how much SRF need to be present to warrant other treatment options. Generally, we tend to use laser retinopexy in acute breaks with limited SRF ($\leq$1.5 disc area) that is anterior to the equator, and the patient does not perceive field defect from this subclinical retinal detachment (Fig. 1).
- We generally do not treat atrophic retinal holes, retinal tufts, or lattice retinal degeneration, even in the fellow eye of retinal detachment. The risk of retinal detachment is very small with these pathologies, and evidence to support the benefit of laser in this situation is lacking particularly that the retinal tears may occur in untreated areas or at the edge of the retinal laser. Though the benefit is debatable, some surgeons may consider retinopexy for selective cases or cases deemed at high risk of progression to retinal detachment, particularly if there is a history of retinal detachment in the fellow or retinal detachment associated with syndromes such as Stickler disease [3, 4].
- Asymptomatic retinal detachment is another entity discovered incidentally, and it tends to be chronic with demarcation marks. While there is no consensus on the best treatment approach for this type of detachment, close observation is usually an acceptable initial approach. Certain factors, however, including the extent of fluid, location of the break, degree of chronicity, age of the patient, and patient's commitment to attend follow-up visits, often play an important role in decision-making.

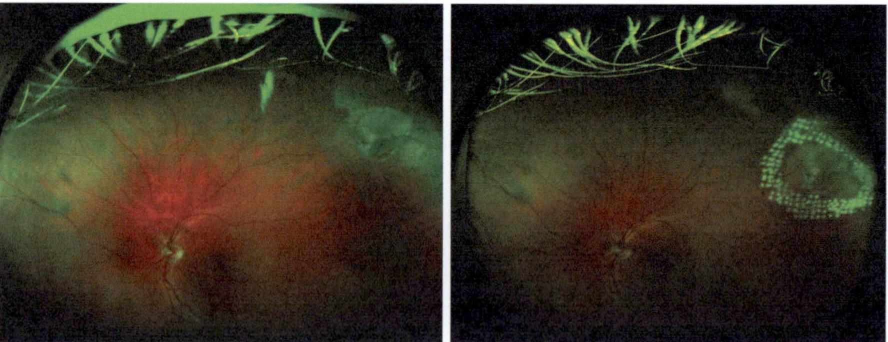

Fig. 1 Retinal tear with limited subretinal fluid treated with laser retinopexy. If no gas is used, laser or cryopexy should be placed outside the subretinal fluid

1.1   Technique of Retinopexy

- **Laser retinopexy**

  - When performing laser retinopexy, 2–3 rows of confluent or near-confluent laser burns should surround the break in a 360° fashion. The first row of laser burns should hug the edges of the break. If there is a cuff of SRF, then the laser should be placed outside the fluid (Fig. 1).
  - In more peripheral breaks where the anterior flap is small or difficult to visualize, the laser should extend up to the ora serrata on both sides of the break (Fig. 2).
  - Although laser indirect ophthalmoscope (LIO) with scleral indentation has been the traditional method for treating retinal tears, with the new models of laser machines, you can also deliver the laser to peripheral tears using the slit lamp.

- **Cryopexy**

  - Laser is more available, easier to use and produces less inflammation than cryo. However, cryotherapy can be helpful in hypopigmented fundi, where laser uptake can be poor.
  - Prior to starting cryotherapy, check if the equipment is functioning by putting a drop of BSS on the tip of the probe to assess its freezing function.
  - Subconjunctival or anterior sub-Tenon's anesthesia should be done at the site intended for cryotherapy.

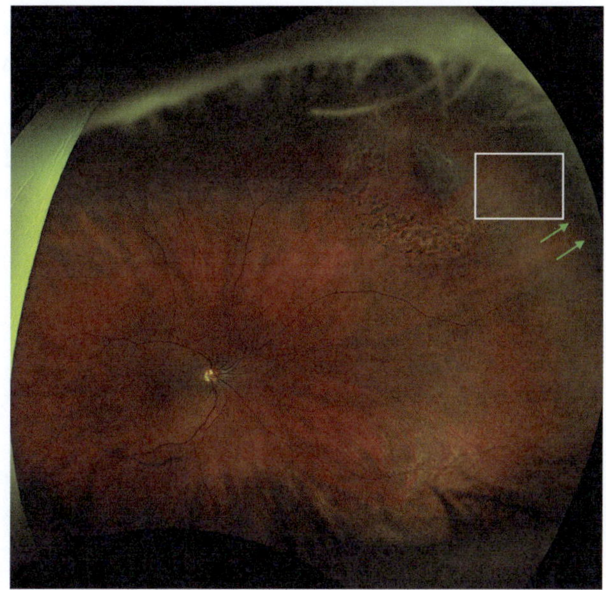

Fig. 2 Peripheral retinal tear. Laser is applied in a U-shaped configuration around the tear, but one horn of the tear is not lasered up to the ora serrata (white rectangle) which may increase the risk for retinal detachment. Arrows mark the ora serrata position

- Similar to laser retinopexy, cryopexy should encircle the break or extend up to the ora serrata on both sides of an anterior break.
- Freezing occurs at the tip of the cryoprobe; thus, it's important to ensure that the tip is at the correct position relative to the edges of the break during scleral depression.
- **NB:** The cryoprobe is bulkier than most scleral depressors, which may cause the shaft of the probe to indent the sclera, giving a false impression of the location of the tip. This may result in inadvertent cryopexy posterior to the target site, which is easy to avoid if you know this fact!

Risk of retinal detachment in the fellow eye

- There is a 10–15% risk of fellow eye RD.
- The risk is higher in aphakia and syndromic retinal detachment such as Stickler's. The presence of hyaloid presentation of the first eye detachment significantly decreases the risk. In one study with OCT imaging of the fellow eye at the time of presentation with an RRD, eyes noted to have a completely detached posterior hyaloid had a 3% risk of RRD, while those with attached haloid had an 8% risk of RRD. For those with attached hyaloid and PVD occurred, the rate of retinal detachment was 24%, and the rate of retinal tears without detachment was 18% [5].

2 Pneumatic Retinopexy

2.1 Introduction

Pneumatic retinopexy (PnR) is a simple, minimally invasive outpatient procedure involving an expansile gas injection into the vitreous cavity and induction of chorio-retinal adhesion around the retinal breaks using cryotherapy or laser photocoagulation. With proper positioning, the gas seals off the retinal break blocking fluid access into the subretinal space and allowing the retinal pigment epithelium (RPE) to pump the SRF out.

2.2 Outcomes

- Although accumulating evidence continues to prove its usefulness, PnR remains an underrated procedure. In two large randomized controlled trials, PnR was associated with only a slightly lower initial success rate compared to pars plana vitrectomy (PPV) [6, 7] or scleral buckle [8]. However, it showed superior visual outcomes compared to the latter procedures. Furthermore, failed PnR does not negatively affect the final visual outcome if further vitreous surgery is to be performed [4].

- The PIVOT trial was a randomized controlled trial that compared PnR to PPV for patients with RRD that met specific inclusion criteria (patients with retinal detachments with one or more breaks in the detached retina all within 1-clock hour and located in the superior 8-clock hours). The percentage of eyes with 20/40 vision or better was 90% in the pneumatic retinopexy group compared to 75% in the vitrectomy group. The primary single-surgery anatomic success rate was about 80% in PnR and 93.2% in the PPV group. However, a pneumatic failure did not affect the final visual acuity, with secondary reattachment rates of 99% in both groups. One major benefit for the PnR group was that cataract surgery at 1 year was 16% compared to 65% in the PPV group [6]. More recently, the INTEGRITY study was a multicenter retrospective case series suggesting that retinal displacement may be higher and more severe with PPV (44%) compared to PnR (7%) for RRD repair [7].

2.3   Indications

- The classic criteria described by Hilton and Grizzard [9] remain the gold standard for selecting candidates for PnR. The ideal candidate should have:

    - A single break ($\leq$1-clock hour in size) or multiple breaks within 1-clock hour in the detached retina.
    - Break(s) should be located above the 8- and 4-clock positions.

- Although there is paucity of evidence on the use of PnR in eyes of young patients with no PVD retinal breaks [10], results appear not to be different from eyes with PVD- related tears, but most eyes go on to develop PVD afterwards.
- Breaks or lattice degeneration in the attached retina may be included as well. However, breaks in the inferior detached retina (i.e., between 5 and 7 o'clock), large (>1-clock hour) or giant retinal tears, proliferative vitreoretinopathy (PVR) > grade B, glaucoma, media opacity, and inability to maintain postoperative posturing are associated with lower success and therefore may be excluded.

2.4   Preoperative Assessment

- Anterior segment examination is necessary to check for media clarity, anterior chamber (AC) depth, and the integrity of intraocular lens-capsular bag complex if prior cataract surgery was done.
- Meticulous scleral depressed exam of the peripheral retina to identify all retinal breaks is a crucial step, as missing any break will likely lead to treatment failure. It is best to draw a fundus diagram before injecting the gas bubble. Determining the location of the breaks and nearby landmarks (e.g., blood vessels, pigments, or scars) is extremely helpful during laser since it is challenging to find small breaks when the retina reattaches and the view is suboptimal due to the gas bubble.

- The patient should be counseled about air travel restrictions and the need for prolonged head positioning. The latter is very important for the success of the procedure.

2.5   Procedure

Anesthesia and Antispesis

- Topical anesthesia may be appropriate for this procedure. However, we recommend subconjunctival or sub-Tenon's anesthesia for better analgesia, particularly if cryotherapy is intended in the same session.
- We instill a drop of povidone-iodine before and after placing the speculum on the sites intended for paracentesis and gas injection.

Paracentesis

- *In phakic eyes*, there is a risk of iatrogenic injury of the crystalline lens since the pupil is pharmacologically dilated. In these cases, it is safer to drain the aqueous passively, with 30-g or preferably through a wider-bore 27-g with plunger taken out.

    - Bend the needle to allow easy access to the AC from either the nasal or the temporal limbus.
    - Have the patient look in the primary position to keep the eye central.
    - The needle should be held with your dominant hand, taking care not to obscure the syringe markings while holding it, and the plunger should be held with the other hand.
    - Use the plunger on one side to fixate the globe while introducing the needle into the AC on the other side.
    - Introduce the bent needle with its bevel up and aim it to lie above the inferior iris. Press on the globe with the plunger on the other side to allow the aqueous to egress out of the AC into the needle. The pressure with the plunger helps to deepen the AC near the needle tip as it starts to shallow (Videos 1 and 2).

- *In pseudophakic eyes*, paracentesis can be done using the latter technique or by active suction using a 30-g bent needle introduced toward the central, deepest part of the AC. If active suction is to be performed, it is important to break the vacuum seal of the syringe before using it to avoid sudden collapse of the AC.
- The amount of aqueous obtained often determines the amount of gas to be injected. We typically drain as much aqueous as possible to an almost flat AC. A volume of 0.3 mL is sufficient in most cases; however, the more, the better!

- The volume of the anterior and posterior chamber is about 0.3 mL. Nevertheless, draining 0.3 mL or more is attainable since some liquefied vitreous behind the lens often comes forward and contributes to the yield.
- Avoid keeping the eye soft for a long time after paracentesis; thus, it's important to load the gas in the syringe before paracentesis and inject it soon after. Pressure by the plunger will keep the eye pressurized during the paracentesis.

    - Paracentesis can be done before or after gas injection; however, softening the eye before gas injection increases the chances of obtaining a single bubble.

2.6   Gas Injection

- A gas bubble of 1 mL covers approximately 130° of the retina; however, this may vary with the axial length of the eye [4]. A bubble of this size is often sufficient to cover one quadrant of the retina where the break resides without the need for exact head positioning.
- Both perfluoropropane (C_3F_8) and sulfur hexafluoride (SF_6) can be used. SF_6 doubles its size within 24 h and lasts for about 2 weeks, whereas C_3F_8 expands to four times its size and lasts for 6–8 weeks.

Type of Gas

- SF_6: we aim to inject a 0.5–0.6 mL bubble into the vitreous cavity. This volume is significantly disproportionate to the amount of aqueous being drained from the AC, which may cause a significant rise in the intraocular pressure (IOP) to block the central retinal artery perfusion.
- C_3F_8: a smaller bubble (0.3 mL) is needed to achieve a volume >1 mL. This obviates the need for repeat paracentesis and is especially useful in patients with glaucoma to avoid the harmful effect of IOP spikes on the optic nerve. However, it lasts longer and is therefore associated with a prolonged recovery period.
- **NB**: Typically, an equivalent volume needs to be drained with intravitreal injections of fluids of more than 0.05 mL to avoid a substantial rise in IOP. However, unlike fluids, gases are compressible, which permits a slightly higher volume to be injected without a substantial rise in IOP.

Site of Injection

To obtain a single bubble of gas, the injection must be at the globe's highest point. In this way, the bubble will stay within the needle while expanding. The site of injection varies with surgeons' preferences.

- **Injection at 12 o'clock** is performed while the patient is sitting up and looking downward to expose the superior quadrant (Video 1).

- **Injection at 6 o'clock** is undertaken while the patient is lying supine. The injection is performed by asking the patient to elevate his chin up and look upward so that the inferior quadrant of the globe is exposed and at the highest point of the globe (Video 2).
- Following the same principle, the injection can be performed at other sites, but we generally favor the 12 o'clock position.
- In aphakic eyes and those with comprised capsular bag, it's advisable to inject the gas while the patient is sitting up to avoid migration of the bubble to the AC and to use cryotherapy instead of the laser since the bubble may migrate to the AC during laser which will hinder a good view to the fundus.
- We prefer to have another 1 cc TB syringe without needle in the non-dominant hand. It comes in handy; it fixes the globe during injection, acts as a caliper to measure the distance from the limbus (the outer diameter of the syringe's tip is about 3 mm), and seals off the puncture site to avoid gas leak after withdrawing the needle. Alternatively, an injection package containing a disposable plastic caliber and Q-tip can be used instead.
- After introducing the needle into the vitreous cavity, withdraw the needle slightly so that the tip of the needle is barely inside the vitreous cavity.
- Injection should be done so that the plunger is pushed in a relatively slow continuous movement. Too fast, too slow, or interrupted movement of the plunger often results in multiple bubbles.
- Withdraw the needle quickly while maintaining pressure on the plunger to avoid gas reflux in the syringe, and massage the puncture site with the TB syringe or Q-tip to prevent a gas leak from the vitreous cavity (Videos 1 and 2).

2.7 Postoperative Assessment and Positioning

- Immediately after injection, we check the vision, the optic nerve perfusion, and the size and number of gas bubble(s) with the indirect ophthalmoscope. If the central retinal artery is not perfused and the vision is below HM, we ask the patient to assume a face down position for 1 min to help reform the AC and then perform another paracentesis through the original needle track. If the artery remains unperfused, we proceed with a vitreous tap with active controlled aspiration of 0.1-0.2 mL of the injected gas going through the same pars plana point we used for the gas injection or just next to it. This restores the patency of central retinal artery though comprises the gas fill. Postoperative IOP-lowering drops are usually not needed.
- We recommend head positioning for 45 min of every hour for 3–7 days! During the 15-min break, the patient should behave normally, avoiding vigorous head movements, supine position, and straining. Positioning may be revised when the gas bubble is larger to allow a more comfortable position for the patient's neck!

- We instruct the patient to continue positioning during sleep, at least in the first couple of days, until the bubble is large enough to allow sleeping on one side.
- Some surgeons adopt a steam roller maneuver to prevent fluid from involving the macula and to aid in SRF drainage; however, it's not mandatory for PnR success.
- We find topical steroids very useful in reducing eye soreness post-PnR. This helps to increase the patient's compliance during subsequent scleral indentation and laser.
- We ask the patient to return 1–2 days after the procedure for the evaluation of the retina and to administer laser.

2.8 Retinopexy (by Laser or Cryotherapy)

Laser Retinopexy

- Laser retinopexy can be done using LIO or on the slit lamp. However, in the presence of gas inside the eye, the former is preferred as it allows scleral depression, provides a superior view through the gas bubble, and permits manipulation of the patient's head during laser.
- Topical anesthesia may be sufficient in some cases; however, most patients in our view require subconjunctival or anterior sub-Tenon's injection at the quadrant where the break resides. These blocks preserve the ocular movements while blocking the sensation, facilitating the retinopexy procedure.
- Using LIO requires a great deal of maneuvering; moving the bubble out of the way requires frequent manipulation of the patient's head and some acrobatic movements by the surgeon.
- The gas bubble provides a more peripheral view of the fundus, allowing lasering up to the ora serrata without scleral depression.
- Chorioretinal adhesions start to form within 1-day post-laser, and adequate adhesions form within 1 week.

Cryotherapy

- After proper anesthesia (see above), cryotherapy is performed before injecting the gas into the vitreous cavity.
- Following cryotherapy, the eye is often too sore to allow scleral indentation, and only limited examination is possible in the first week.
- We tend to use cryotherapy for small holes and breaks as they are hard to find after retinal reattachment and do not require excessive cryotherapy.
- In contrast to laser retinopexy, cryo-retinopexy is completed in one visit. However, it is associated with increased patient discomfort, pigment dispersion, and corneal haze that can make postoperative examination troublesome.

- Chorioretinal adhesions start to form within 2-days post-cryotherapy, with adequate adhesions forming within 12 days. The delayed retinal adherence with cryopexy compared to laser is a disdvantage.

2.9 Complications

1. **Fish eggs**: Improper injection technique may result in numerous small bubbles instead of a single large bubble. These bubbles usually coalesce with each other as they expand. To avoid the escape of these bubbles through the break into the subretinal space (not common), the patient should remain facedown until they notice that the bubbles coalesce into one or two large bubbles before starting positioning.
2. **Subretinal gas**: This often occurs in the context of fish eggs and large retinal breaks. It's prudent to tease the bubble from underneath the retina before it expands. The scleral depressor can be used to tease the bubble out; however, if this fails, PPV should be performed.
3. **Gas migration into the AC**: This tends to occur in aphakia or compromised capsular bag- IOL complex cases. It can be avoided by injecting the gas while the patient sits upright. Assuming facedown position may cause the bubble to go back to the vitreous cavity. However, if this is not successful while the patient is sitting upright, aspiration of the gas through the paracentesis and reinjection can be performed.
4. **New retinal break formation:** In a non-vitrectomized eye, the expanding gas bubble may cause vitreous traction or push the SRF at areas of retinal thinning or lattice, causing a new break. While this complication is a common concern for retina specialists who are unfamiliar with PnR, in our experience, it's a rare complication, and it should not preclude surgeons from performing PnR.

   Areas of lattice or atrophic holes in the attached retina are best lasered prior to gas injection to minimize the likelihood of new break formation.
5. **Persistent fluid:** The rate of persistent subreitnal fluid after PnR is approximately 15%, which is not higher than after PPV [11]. In a few cases, SRF may collect inferiorly and take a long time to resorb. It is important to differentiate these cases from failed PnR due to new/missed breaks. Certain clues are helpful to make this distinction: (1) the amount of SRF is rather stable or decreasing but has not increased; (2) the SRF is limited to the posterior to mid-peripheral retina but doesn't extend up to the ora serrata, and the retina doesn't undulate with scleral depression as with cases of RRD; and (3) scleral depression shows that the SRF doesn't track back to the original break, and no new break can be detected in the area of the SRF. These findings indicate that the SRF is likely to be persistent rather than new. Observation is recommended in these cases keeping in mind that it may take up to 2 years for the SRF to resolve.
6. **Injection-related complications** include cataracts, vitreous hemorrhage, retinal tears, and endophthalmitis.

3   Final Note

PnR is the most physiological technique to treat RRD. With proper selection, the results are great. However, the technique can be time-consuming if a proper setup is not established. The required gas and filters should be readily available in the clinic to save time and avoid the disruption of a busy clinic. Also, laser retinopexy may take a long time, especially in very sensitive patients. Patients who often feel a lot of discomfort during scleral indentation in the clinic may not be the best candidates for office-based PnR.

4   Case Scenario

A 54-year-old male with macula on superotemporal RRD (Fig. 3a) and horseshoe tear at 10 o'clock within 2 areas of lattice degeneration. On indentation, no other retinal pathology was noted. This patient was treated with a two-stage pneumatic retinopexy using 0.6 mL of 100% SF_6 gas followed by laser retinopexy 1 day later (Fig. 3b–d).

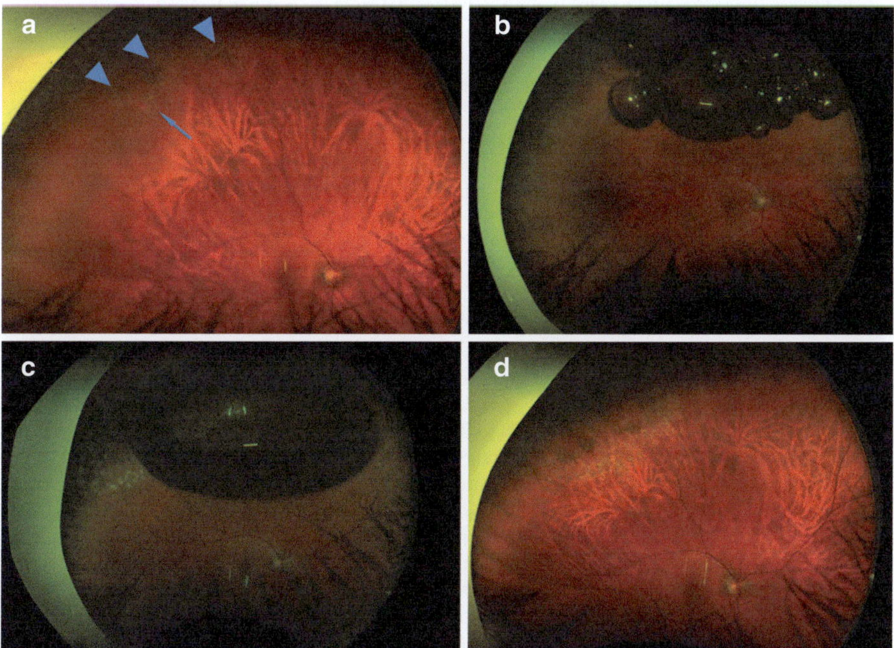

Fig. 3 Pneumatic retinopexy for a macula on superotemporal retinal detachment and a horseshoe tear at 10 o'clock (arrow) within two areas of lattice degeneration (arrowhead) (**a**). Note fish egg gas bubbles after the gas injection (**b**) that coalesced completely on day 3 (**c**). The retina remains flat at day 10, with no gas remaining (**d**)

Key Points

- PnR is a useful outpatient procedure to repair RRD in select patients.
- PnR teaches the new retina surgeon excellent skills including indirect ophthalmoscopy, meticulous retinal examination for retinal tears as well as lasering of the retina under gas.
- Retinal breaks should be in the superior 8-clock hours (8–4 o'clock). The presence of inferior retinal pathology, PVR, or a history of glaucoma are relative contraindications that are associated with poor outcomes.
- In pneumatic retinopexy, compared to PPV, the size of the gas bubble is small, and vitreous traction remains on the retinal break. Postoperative positioning is therefore essential to maximize gas contact with the retinal tear.
- A pneumatic failure does not affect the final visual outcome, with high secondary reattachment rates after subsequent pars plana vitrectomy.

References

1. Goh YW, Ehrlich R, Stewart J, et al. The incidence of retinal breaks in the presenting and fellow eyes in patients with acute symptomatic posterior vitreous detachment and their associated risk factors. Asia Pac J Ophthalmol (Phila). 2015;4:5–8. 6. Brod RD, 10.
2. Mitry D, Singh J, Yorston D, et al. The fellow eye in retinal detachment: findings from the Scottish Retinal Detachment study. Br J Ophthalmol. 2012;96:110–3.
3. Fincham GS, Pasea L, Carroll C, McNinch AM, Poulson AV, Richards AJ, Scott JD, Snead MP. Prevention of retinal detachment in Stickler syndrome: the Cambridge prophylactic cryotherapy protocol. Ophthalmology. 2014;121(8):1588–97. Epub 2014 May 1. PMID: 24793526.
4. Khanna S, Rodriguez SH, Blair MA, Wroblewski K, Shapiro MJ, Blair MP. Laser prophylaxis in patients with stickler syndrome. Ophthalmol Retina. 2022;6(4):263–7. Epub 2021 Nov 11. PMID: 34774838.
5. Wallsh JO, Langevin ST, Kumar A, Huz J, Falk NS, Bhatnagar P. Fellow-eye retinal detachment risk as stratified by hyaloid status on OCT. Ophthalmology. 2023;130(6):624–30. S0161-6420(23)00105-7.
6. Hillier RJ, Felfeli T, Berger AR, Wong DT, Altomare F, Dai D, Giavedoni LR, Kertes PJ, Kohly RP, Muni RH. Pneumatic retinopexy vs. vitrectomy for the management of primary rhegmatogenous retinal detachment outcomes randomized trial (PIVOT). Ophthalmology. 2019;126(4):531–9.
7. Brosh K, Francisconi CLM, Qian J, Sabatino F, Juncal VR, Hillier RJ, Chaudhary V, Berger AR, Giavedoni LR, Wong DT, Altomare F, Kadhim MR, Newsom RB, Marafon SB, Muni RH. Retinal displacement following pneumatic retinopexy vs pars plana vitrectomy for rhegmatogenous retinal detachment (INTEGRITY). JAMA Ophthalmol. 2020;138(6):652–9.
8. Tornambe PE, Hilton GF. Pneumatic retinopexy. A multicenter randomized controlled clinical trial comparing pneumatic retinopexy with scleral buckling. The Retinal Detachment Study Group. Ophthalmology. 1989;96(6):772–83.
9. Hilton GF, Grizzard WS. Pneumatic retinopexy. A two-step outpatient operation without conjunctival incision. Ophthalmology. 1986;93(5):626–41.
10. Figueiredo N, Warder DC, Muni RH, Lee WW, Yong SO, Kertes PJ. Pneumatic retinopexy as a treatment for rhegmatogenous retinal detachment in pediatric patients meeting PIVOT criteria. Canadian Journal of Ophthalmology. 2022;57(6):359–63.
11. Bansal Wei A, Lee W, Sarraf D, Sadda SR, Berger AR, Wong DT, Kertes PT, Kohly RP, Hillier RJ, Muni RH. Persistent subfoveal fluid in pneumatic retinopexy versus pars plana vitrectomy for rhegmatogenous retinal detachment: posthoc analysis of the PIVOT randomised trial. British Journal of Ophthalmology. 2023;107(11):1693–7.

Primary Retinal Detachment: Pars Plana Vitrectomy

Abdallah A. Ellabban, Mohamed Kamel Soliman, Ahmed B. Sallam, and Giampaolo Gini

1 Introduction

Pars plana vitrectomy (PPV) has become a popular option for rhegmatogenous retinal detachment (RRD) surgery over the past two decades. This is mainly because of the following:

1. The development of the new wide-field viewing systems.
2. The development of the small-gauge (g) (23-, 25-, or 27-g) vitrectomy systems that offer microinvasive surgery with less conjunctival manipulations leading to faster rehabilitation and less pain and inflammation after surgery.
3. The improvement of machine technology, including better illumination, cutters, and fluidics, alongside a wider range of instrumentations.

Supplementary Information The online version contains supplementary material available at https://doi.org/10.1007/978-3-031-47827-7_8.

A. A. Ellabban
Department of Ophthalmology, Hull University Teaching Hospitals, Hull, UK

M. K. Soliman
Department of Ophthalmology and Visual Sciences, University Hospitals Eye Institute, Cleveland, OH, USA

Department of Ophthalmology, Assiut University Hospitals, Assiut, Egypt

A. B. Sallam (✉)
Jones Eye Institute, University of Arkansas for Medical Sciences, Little Rock, AR, USA

G. Gini
Department of Ophthalmology, University Hospitals Sussex NHS Foundation Trust, Worthing, West Sussex, UK

4. The flexibility of the technique to deal with a wide range of retinal detachment scenarios and any associated pathology.
5. Most procedures can be performed under local anesthetics as day-case surgery.

In our practice, we tend to use PPV (23-g or 25-g) in most cases of RRD with posterior vitreous detachment (PVD) related tractional tears, particularly if the patient's age is over 50 years, or pseudophakic. In cases of no PVD RRD due to retinal dialysis or atrophic holes in young patients, our preferred surgery is segmental scleral buckle. We also consider the use of pneumatic retinopexy in co-operative patients with straightforward, phakic retinal detachment, and 1–2 superior retinal breaks.

2   Timing of Surgery

- We operate acute macula-on RRD within 24 hours. Until the surgery, we advise patients to limit their activities and posture their heads so that the retinal tear is in a dependent position to decrease the risk of detachment progression.
- For acute macula-off RRD (Fig. 1), we aim to operate them within <1 week, usually within 3 days, to decrease the time of macular detachment. In general, it is advisable to operate on RRD as early as possible, whether macula-on or macula-off, to avoid the risk of photoreceptor damage. The appearance of outer retinal corrugation can help estimate the duration of the sensory retinal detachment from the retinal pigment epithelium (RPE) and the risk of postoperative poor vision [1, 2].
- Chronic RRD is scheduled as non-urgent.

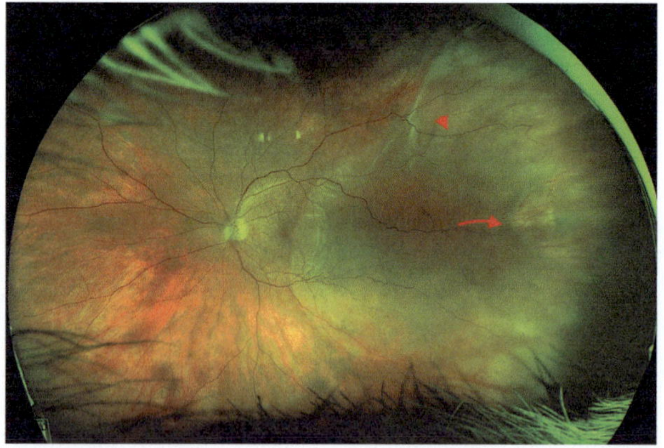

Fig. 1 Macula-off rhegmatogenous retinal detachment with fovea splitting. Note the presence of a large temporal tear (arrow) and a very small tear superiorly (arrowhead above the tear)

3 Principles of Surgery

Vitrectomy for RRD has five main steps:

1. Relieving vitreoretinal traction.
2. Finding the retinal break(s).
3. Drainage of the subretinal fluid (SRF).
4. Sealing the break (retinopexy).
5. Tamponade to support the retinal break until the retinopexy effect takes place.

3.1 Reliving Vitreoretinal Traction

- PPV is performed in the usual manner with smaller-gauge instrumentation (23-, 25-g, or 27-g) according to the surgeon's preference.
- The main aim is to remove the vitreous to relieve traction on the retina and create a space for the tamponade.
- In general, most cases of RRD due to horseshoe retinal tears would have PVD. It is, however, worth checking with triamcinolone, if required, that there is no vitreoschisis, particularly in myopic patients (Video 1).
- We advise using the "shaving mode" with a high cutting rate (low duty cycle) and low vacuum near the retina if the retinal detachment is mobile to avoid "sucking" the retina inadvertently and causing iatrogenic retinal tears (Video 2).

3.2 Finding the Retinal Breaks

- The success of RD surgery depends on finding and treating all retinal breaks. It is important to note that more than half of RDs may have more than one break.
- The Lincoff rule is a good guide (Fig. 5 in chapter "Scleral Buckle Surgery") that indicates the location of the primary break.
- Searching for breaks intraoperatively can be done by several ways:
  - Performing 360° dynamic indentation of the retina by a blunt instrument, rolling the depressor on the sclera from anterior to posterior, starting just anterior to the ora serrata, and moving down posteriorly to the posterior extent of the vitreous base, over each clock hour. It is important to perform this step meticulously and not to skip any areas, under high magnification and sharp focus. With dynamic indentation, the break will pout, as there is usually some traction over the break.
  - Look for a "the schlieren phenomenon", the track of viscid SRF coming off the break, when the aspiration port comes close to the break.

- Sometimes, there is a small anterior hole or tiny horseshoe tear that is covered with the peripheral vitreous near the vitreous base. Lifting this vitreous skirt up with the cutter tip may reveal the tear.
- When there is a suspicious small break, the surgeon can check this area with dynamic indention or perform gentle suction over a flute needle or vitreous cutter (on gentle suction mode) to check if any SRF coming out of it.
- Another strategy is to try to apply cryotherapy over it, and if there is a small hole, it will show up.

- It is important to remove the traction from the anterior margin of the break, and therefore, we often trim the retinal tear flap. This can often be done while shaving the vitreous anterior to the break. The easiest way to do this is to use only the suction mode until the flap is in the mouth of the cutter and then cut. This can be helped by scleral indentation to stabilize the retina if very mobile.
- Next, all breaks in the detached retina should be marked with gentle endodiathermy (Video 3) to allow better visualization after draining the subretinal fluid, and the eye is filled with air. One or two corners of the breaks are enough as diathermy can shrink the retina. The surgeon may opt to remember the break by some adjacent landmarks as blood vessels or scars or map the breaks in clock hours on a theatre board or to mind. In our experience, this often does not work every time, especially if there are multiple breaks or small breaks. The surgeon may end up overusing the cryo- or laser retinopexy treatment. In short, mark all breaks in the detached retina.
- Breaks in the attached retina do not need to be marked if they are to be treated with laser or cryopexy before placing air in the eye.

3.3 Drainage of the Subretinal Fluid (SRF)

- After all breaks have been identified and marked, the surgeon can plan to start removing the SRF. There are different strategies of removing the SRF depending on the geometry of the detached retina and the surgeon's preference including drainage from the retinal break, drainage retinotomy, and drainage with the help of perfluorocarbon liquid (PFCL).
- Drainage from the retinal break

  - It often helps to rotate the eye to make the break, and hence the SRF, in the dependent position (e.g., for inferior breaks, rotate the eye downward, and in superior breaks, rotate the eye upward).
  - You can use the vitreous cutter or the flute/extrusion/backflush needle. The latter helps in better drainage as the opening is at the tip and not on the side as in the cutter (Video 4).
  - Subretinal fluid aspiration can be passive or active. Passive can be very slow if using a gauge smaller than 23-g. Extrusion needle can also be soft or non-soft tipped (conventional). The former is less traumatic and can go more under the edge of the tear for better drainage, but it is slower.

- Using the cutter at the beginning of the exchange until the air reaches the break can be useful if you think there are some vitreous remnants anterior to the breaks, as it gives you a chance to deal with this (switching to cut mode as needed).
- Fluid/air exchange. A safe way is to keep the extrusion tip in the anterior vitreous cavity until the air bubbles coalesce and the view becomes clear. There will be a momentary loss of view that will quickly pass, and the view will come back as the air gets more into the eye. Then we advance the tip toward the break slowly. Don't go directly to the break but instead advance the tip along the interface between the air and fluid and move posteriorly as the interface moves until you reach the break. This causes the air to stabilize the retina by the time the tip reaches the break, which prevents repeated jumping of the retina to the aspiration tip (Video 5).
- Continue to drain the SRF till the retina is attached back and the break is flat (the retina is stuck down to the RPE). You may notice some bubbling sounds if the flute is only aspirating air. Also, further titling of the eye toward the break at this stage may help to drain some of the remaining fluid in the vitreous cavity.
- Assess the remaining fluid level in the vitreous cavity. If you decide to drain this fluid to get a bigger gas fill, follow the fluid to the optic disc cup. Ensure you see well (adjust the focus), and avoid touching the disc. We often recommend that you avoid going back to drain the remaining fluid over the disc or macula, as this may cause the SRF to move posteriorly under the macula (Video 5) and increase the risk of retinal displacement.
- Occasionally, the retina may be caught or sucked in by the aspiration tip if the hole is small. To deal with this, you can reflux some fluid to disengage the retina. Some surgeons opt to slightly enlarge the break during vitrectomy, especially if the break is small, to allow the easier removal of SRF during fluid/air exchange and to ensure that all the traction has been cleared. Always aim the extrusion tip to the middle of the break, away from retinal edges and any remaining vitreous near the anterior edge.
- Sometimes, in the case of anterior breaks, the retina may become prematurely attached, and there is a remaining cuff of the subretinal fluid posteriorly. The surgeon may find ways to avoid this scenario as:

  Making sure the eye is in the dependent position before starting fluid/air exchange.

  Placing a soft tip needle under the break to remove as much SRF as possible before the retina comes close to the RPE.

  If feasible, tilting the head so that the break is in the most dependent position. This will move the subretinal fluid toward the break.

  Leaving the subretinal fluid and ending up with a smaller gas fill. However, it is important to note that if you drain the fluid in the vitreous cavity by moving the aspiration tip toward the optic disc, this subretinal fluid will move more centrally.

- Drainage retinotomy

  - May be needed occasionally when access to the retinal break is difficult as in very anterior breaks, especially in phakic patients or when fluid/air exchange is performed and still a remaining lot of SRF at the macula and you need to have a big gas fill as in RRD due to inferior retinal tears (Video 6).
  - Choose the site of the retinotomy, preferably outside the arcade at the most posterior extend of SRF, often nasal is better than temporal and superior better than inferior.
  - Mark the site of the retinotomy by a gentle endodiathermy burn and take care to avoid areas of blood vessels because these may bleed while creating the retinotomy.
  - Poke the retina in the middle of the mark with the pointed diathermy tip. This makes the next step easy.
  - The retinotomy is made by a gentle suction using the extrusion needle or a single side cut with the vitreous cutter.
  - Gentle laser is placed around the retinotomy at the end after all SRF have been cleared. Some surgeons elect not to laser a small non-enlarged retinotomy as it is posterior and there is no vitreous traction on it. A polytip 25g/33g cannula can be used for penetration through the retina, allowing drainage of subretinal fluid through a minimally traumatic drainage retinotomy. Thin wall tip of the cannula has a flow rate similar to a 25g soft tip but with a smaller retinotomy.
  - Drainage retinotomy may be associated with intraoperative bleeding, may cause a visual field defect, and may increase the risk of postoperative epiretinal membranes.

- PFCL (heavy liquid)

  - PFCL can help push the fluid from the posterior to the anterior to the exit through the anterior retinal tear.
  - Refer to chap. 4 "Vitreous Substitutes" for the discussion on the physical properties and technique of injection and removal of PFCL.
  - We do not routinely use PFCL in primary RRD repair as in most cases the retina can be successfully flattened without the use of heavy liquid. We mainly use heavy liquid in the following scenarios:

    1. For giant retinal tear detachment: this is our main indication and details can be found in chapter "Giant Retinal Tears".
    2. For bullous RRD where the retina is not settling down even after cutting and sucking the vitreous near the break to decrease the volume of SRF (Video 7).
    3. For pseudophakic eyes with open posterior capsules and multiple tears: the view can get difficult when trying to apply laser under air. However, the problem with "fogging" may come back to "haunt you" as you are exchanging PFCL for air. Also, PFCL itself may exacerbate condensation on acrylic, silicone, and PMAA IOLs by acting as a buffer between water droplets and the surface of the IOL. If there is only 1 or 2 tears, it is best to do cryopexy under air.

4. As an intraoperative tool for finding a retinal break that could not be identified on internal search (see later).
5. For vitreous or retinal incarceration in the sclerotomy: a very rare indication now in the era of valved small gauge trocars. This problem was encountered more often during the era of non-valved 20-g trocars.

3.4 Sealing the Break(s) (Retinopexy)

- The aim of retinopexy is to create a chorioretinal scarring that will create firm adhesions between the retina and the RPE around the break.
- The two main options for retinopexy during vitrectomy are cryotherapy or laser.
- For breaks in the detached retina, we will perform this step after all the subretinal fluid has been removed and the retina is reattached under air.
- We use cryopexy if there is a single or few retinal tears particularly if the tears are anterior in phakic eyes [3]. As such, it does not appear to increase the risk of RRD failure/ development of proliferative vitreoretinopathy (PVR). Cryopexy is quick and simple, and the retina does not need to be completely dry for the cryo to take up as compared to laser. It is also helpful if the retinal view is compromised due to corneal or lens problems as it is less visually demanding especially with air inside the eye compared to applying endolaser. We apply it directly over the break to avoid multiple cryo applications. We avoid excessive freezing and aim for gentle change in the color of the RPE (orange white) and retina (white).
- We use laser if there are posterior breaks or multiple breaks to avoid excessive use of cryotherapy that may potentially increase the risk of PVR. The use of directional/curved laser probes also helps for better access to the peripheral retina and minimizes the risk of lens damage in phakic eyes.

3.5 Tamponade

- For primary RRD, the usual tamponade used is SF_6 gas for RRD due to tears in the upper 2/3 of the eye and long-acting gas C_2F_6 or C_3F_8 for RRD due to tears in the lower 1/3.
- Silicone oil (SO) is rarely used in primary RRD. Refer to Chap. 5 "Vitreous Substitutes." The indications are mainly social—a patient who needs to fly directly after surgery.

4 Note on PPV Technique: What Do We Do in Primary RRD?

- Our management is different based on the geometry of RRD and the position of retinal tears in relation to the retinal detachment.

- RRD due to retinal tears in the upper 2/3 of the retina do not need a big gas fill, compared to RRD due to retinal tears in the lower 1/3 of the retina, as breaks are easily supported with gas but are at a higher risk of retinal displacement/folds. Inferior retinal breaks and inferior detachment are risk factors for failure [3].
- Therefore, for upper tears RRD (including RRD with inferior tears in the attached retina), we do what we call "minimal drainage, minimal gas vitrectomy" (Video 8). As most of the retinal displacement happens when the surgeon moves over the disc to drain the vitreous fluid and replace it with air, we avoid this step by only draining from the retinal tear and not moving to the disc. Less air fill and, hence, less gas fill later are expected; so, in this case, use 30% SF_6. Postoperatively, with this technique, you usually have approximately 70–75% gas fill the next day. The technique is also quick and avoids the cost and complications of PFCL and the risks associated with drainage retinotomy.
- For lower breaks detachment, we aim to drain SRF as much as we can, and if this is not achieved by draining from an existing peripheral tear, we perform a posterior drainage retinotomy. We use a long-acting gas bubble, 14–16% C_3F_8 (Video 6)

5 Additional Debatable Steps

5.1 Combined Cataract PPV Surgery

We do not perform combined surgery unless there is a significant cataract that may impair the visualization during the surgery. We prefer to deal with the cataract later after successful RRD repair. More discussion can be found in Chap. 34 "Cataract Surgery and Vitreoretinal Surgery".

5.2 Vitreous Base Shaving

- We are not so obsessed with vitreous base shaving (unless there is anterior PVR).
- As far as we know, there is no proof that vitreous base shaving improves RRD outcomes [4].
- This technique is also not without risks, including lens touch and iatrogenic retinal tears.
- We remove the peripheral vitreous as far as we can see, with emphasis on indentation vitrectomy over retinal breaks and removing all the vitreous traction over the breaks(s).
- Placing a chandelier is helpful but not necessary if an assistant is present to perform scleral indentation.

5.3   360° Laser

- Some surgeons perform a circumferential 360° laser in cases with multiple peripheral breaks or in cases where no break is found or even routinely in all cases. We believe this is unnecessary as the chance of not finding the breaks with modern viewing systems is as low as 0.5%, and studies showed that 360° laser does not improve the surgery outcome as compared to focal laser [5].
- Disadvantages of 360° laser are:
- Retinopexy can cause further intraocular inflammation and scarring, increasing the risk of PVR or ERM.
- Postoperative hypotony, anterior segment ischemia, and loss of pupil tone have been reported as complications of 360° laser due to damage to the long ciliary nerves or vessels.
- Another disadvantage is that if re-detachment occurs, it can be very challenging to find the retinal break or you may have many tears at the areas of laser-induced chorioretinal atrophy.

5.4   Additional Encirclement Buckle

Some surgeons add a circumferential band with PPV for primary RRD to support missed breaks. Additional of an encirclement buckle with PPV is time-consuming, and is associated with an increased risk of complications and significant refractive changes. Current evidence does not show an overall higher success rate in combined PPV with buckle vs. PPV alone [6]. However, studies found improved outcomes in cases with inferior retinal tears in phakic eyes [7, 8].

6   Postoperative Posturing

There is no agreement on the best posturing position after surgery [9]. The two main points to consider are:

1. What is the best position to avoid retinal displacement or retinal folds?
2. What is the position needed for the gas which supports the break?

   The answer to the first question is not simple, and we are still unsure whether the supine or prone position is less likely to cause retinal displacement. If a prone position is to be used, it is best to be immediate without any time of sitting up to avoid gravity-dependent displacement of the subretinal fluid and the retina inferiorly [10].

   We prefer to position the patient supine for 1–2 hours post-surgery without sitting up at all whatsoever. We feel this avoids retinal displacement and folds that can happen just after a few seconds of sitting up if SRF is still present under the macula. This is important, particularly if some SRF is left under the retina at the end of the surgery. A supine position for 1–2 hours post-surgery will give a chance for the RPE pump to absorb some of the residual SRF and help the retina to stick at the area of the break (Video 8).

Following this time, the patient can sit up, dress, and leave the surgery facility. We advise positioning to support the break mainly during night sleep only if the detachment is caused by breaks below the horizontal meridian. Otherwise, we advise not lying flat on their back. We do not advise day positioning. We think it is not needed if there is a good amount of gas in the eye [11].

7 Special Categories of RRD

7.1 RRD and No Detectable Break

- There may be no detectable break pre-operatively in about 5% of RRD. Therefore, it is important to ensure you are not misdiagnosing exudative RD as RRD.
- Intraoperatively, you will usually find the break(s) by dynamic internal search as detailed before. In many times, there is a small tear near an area of retina degeneration or previous retinopexy scar.
- If this fails:

  - The next step is to use PFCL. Filling the eye with PFCL till the equator forces the SRF peripherally and can make a hidden tear 'pout'; a schlieren may also be seen coming out from the break.
  - If still the break cannot be located, we inject diluted trypan blue dye, 0.06%, with a 38-gauge needle under the retina outside the PFCL bubble [12]. This forces the SRF containing the blue dye to egress from the small break (Video 9).
  - Finally, if no break can be located, we perform a drainage retinotomy to aspirate the SRF, then apply the laser to the drainage retinotomy and posterior to the anterior limit of the vitreous base, from dry retina to dry retina (Video 10).

7.2 Bullous RRD

There are some additional surgical challenges when dealing with bullous RRD (Fig. 2) as follows:

1. Risk of placing the infusion under the retina, particularly if the ciliary body epithelium is also detached.
2. Very mobile retina, which is difficult to flatten, and higher risk of iatrogenic retinal tears during vitrectomy.
3. Risk of retinal incarceration if using large sclerotomies or non-valved trocars.

Fig. 2 Bullous rhegmatogenous retinal detachment. The macular region is concealed with the hanging retinal bullous detachment. In most of these cases, the macula would be detached

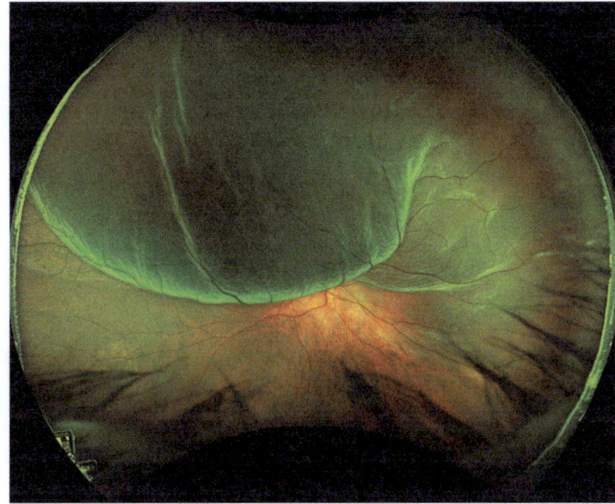

- Surgical tips:
  - Always use valved trocars.
  - The retina settles down when the patient lies flat on their back so they can do this for a few hours before the surgery.
  - Consider placing the infusion in a quadrant where the retina is not bullous, for example, moving it to an inferonasal quadrant.
  - Make sure the infusion *is inside the vitreous cavity* before switching it on.
  - The aim is to stabilize the retina at the beginning of the vitrectomy:

    Use lower vacuum, high cutting at the begining of surgery (e.g. shave mode). Start cutting near the retinal break or in the quadrant where you expect the break to be. This will draw some of the SRF out and will help stabilize the retina.

    If the above is not working, you could use PFCL. To do this, you need to have a view of the disc to inject nasal to it. Remove some of the central vitreous, and then inject the PFCL. The aim is to only get a partial fill till the vascular arcade at this stage (Video 7).

    Rarely, in some of these bullous RRD cases, if you cannot find the break and the disc is not visible to put the PFCL, you could simply do a superior peripheral drainage retinotomy to partially flatten the retina.

7.3 *RRD Due to Posterior Break*

- Breaks usually happen anterior to the equator and close to the posterior border of the vitreous base.

- Sometimes, posterior tears can be present. Surgeons should therefore keep this in mind at all times. These breaks are usually helpful to drain from (if they are not in the macula) and are lasered.
- For breaks in the macular area, we advise no laser and using gas.

7.4 RRD Due to High Myopia [13]

- In young patients with RRD due to atrophic myopic holes, these cases are best treated with scleral buckles and not PPV. There is difficulty of PVD induction in young patient as the posterior hyaloid is very adherent to the retina. Also inducing PVD in detached retina is challenging and associated with increased risks of iatrogenic breaks. PPV may induce more inflammatory response in these eyes, more risk of cataract and possibly a higher PVR risk.
- In older patients with horseshoe retinal tears, vitreoschisis is common. Triamcinolone staining of the vitreous is therefore important during PPV (Video 1).
- A good number of myopic eyes may have had prophylactic laser for lattice or atrophic holes, a practice that we do not recommend. Retinal tears may happen at the posterior edge of laser and can be multiple and small making it difficult to find.
- Instruments may be difficult to reach the macular/disc area in very long eyes. This poses a challenge when macular work such as ILM peel is needed or when tears are posterior. Longer, extended reach, instruments are now available. Removing the trocars may also help. In eyes >31 mm in length, moving the trocar from 3.5–4.0 mm to 5.0–6.0 mm away from the limbus may provide a safe entry in the pars plana and easier access to the posterior pole. Still, one is to affirm the entry position before placing the trocar by depressing the sclera at the planned position while illuminating the pars plana area from the other superior trocar [14].
- The vitreous base can be inserted more posteriorly than in emmetropic eyes limiting further anterior extension of the posterior hyaloid. This needs to be taken in consideration to avoid aggressive pull on the hyaloid that can result in retinal tears (Video 1). Some studies suggested placing an additional broad encirclement buckle with PPV in eyes with RRD and posterior vitreous base insertion [15]. We usually do not do this.
- Breaks can be present posterior to the equator and at the edge of a posterior staphyloma.
- RPE and choroid pigmentation may be lacking (Fig. 3), making laser retinopexy difficult. Cryopexy for peripheral breaks can be an alternative. Amniotic membrane stuffing with posterior holes can be an option if there is no laser uptake.
- There is a higher risk of suprachoroidal hemorrhage, so intra- and postoperative hypotony should be avoided.
- Decreased scleral rigidity may limit sclerotomy port closure, and sutures may be needed.
- Unlike senile (primary) macular holes (MH), myopic macular holes can cause RRD.

Fig. 3 (**a**) Superior rhegmatogenous retinal detachment in high myopia treated with (**b**) vitrectomy, laser and SF$_6$ gas. Note the hypopigmented fundus and the relative posterior location of the retinal tear

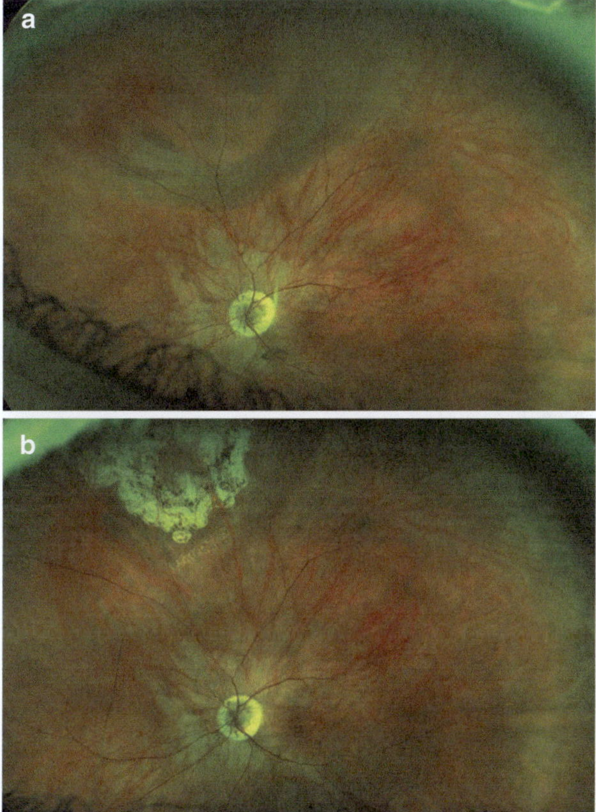

7.5   RRD with Coexisting Choroidal Detachment (CD)

- Choroidal detachment may exist with RRD in up to 5% of cases in the Western countries, but rates are higher in other countries such as China (15%) [16].
- Most cases have co-existing hypotony.
- It is important to rule out other causes of CD, most important being exudative retinal detachment. Refer to Chap. 26 "Vitreoretinal Surgery in Uveitis".
- Risk factors for CD in the context of RRD include high myopia, ocular trauma, older age, and pseudophakia [16].
- During surgery, we usually do not drain the choroidal detachment unless the RRD is due to inferior breaks and a bigger gas fill is needed (Video 11). One of the most important points to be wary of in eyes with choroidals is where to place the infusion cannula. To avoid subretinal infusion of fluids, avoid putting the infusion cannula in the quadrants that have the choroidals. Also make sure you can see the tip of the cannula inside the vitreous cavity before opening it. If there is ciliary body tissue covering the tip, it can be incised using a needle through one of the superior ports. You could also use a 6 mm cannula or put the infusion cannula in the anterior chamber in pseudophakic eyes.

7.6 Giant Retinal Tear Detachment

Please refer to Chap. 10 "Giant Retinal Tears".

8 Primary Retinal Detachment Failure

- The single-operation success rate is in the range of 80–85% in big series of RRD (not as high as 90% as reported in small series) [3, 6].
- Only a small number of patients (<5%) need three or more retinal reattachment surgeries [17].
- The multiple-operation success rate is in the range of 95%.
- Visual recovery is not complete in macula-off detachments, and distortion may be present. This may result from damage to the apical villi of RPE, photoreceptors' outer segments, and possibly bipolar cells. Part of this decreased visual function could be due to retinal displacement from surgery [18].
- While an increased number of RRD repair surgeries do not correlate with decreased final anatomic success rates, it does correlate with final acuity. After three RRD repairs, vision is usually poor (<20/200) and is not different from baseline vision [17].
- There appears to be an association between drainage technique and discontinuity of the external limiting membrane, ellipsoid zone (PRB), and interdigitation zone with rates being higher in the range of 1.5–2-folds with the use of PFCL as compared to drainage from a peripheral break or drainage retinotomy [19].
- Risk factors for retinal re-detachment are age <45 or >79 years, inferior retinal breaks, total detachment, inferior detachment, and presence of grade C PVR before surgery [3] Prior cataract extraction [3] and the use of cryopexy compared to laser and the presence of inferior tears do not appear to be consistent risk factors for failure [3, 20].
- RRD with CD has a poor prognosis, primarily due to poor visualization, difficult identification of causative retinal breaks that may cause delay in treatment, difficult application of retinopexy, tamponade underfill, and higher rates of PVR rates of up to 50% [21].
- Most initial RRD surgery failures occur in the first year and particularly in the first 6 months. Reasons for failure (Fig. 4) include:

  - PVR is the most common reason for failure in about 75% of cases. Treatment is discussed in the PVR chapter but usually entails PVR membrane peel which may require extra maneuvers such as additional retinectomy or buckle with SO tamponade.
  - Missed/new breaks causing re-detachment without PVR can be treated with PPV, laser, and gas. Most new breaks happen at the edge of the retinopexy scar.
  - An opened original break may result from insufficient retinopexy, overzealous retinopexy with retinal necrosis, and insufficient tamponade (Fig. 5).

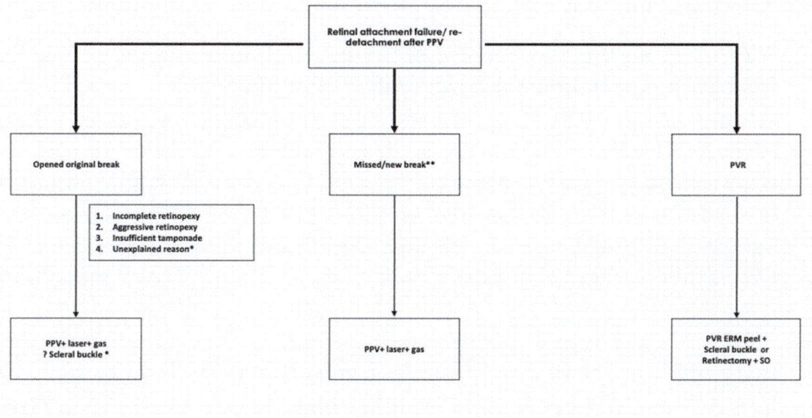

Fig. 4 Flowchart for the causes of retinal attachment failure

Fig. 5 Retinal attachment failure due to silicone oil underfill and poor support of an inferior break

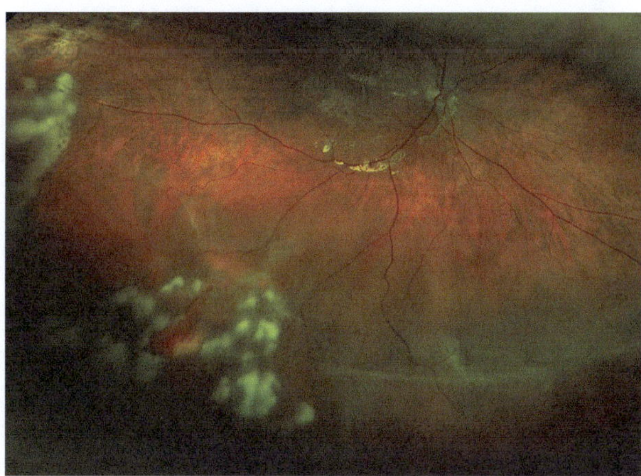

Treatment is usually along the line of PPV with laser around the previous laser and gas. Make sure the break is well supported by the tamponade and use a long-acting gas for inferior tears. With repeat failure to close a break or poor laser uptake, consider adding a buckle.

9 Complications

1. Anterior segment complications such as high intraocular pressure and cataract. Further discussion can be found in chapters 24 and 34.
2. Posterior segment complications.

1. Epiretinal membrane (ERM)

   - The risk is higher with the use of drainage retinotomy than with draining from the peripheral retinal break or the use of PFCL [19].
   - Additional internal limiting membrane peel during PPV for primary RRD was advocated by some authors for decreasing the risk of ERM. However, this was found to negatively affect the vision [22] and we do not recommend it.
   - In many situations, the secondary ERM has a limited impact on vision. Surgery is only indicated for visually significant ERMs.
   - We usually prefer to wait for 3 months or more as the risk of PVR decreases.

2. Macular hole

   - RRD with concomitant, non-causal macular hole (MH) is a rare association in 1–4% of RRD cases. This excludes high myopic eyes where MH can cause a RRD [23].
   - We usually use long-acting gas in these cases and advise no supine position for 1 week to help MH closure.
   - Data from a large retrospective study suggests that ILM peeling during the repair of RRD + MH is more successful in closing the MH (91%) than vitrectomy without ILM peeling (33%) [23].
   - ILM peeling is particularly difficult with a detached retina since the membrane is hard to grasp and separate from the mobile macula. To overcome this, we stain the ILM with trypan blue and stabilize the macula with PFCL.
   - Bacillary layer detachment is a splitting in the inner myoid segment of the retinal photoreceptors. In the context of RRD, it occurs in 20% of cases. Of note, bacillary layer detachment in 15% of cases can result in a lamellar hole formation progressing to full thickness MH [24].

3. Retinal displacement/retinal fold

   - Some retinal displacement happens in up to 45% (Fig. 6), but retinal folds are rare [18].
   - Retinal displacement is more common/significant in RRD due to retinal tears in the upper part of the retina particularly in bullous macula-off superior RRD.
   - Due to a combination of several factors: persistent SRF, gas buoyancy, and the effect of gravity on the residual subretinal fluid movement.
   - Drainage retinotomy and use of PFCL do not decrease the risk of retinal displacement.
   - As its buoyancy is near to water, displacement is less with silicone oil (SO) as compared to gas tamponade [25].
   - Our suggested technique of minimal gas, minimal drainage vitrectomy and immediate supine position 1–2 hours after the surgery may help decrease displacement of the subretinal fluid.
   - Treatment of retinal folds:

     Mild inner retinal folds can be observed.
     Significant outer or full-thickness folds need to be addressed in the first 1–2 weeks post-surgery.

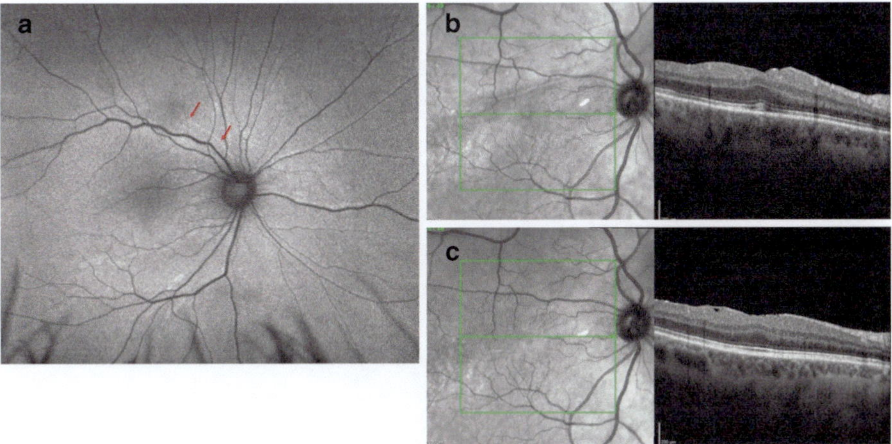

Fig. 6 Inferior retinal displacement after pars plana vitrectomy (PPV) for macula-off rhegmatogenous retinal detachment. Note the retinal vessel printings (arrows) at the site of the original retinal position. Outer and inner retinal folds in another patient post-surgery (**b**). This patient had mild distortion and 20/40 vision. The retinal folds resolved without surgery after 3 months with some vision improvement (**c**). (**a**) PPV, (**b**) drainage retinotomy, (**c**) laser and 12% C_3F_8 for retinal detachment due to inferior retinal breaks

> The technique involves detaching the macula with subretinal BSS injection, stretching the retina with PFCL injection, as well as gentle manipulations by diamond scrapper or finesse loop to get the fold out of the center followed by a peripheral drainage retinotomy, PFCL/air exchange, and gas (Video 12).

4. Persistent subretinal fluid.

   - Occurs in up to 10% of cases [26].
   - Rates are lower in PPV as compared to scleral buckles and more or less similar to pneumatic retinopexy.
   - Persistent SRF usually does not progress and does not communicate with a peripheral tear (differentiating features from recurrent detachment). Another important differential diagnosis in this context is central serous retinopathy due to triamcinolone use to stain the vitreous during PPV [27].
   - Persistent SRF usually settles with treatment but can take up to several months (Fig. 7).

5. Vitreous hemorrhage.
6. Suprachoroidal hemorrhage

   - Usually self-limiting but can be painful in the postoperative period.
   - Hypotony is an important precursor.
   - Refer to chapter 20 for more discussion.

7. Endophthalmitis.
8. Complications related to PFCL include retained PFCL and subfoveal PFCL.
9. Complications related to SO.

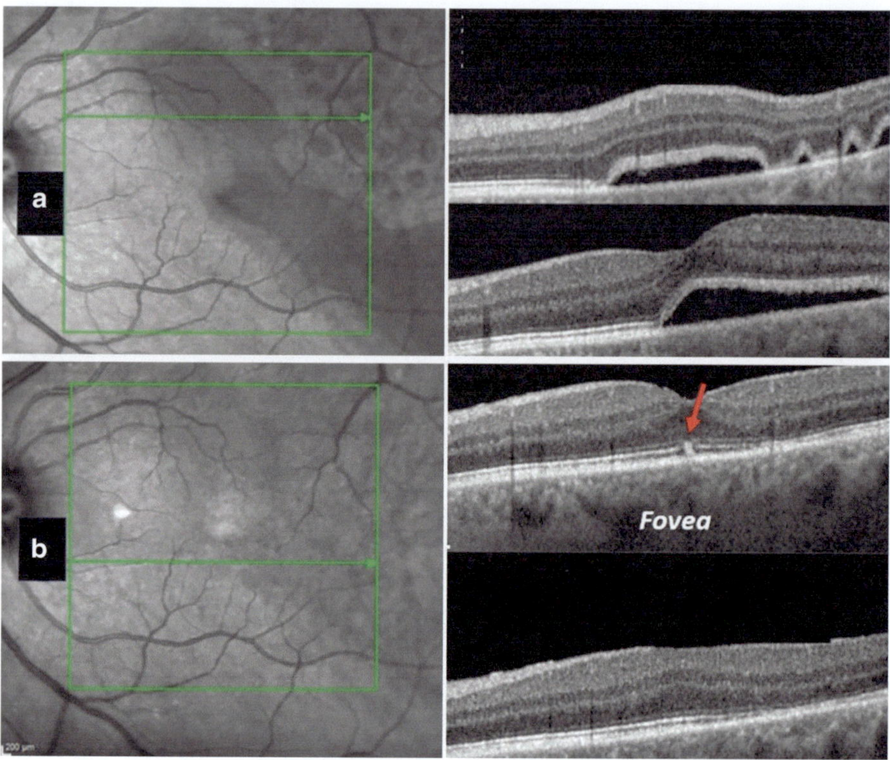

Fig. 7 (**a**) Two cases of retinal detachment surgery where perfluorocarbon liquid (PFCL) was used to uncurl a giant retinal tear flap and flatten a very bullous retinal detachment. (**b**) In the second case, the injection of PFCL was not ideal being rapid and without submerging the tip of the cannula in the formed PFCL bubble resulting in numerous PFCL bubbles 'fish eggs.' These bubbles may migrate into the subretinal space through an opened tear

10. Risk of sympathetic ophthalmitis.

- Vitreoretinal surgery is currently the main inciting event. Penetrating trauma comes second [28].
- The risk of sympathetic ophthalmitis is small after one surgery (0.008%) but increases by ten times with the second surgery. After three surgeries, the risk is nearly 1%, 2% after six surgeries, and 6.5% after seven surgeries [28].

10 Case Scenario (Video 12)

A 50-year-old male with significant visual distortion and reduced vision 10 days after right eye vitrectomy with SF_6 gas tamponade for a superior macula-off retinal detachment. Fundus examination shows a large fold crossing directly into the macula and a few smaller ones associated with it. Under high magnification, using a diamond-dusted scraper stiffness of the fold is highlighted. Internal limiting membrane peeling was carried out. This step is not strictly necessary in obtaining resolution of the macular fold, but it may be useful in preventing future complications such as a macular pucker. BSS was injected under the retina directly into the main fold. This maneuver is key to resolving macular folds provided it is performed soon after the folds are detected. Repositioning of the retina is obtained with gentle strokes carried out with the diamond-dusted scraper tip under BSS first and then under PFCL injection to obtain further distension of the smaller folds. PFCL injection/air exchange was performed followed by 20% SF_6 and 3-day face-down positioning.

Key Points

- Once a retinal break is found, it is important for the surgeon to check that the break matches the configuration of the RD; otherwise, there may be another break(s).
- Avoid heavy laser or cryopexy as this could result in retinal necrosis and new tears and ERM.
- Cryotherapy is a fantastic tool if there are only one or two retinal tears.
- Keep surgery for primary RRD simple and avoid the routine use of PFCL.
- Be wary of retinal displacement that happens with RRD surgery.
- After 3 RRD surgeries, the vision does not improve from baseline, and the risk of sympathetic ophthalmia increases by 100 times as compared to primary surgery.

References

1. Muni RH, Darabad MN, Oquendo PL, et al. Outer retinal corrugations in rhegmatogenous retinal detachment: the retinal pigment epithelium-photoreceptor dysregulation theory. Am J Ophthalmol. 2023;245:14–24.
2. Martins Melo I, Bansal A, et al. Morphologic stages of rhegmatogenous retinal detachment assessed using swept-source OCT. Ophthalol Retina. 2023;7(5):398–405.
3. Yorston D, Donachie PHJ, Laidlaw DA, Steel DH, Aylward GW, Williamson TH. BEAVRS database study group. Stratifying the risk of re-detachment: variables associated with outcome of vitrectomy for rhegmatogenous retinal detachment in a large UK cohort study. Eye (Lond). 2023;37(8):1527–37.
4. Tabandeh H, London NJS, Boyer DS, Flynn HW Jr. Outcomes of small-gauge vitreoretinal surgery without scleral-depressed shaving of the vitreous base in the era of wide-angle viewing systems. Br J Ophthalmol. 2019;103(12):1765–8.
5. Mathai M, Godwin KS, Albarracin J, Levinson J, Broderick K, Melamud A. 360 degree endolaser versus focal endolaser in primary rhegmatogenous retinal detachment repair. Retina. 2022;42(11):2046–50.
6. Sallam AB, Donachie PHJ, Yorston D, Steel DHW, Williamson TH, Jackson TL, Sparrow JM, Johnston RL. Royal College of Ophthalmologists' National Database Study of Vitreoretinal Surgery: report 7, intersurgeon variations in primary rhegmatogenous retinal detachment failure. Retina. 2018;38(2):334–42.
7. Starr MR, Obeid A, Ryan EH, Ryan C, Ammar M, Patel LG, Forbes NJ, Capone A, Emerson GG, Joseph DP, Eliott D, Gupta OP, Regillo CD, Hsu J, Yonekawa Y. Retinal detachment with inferior retinal breaks. Retina. 2021;41(3):525–30.
8. Baumgarten S, Schiller P, Hellmich M, Walter P, Agostini H, Junker B, Helbig H, Lommatzsch A, Mazinani B. Vitrectomy with and without encircling band for pseudophakic retinal detachment with inferior breaks: VIPER Study Report No. 3. Graefes Arch Clin Exp Ophthalmol. 2018;256(11):2069–73.

9. Sverdlichenko I, Lim M, Popovic MM, Pimentel MC, Kertes PJ, Muni RH. Postoperative positioning regimens in adults who undergo retinal detachment repair: a systematic review. Surv Ophthalmol. 2023;68(1):113–25.

10. Shiragami C, Fukuda K, Yamaji H, Morita M, Shiraga F. A method to decrease the frequency of unintentional slippage after vitrectomy for rhegmatogenous retinal detachment. Retina. 2015;35(4):758–63.

11. Angunawela RI, Azarbadegan A, Aylward GW, Eames I. Intraocular fluid dynamics and retinal shear stress after vitrectomy and gas tamponade. Invest Ophthalmol Vis Sci. 2011;52(10):7046–51.

12. Wong R, Gupta B, Aylward GW, Laidlaw DA. Dye extrusion technique (DE-TECH): occult retinal break detection with subretinal dye extrusion during vitrectomy for retinal detachment repair. Retina. 2009;29(4):492–6.

13. Coppola M, Rabiolo A, Cicinelli MV, et al. Vitrectomy in high myopia: a narrative review. Int J Retina Vitreous. 2017;3:37.

14. Iwama Y, Ikeda T, Nakashima H, Matsumoto E, Inoue R, Emi K. Extending the limbus-to-cannula distance to 6.0 mm during pars plana vitrectomy in highly myopic eyes. Retina. 2022;42(6):1199–202.

15. Sohn EH, Strohbehn A, Stryjewski T, Brodowska K, Flamme-Wiese MJ, Mullins RF, Eliott D. Posteriorly inserted vitreous base. Retina. 2020;40(5):943–50.

16. Seelenfreund MH, Kraushar MF, Schepens CL, Freilich DB. Choroidal detachment associated with primary retinal detachment. Arch Ophthalmol. 1974;91(4):254–8.

17. Stenz EC, Yu HJ, Shah AR, Wong TP, Major JC, Benz MS, Wykoff CC, Patel SB. Outcomes of eyes undergoing multiple surgical interventions after failure of primary rhegmatogenous retinal detachment repair. Ophthalmol Retina. 2022;6(5):339–46.

18. Brosh K, Francisconi CLM, Qian J, Sabatino F, Juncal VR, Hillier RJ, Chaudhary V, Berger AR, Giavedoni LR, Wong DT, Altomare F, Kadhim MR, Newsom RB, Marafon SB, Muni RH. Retinal displacement following pneumatic retinopexy vs pars plana vitrectomy for rhegmatogenous retinal detachment. JAMA Ophthalmol. 2020;138(6):652–9.

19. McKay BR, Bansal A, Kryshtalskyj M, Wong DT, Berger A, Muni RH. Evaluation of subretinal fluid drainage techniques during pars plana vitrectomy for primary rhegmatogenous retinal detachment-ELLIPSOID study. Am J Ophthalmol. 2022;241:227–37.

20. Wickham L, Bunce C, Wong D, Charteris DG. Retinal detachment repair by vitrectomy: simplified formulae to estimate the risk of failure. Br J Ophthalmol. 2011;95(9):1239–44.

21. Sharma T, Gopal L, Reddy RK, Kasinathan N, Shah NA, Sulochana KN, et al. Primary vitrectomy for combined rhegmatogenous retinal detachment and choroidal detachment with or without oral corticosteroids: a pilot study. Retina. 2005;25(2):152–7.

22. Eissa MGAM, Abdelhakim MASE, Macky TA, Khafagy MM, Mortada HA. Functional and structural outcomes of ILM peeling in uncomplicated macula-off RRD using microperimetry & en-face OCT. Graefes Arch Clin Exp Ophthalmol. 2018;256(2):249–57.

23. Ryan EH Jr, Bramante CT, Mittra RA, Dev S, et al. Management of rhegmatogenous retinal detachment with coexistent macular hole in the era of internal limiting membrane peeling. Am J Ophthalmol. 2011;152(5):815–9.

24. Melo IM, Bansal A, Lee WW, Oquendo PL, Hamli H, Muni RH. Bacillary layer detachment and associated abnormalities in rhegmatogenous retinal detachment. Retina. 2023;43(4):670–8.

25. Dell'Omo R, Scupola A, Viggiano D, et al. Incidence and factors influencing retinal displacement in eyes treated for rhegmatogenous retinal detachment with vitrectomy and gas or silicone oil. Invest Ophthalmol Vis Sci. 2017;58(6):BIO191–9.

26. Fouad YA, Habib AM, Sanders RN, Sallam AB. Persistent subretinal fluid following successful rhegmatogenous retinal detachment surgery. Semin Ophthalmol. 2022;37(6):724–9.

27. Imasawa M, Ohshiro T, Gotoh T, Imai M, Iijima H. Central serous chorioretinopathy following vitrectomy with intravitreal triamcinolone acetonide for diabetic macular oedema. Acta Ophthalmol Scand. 2005;83(1):132–3.

28. Anikina E, Wagner SK, Liyanage S, Sullivan P, Pavesio C, Okhravi N. The risk of sympathetic ophthalmia after vitreoretinal surgery. Ophthalmol Retina. 2022;6(5):347–60.

Scleral Buckle Surgery

Ahmed Roshdy Alagorie, Ahmed B. Sallam, and Sherif A. Dabour

1 How Does Scleral Buckle Surgery Work?

- The scleral buckle supports the retinal break from the outside by pushing the sclera, choroid and retinal pigment epithelium in toward the sensory retina.
- The height of the buckle (buckle effect) depends on several factors:

  - Tightness of the buckle—dictated by the tension of the sutures holding the buckle to the sclera, suture distance separating the suture bites, and, in encircling buckles, how much the buckle is shortened
  - Presence of subretinal fluid (SRF) around the tear
  - Intraocular pressure (IOP)

- If the buckle effect goes away, the support of the retinal tear will decrease. Therefore, permanent chorioretinal adhesion around the retinal tear is needed.

Supplementary Information The online version contains supplementary material available at https://doi.org/10.1007/978-3-031-47827-7_9.

A. R. Alagorie
Faculty of Medicine, Department of Ophthalmology, Tanta University, Tanta, Egypt

A. B. Sallam
Jones Eye Institute, University of Arkansas for Medical Sciences, Little Rock, AR, USA

S. A. Dabour (✉)
Department of Ophthalmology, Zagazig University, Zagazig, Egypt

A. B. Sallam et al. (eds.), *Practical Manual of Vitreoretinal Surgery*, https://doi.org/10.1007/978-3-031-47827-7_9

2   Classification of Scleral Buckles

- Scleral buckles can be further divided into segmental buckles and encircling (360°) buckles. A segmental buckle can be further divided according to its orientation into a radial or circumferential buckle.
- Buckles can also be classified according to the material they are made from, most commonly silicone. These include (1) hard silicone (tires, wedges, and bands) or (2) soft silicone sponge and (3) other buckles types and modifications including suprachoroidal buckles attained by the injection of a viscoelastic device in the suprachoroidal space or balloon buckle using a balloon after inflation to press on the sclera from the outside to create a temporary buckle effect [1–3].
- It is of note that the solid buckle has less rate of extrusion than the sponge buckle because of the higher rate of infection of the sponge due to its porous nature, which might be more conducive to bacterial growth [4–7]. The buckling effect achieved by the sponge is, however, higher.

3   How Is the Buckle Effect Achieved?

- Segmental buckle:
  - The buckle height depends mainly on the tension of the anchoring suture, which is dictated primarily by the distance between the sutures' bites around the buckle.
  - The buckle effect usually decreases after 6 months as the tension of the sutures wanes.
- Encircling buckle:
  - The buckle height depends mainly on the amount of shortening of the encircling element rather than the distance between the sutures bites, e.g., 12 mm shortening produces about 2 mm indentation.
  - In contrast to segmental buckles, the effect is usually permanent as long as the buckle remains in place.

4   Encircling Buckle "360°"

- We prefer a segmental buckle as it achieves the purpose with the least amount of tissue manipulation/distortion.
- Our indications of encircling buckles are very limited and include (1) rhegmatogenous retinal detachment (RRD) in children with or without nonextensive proliferative vitreoretinopathy (PVR) where the breaks are multiple in ≥3 quadrants or there is no detectable break and (2) PVR retinal detachment in adults that is not severe enough to mandate a retinectomy (Fig. 1). The aim in this case is to relax the peripheral retina and alleviate the need for an extensive retinectomy.

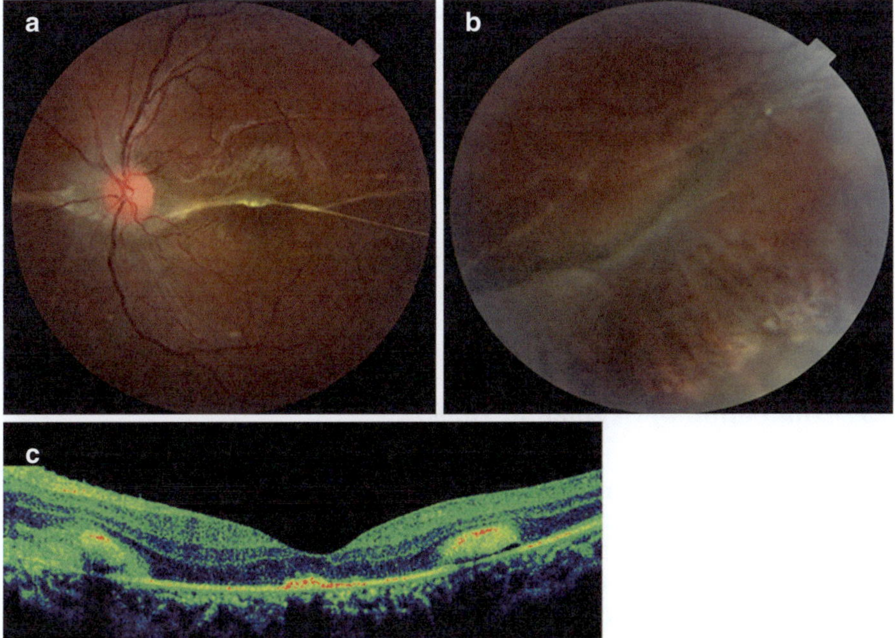

Fig. 1 A 16-year-old patient presented with chronic lower retinal detachment, demarcation line, proliferative vitreoretinopathy with short retina, and subretinal bands. Postoperative images show attached central and peripheral retina with a good buckling effect of the 41-encircling band (**a, b**). (**c**) Horizontal optical coherence tomography scan shows a subretinal band passing around the fovea that did not interfere with macular attachment

- For encirclement, we use a band. Our choices are mainly a 41 band (3.5 mm width) or a narrower 240 band (2.5 mm width). A tire segment (e.g., no 276 or 287) can be added to the band to support larger breaks, but this is rarely needed.
- We place one horizontal mattress suture in each quadrant to hold the buckle (Video 1). Alternatively, a scleral belt loop (Video 2) can be used [8, 9].
- Because most breaks are located at the posterior aspect of the vitreous base and anterior to the equator, we usually place the anterior limb of the anchoring suture 4 mm behind the insertion of the recti muscles. The posterior limb is usually placed 1 mm behind the posterior edge of the band. However, the exact positioning of the suture site depends on the location of the break, with attention to the encirclement placement to support breaks.
- It is of note that the scleral loops are easier to do and more elegant with no suture problems later on, e.g., extrusion or protrusion. However, if a scleral perforation happens, it is more difficult to manage than a needle perforation.
- We usually secure the ends of the buckle using a 70 Watzke sleeve or clove hitch knot using a non-absorbable suture (Video 3).
- We shorten the band by about 10 mm, but a range between 8 and 12 mm can be used. From the outside, it looks like a gentle indent to the sclera resembling a stretched 'oud string'.

– The height of the encircling buckle depends on the specific indication for its usage, e.g., for retinal dialysis, we need a low, broad buckle to support the vitreous base and prevent fish mouthing.

5 Segmental Scleral Buckle

Our philosophy is to use the minimal buckle required and not to overdo it—we treat the detachment of today, not of tomorrow!

5.1 Indication of Segmental Buckle

1. The primary use of segmental buckle is now predominantly confined to managing RRD in phakic eyes. In our practice, a prevalent indication for this approach is non-posterior vitreous detachment (PVD) retinal detachment observed in young patients and children. This condition commonly arises due to atrophic hole(s) or retinal dialyses. In these cases of non-PVD retinal detachment, the segmental scleral buckle emerges as a straightforward and effective surgical option. Performing a pars plana vitrectomy (PPV) in these cases can present challenges, as inducing PVD proves difficult due to the adherent nature of the posterior hyaloid. Furthermore, myopic patients often exhibit peripheral retinal thinning and lattice degeneration, increasing the risk of iatrogenic retinal tears during PPV.
2. Eyes with a single tear localized PVD detachment are also good candidates for segmental buckles. Because the presence of inferior retinal tears is a risk factor for failure of PPV, [10] we use them more commonly in patients with inferior tears but they could also work well for superior tears.

Surgical Tips

1. If the retinal tear is anterior to the surgical equator, which corresponds to the ampulla of the vortex veins, then it should not be difficult to get a segmental buckle on the retinal tear (Fig. 2). Also, if you can reach the retinal tear during scleral indentation in the clinic, it is easy to place a buckle on.
2. Large retinal dialysis with a posteriorly displaced or folded edge may not sit well on a buckle (Fig. 3). A scleral buckle can still be tried, but these cases may need PPV.

5.2 Buckle Choice "Radial vs. Circumferential"

– It is generally easier to place a segmental circumferential buckle than a radial buckle. There is more leeway for localization errors with the former.

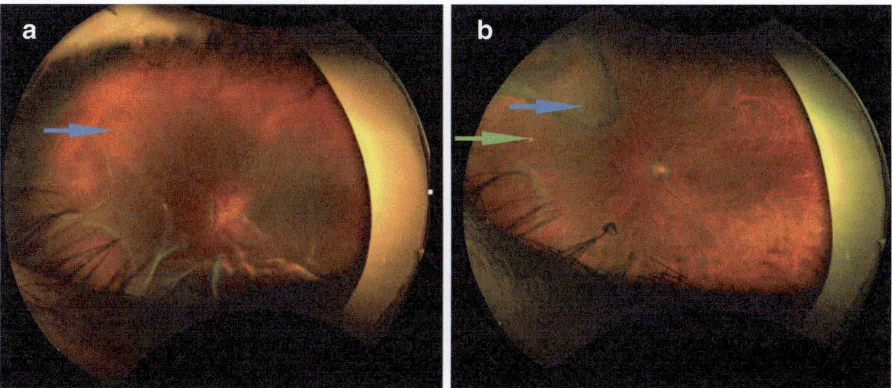

Fig. 2 Chronic retinal detachment due to a retinal hole in a young patient with no posterior vitreous detachment (**a**), treated with a 5 mm radial sponge (**b**). The blue arrow points to the location of the retinal hole, which is at the equator, near a vortex vein. The green arrow points to a spot of choroidal depigmentation at the site of the subretinal fluid drainage. (Courtesy of Assem Mejaddam, MD, Sweden)

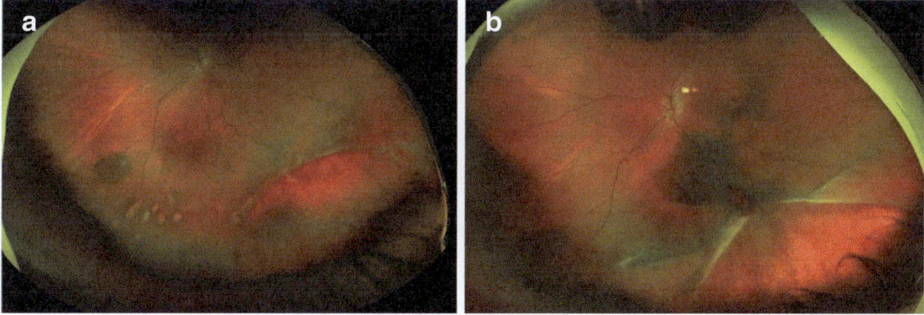

Fig. 3 Chronic retinal detachment from a retinal dialysis in a 23-year-old patient. Note the large size of the dialysis and the posterior sagging of its edges (**a**). This limited a good buckle-tear relationship after a circumferential sponge and subretinal fluid drainage, with the center of the tear remaining open (**b**). Also, note the presence of subretinal hemorrhage complicating drainage (**b**). Pars plana vitrectomy with laser and C_3F_8 gas was required to treat the persistent detachment with success

- Usually, we resort to a segmental radial buckle if the break is posterior or large, as it closes the tear more effectively with fewer chances of radial folds and fish mouthing. A radial buckle is easier to place if the retinal tear is in the middle of the quadrant as compared to under the muscle.
- The size of the buckle material is determined by the dimensions of the retinal tear, with the chosen buckle being just slightly larger than the tear itself. This approach ensures a buckling effect that extends approximately 2 mm beyond the edges of the tear. We aim to use the minimum buckle element required– typically 4 or 5 mm in width– which usually suffices. Our preferred choices are 510, 504, 505, and 506 (Table 1).

Table 1 Commonly used buckle elements

Types	Shape/size in mm
Silicone Sponges	
504	4.0
505	5.0
506	3.0 × 5.0
510	2.5 × 5.0
Bands	
240	0.60 × 2.5
41	0.76 × 3.5
40	0.75 × 2.0
Tires	
276	2.5 × 7.0
287	2.5 × 7.0
Sleeves	
70 (Watzke)	1.0 × 2.2

5.3 *Landmarks and Suture Placement*

- For localized buckles, the precise localization of the retinal break(s) is crucial for successful surgery.
- We usually mark the apex and the two horns of a retinal tear or the middle of the break if it is a small retinal hole.
- The separation of the sutures primarily dictates the indentation of a segmental buckle and this distance is usually calculated as 1.5× the width of the buckle used. That is, for a 5 mm buckle, we separate the suture bites by 7.5 mm.
- For a segmental circumferential buckle, after we localize the retinal break on the sclera, we place the suture bites circumferentially on either side of the external mark putting in mind to support the posterior aspect of the break more than the anterior one, as the circumferential buckles tend to migrate anteriorly with time and also because the buckling effect is less that of a radial buckle. For example, if we use a 4 mm sponge, we take the anterior bite 2 mm in front of the mark and the posterior one 4 mm behind it with a suture width of 6 mm. Placing the anterior suture just behind the muscle insertion usually achieves this concept. Also, it

prevents the development of anterior SRF gutter. This technique for placing the buckle is called the "break-ora-occlusive-buckle."

- For a radial buckle, the sutures are centered on the middle of the tear. One or two sutures could be placed radially depending on the size of the tear, but usually, one long suture (4 mm) parallel to the tear is enough.
- We use non-absorbable 5-0 sutures such as Ethibond, Nylon, or Mersilene suture to anchor the buckle.
- Fig. 4 and Video 4 shows the technique of placing *radial and circumferential segmental buckles.*

6 Subretinal Fluid Drainage

- Drainage of the SRF allows for a higher buckle indent and a better tear-buckle relationship. However, it is not without a risk!

6.1 Indications

1. Chronic RRD where the fluid is very thick and will take a long time to resolve
2. Poor retinal tear-buckle relationship at the end of the surgery

    (a) At the end of the surgery, you should see a good relationship with the buckle well supporting the break. You might see more fluid posterior to the buckle

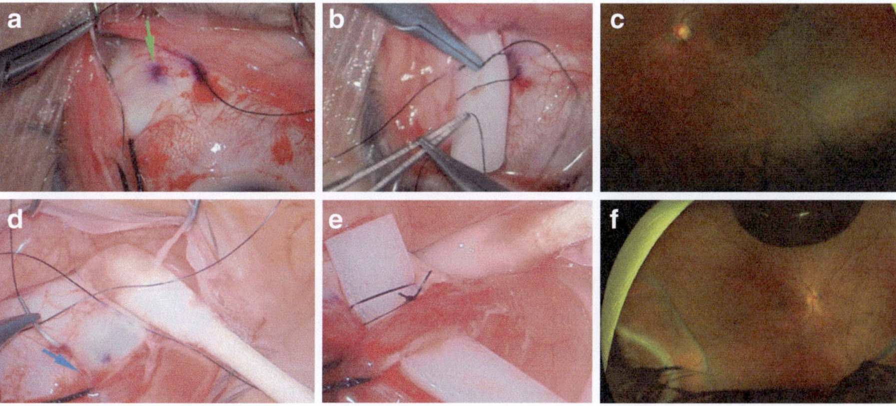

Fig. 4 The strategic landmarks for precisely placing scleral sutures in segmental buckles. The first case is a chronic detachment due to an inferotemporal retinal hole treated with a radial sponge. The sutures are centered on the retinal tear. Note the green arrow highlighting the scleral purple marking of the center of the tear (**a**). The buckle is radially placed (**b**) with a good buckle-tear relationship and retinal attachment (**c**). Another case of an inferotemporal retinal dialysis detachment was treated with a circumferential buckle. The anterior limb of the suture is placed behind the muscle insertion (blue arrow) (**d**). Note the circumferential placement of the buckle (**e**) with a good buckle-tear relationship and retinal attachment (**f**). In both cases, we employed a 5 mm sponge (#510) affixed with a single 5-0 horizontal mattress suture. The spacing between the suture limbs measures approximately 7.5 mm, equivalent to 1.5 times the width of the explant

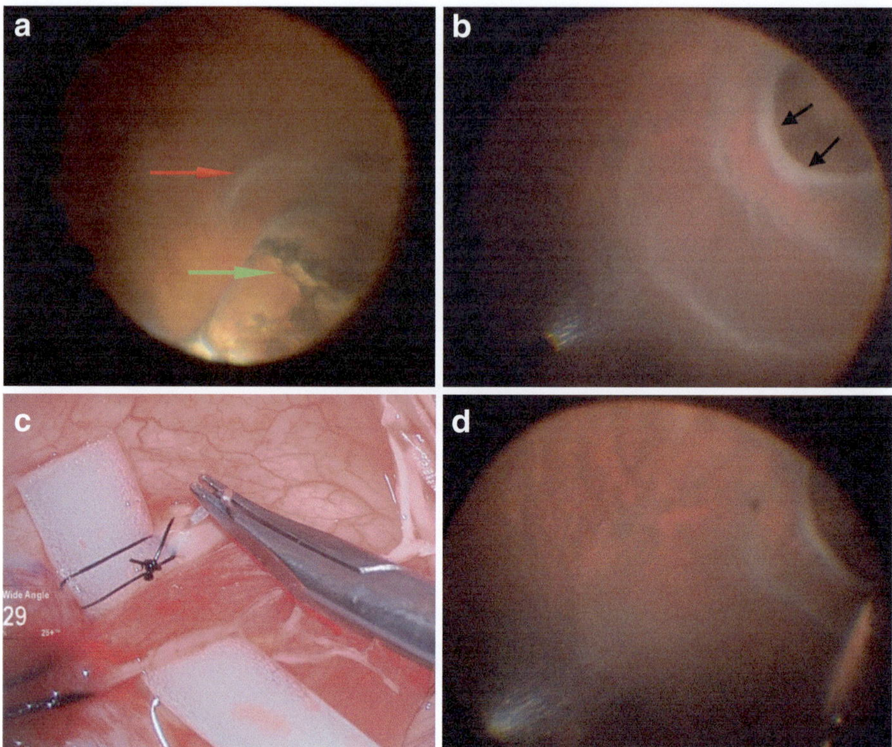

Fig. 5 (**a**) Intraoperative view of 2 cases of segmental circumferential sponge for retinal detachment. In the first case, the detachment was due to laser necrosis at the edge of previous laser retinopexy. This area was well supported and nearly attached after placing the buckle (blue arrow), and hence, there was no need for subretinal fluid drainage. Note the presence of posteriorly displaced subretinal fluid (red arrow) that is expected to absorb (**a**). In the second case, the detachment was due to a retinal dialysis. Although the buckle was in good position to support the dialysis, it was still open with a lot of subretinal fluid between the dialysis and the buckle (arrows) (**b**). External drainge was done (**c**) with the break settling down over the buckle (**d**)

that has been shifted by the buckle, but that is fine, and will go away (Fig. 5). What you do not want to see is an open tear away from the buckle with retina corrugations that are not conforming to the buckle. If so, it is unlikely that the buckle will be successful without drainage.

3. Inferior retinal tear detachment with PVR or stiff retina is a relative indication. This because a delayed absorption of the SRF may hinder the retinal tear to settle down on the buckle and effective chorioretinal adhesions around the retinal break to happen.

6.2   Drainage Site Selection

- The chosen site must be in an area with sufficient SRF to be effective.
- Other factors also need to be considered, including the position of vortex veins, the location of the SRF, and the status of the macula.
- The vortex veins are mostly present toward the vertical meridian, so you want to be draining more toward the horizontal recti at the upper or lower border.
- If subretinal hemorrhage happens, it can reach under the macula easier if the detachment is superior and temporal and if it is a macula-off detachment. It is, therefore, safer to drain inferonasal and macula-on detachments.
- If feasible with the distribution of the fluid, it might be best drain in the bed of the buckle, between the suture bites, incase a retinal perforation happens (Videos 5 and 6).

6.3   Timing of Drainage

- To achieve a good tight buckle, you want to tighten the suture of the buckle when the eye is soft (low IOP).
- If the plan is to do a non-drainage procedure, then do a paracentesis first before tightening the sutures. You still can drain SRF afterward if this appears to be needed.
- If the plan is a drainage procedure, drain the SRF first and then tighten the buckle sutures.

6.4   Techniques of the SRF Drainage (Video 5)

There are basically two techniques:

1. Scleral cut-down: the sclera is cut down until the choroid is exposed. The choroid is treated with diathermy or laser, and the choroid is then incised. Because the choroid has been prepared, the risk of bleeding is less.
2. Prang technique: using a needle to perforate the sclera and the choroid without preparing the choroid. This is a quick technique, but the risk of bleeding is higher as the choroid has not been treated with diathermy.

Important notes:

1. Make the opening of the choroid small to avoid retinal incarceration. Use a suture needle such as that of the 5-0 used to suture the buckle or a needle of 26–28-gauge.

2. Raise the eye pressure to improve the drainage and decrease the risk of bleeding for 1–2 min immediately after drainage. This could be achieved by pressing on the sclera with cotton-tipped applicators or by pulling on the recti muscle sutures.
3. Measure 4 mm from the limbus and be ready with a syringe of sterile air on a 30-gauge needle to inject intravitreally after drainage. It is best to always inject air after drainage of SRF routinely to avoid hypotony (Video 6).

7 Scleral Buckle Surgery Technique

- Conventionally, surgery is performed by the indirect ophthalmoscope.
- Modifications of this technique include using endoillumination with a chandelier light or using a wide-field light pipe to illuminate the eye from the inside as needed.
- Advantages of those modifications include better visualization, better ergonomics, easier to video record the surgery and mentor a trainee.
- The disadvantage of endoillumination includes a higher risk of epiretinal membranes and vitreous prolapse with incarceration in the sclera [11]. There is a possibly increased risk of endophthalmitis due to the intraocular nature of this surgery. The cost of surgery also becomes higher.
- If endoillumination is used, we advise closing the sclerotomy with a suture at the time of the conjunctival closure to decrease the potential risk of endophthalmitis.
- Video 7 shows the technique of using endoillumination and chandelier light for break localization and application of cryopexy.
- The following is the step-by-step order of how we perform a scleral buckle procedure (Video 4):

  - Anesthesia: General or local anesthesia is administered based on the patient's needs and surgeon's preference. Most patients are young, and we choose general anesthesia. Even if the surgery is performed under general anesthesia, local anesthetic is typically administered to avoid oculocardiac reflex and reduce the need for narcotics during and after the procedure.
  - Examination of the retina: Before scrubbing or prepping the eyes, we examine the fundus. The retina is examined using indirect ophthalmoscopy with 360° scleral depression to ensure that the surgical plan remains unchanged. Any additional breaks in the detached retina may necessitate alterations in the surgical plan. Breaks in the attached retina usually do not affect the plan, as they can be treated with cryopexy or laser during or after the surgery. It is important to keep in mind that many cases requiring scleral buckles involve young patients who may not have been amenable to scleral indentation during clinic visits; thus, this step is usually needed.
  - Conjunctival opening: Initially, it is recommended to open the conjunctiva 360°. With experience, you may limit the conjunctival opening to the

quadrant(s) where the scleral buckle will be placed. It is important to dissect the conjunctiva and Tenon's capsule fully off the sclera. This step ensures that the quadrant(s) of interest is free from adhesions, scleral malacia, and vortex veins are not in a position that would interfere with the buckle placement.

- Recti muscle manipulation: The same principle applies to hooking and slinging the recti muscles. Initially, all four recti muscles are slung, but as the surgeon gains experience, the number of recti muscles slung can be limited based on the extent of the scleral buckle required.
- Scleral buckling: If a microscope is used, surgery commences by placing a trocar opposite the quadrant of interest—where the retinal break is located and where the buckle will be applied.
- Tear localization and marking: The tear is located internally using the light pipe, and its position is marked on the sclera. This step is crucial to ensure accurate placement of the buckle.
- Cryopexy: Cryopexy is performed to treat the tear at this stage. Gentle whitening of the RPE reaction is what is needed, and you should avoid overtreatment.
- Suture placement: Sutures are placed for the buckle as discussed previously.
- Buckle insertion: The buckle is passed under the sutures.
- Eye softening: Before tying the buckle sutures, the eye needs to be softened to achieve a good ident. Scleral drainage or anterior chamber paracentesis is performed.
- Suture tying: The buckle sutures are tied and cut short.
- Fundus examination: The fundus is examined to ensure a good tear-buckle relationship and to verify that the central retinal artery is not occluded.
- Buckle trimming and suture knot rotation: The buckle edges are trimmed, and the suture knots are rotated backward.
- Closure: The recti bridal sutures are cut followed by the removal of the trocar and suturing of the scleral port and conjunctival peritomy. Please note that the trocar should gently be pulled without exerting excessive pressure on the eye to minimize vitreous prolapse. Whenever possible and especially in young patients, we prefer to separately close Tenon's layer over the scleral buckle area before closing the conjunctiva.
- We ask the anesthetist to administer intravenous steroids to help reduce postoperative lid edema/swelling that commonly occur post-scleral buckle surgery.

8 Complications of Scleral Buckle Surgery

- The most common complication of scleral buckling surgery is the failure of reattachment or re-detachment in about 10–15%. Most failures occur in the first year and are due to unsupported breaks. This is because of either missed breaks, inadequate or misplaced buckles, or inadequate retinopexy [12].

1. Missed retinal break

   (a) Many patients undergoing scleral buckles are young, and it may have been difficult to perform a thorough examination with scleral indentation in the clinic. It is therefore best to examine the eye with scleral depression after administering anesthesia and before starting the surgery. The aim is to ensure that there are no other breaks, particularly in the detached retina, and, if needed, revise the plan.

   (b) Remember Lincoff's rules for SRF location and retinal tears when looking for breaks (Fig. 6).

2. Inadequate buckle

   (a) Inadequate height or poor buckle alignment

   • Taking wider sutures, 1.5 mm × buckle width, and performing paracentesis before tying the suture usually results in a good buckle indent/ height. If the buckle-tear relationship is still inadequate, SRF drainage is needed.

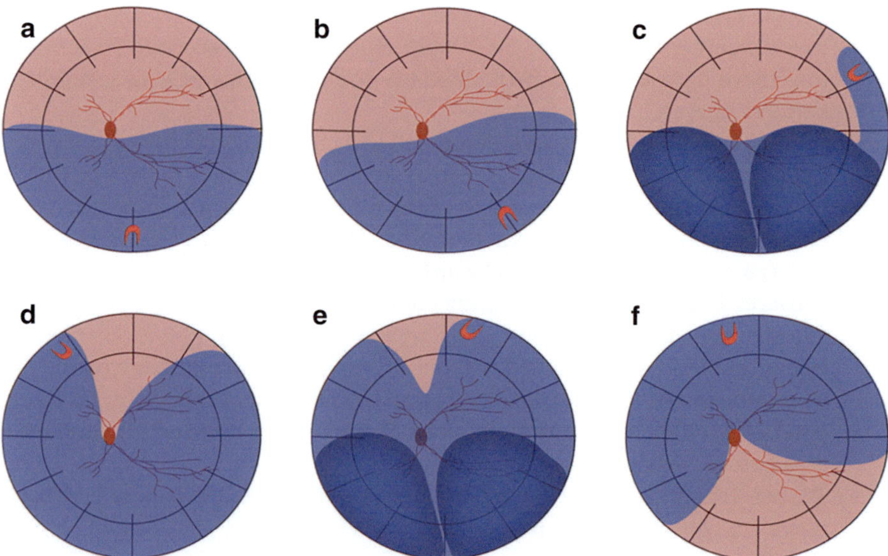

Fig. 6 A primary tear located at 6 o'clock will cause a shallow inferior rhegmatogenous retinal detachment (RRD) with equal fluid levels (**a**). A shallow inferior RRD in which the subretinal fluid (SRF) is higher on one side indicates that the tear is located inferiorly on this side (**b**). A primary tear that is located above the horizontal meridian will cause an inferior bullous RRD (**c**). If the primary tear is in the upper nasal area, the SRF will turn around the optic disc, and the temporal side will rise to the level of the primary tear (**d**). If a subtotal RRD is associated with a superior wedge of the attached retina, the primary tear is in the periphery close to its highest border (**e**). A superior SRF that crosses the vertical midline indicates that the primary tear is located near 12 o'clock toward the lower edge of the RRD (**f**)

- A misaligned buckle is more likely to occur in the surgeon's learning phase and is more likely with radial buckles. It is easy to spot during surgery and rectify by revising the sutures.

(b) Anterior gutter of SRF in a circumferential buckle

- Because of parallax, an anterior tear in a detached retina may appear more posterior than it really is on scleral indentation.
- As such, a segmental buckle may be placed more posteriorly, and the anterior part of the tear may not be supported. This could result in the anterior gutter of SRF and failure of retina reattachment.
- This situation is best avoided by always using a break-ora-occlusive-buckle, with the anterior bite of the suture placed just behind the rectus muscle insertion [13].

(c) Fish mouthing

- This happens when treating a large tear with a circumferential buckle causing retinal redundancy.
- Injecting air can help manage this situation if there is a superior break.

- It is best to avoid using radial and not circumferential buckles for large horse-shoe retinal tears.

3. Retinopexy-related problems

(a) Undertreating is not common. In general, if in doubt whether cryopexy has been applied completely around a tear or if the cryo machine fails to work, the advice is to place the buckle and apply laser later as the retina flattens. Retinopexy is not important in the initial phase as the tear will be closed by the buckle.

(b) Overtreating with cryopexy (and laser) can result in pigment liberation with an increased risk of PVR (Fig. 7). Also, it can lead to retinal necrosis and new breaks at the edge of the retinopexy scar (Fig. 8).

(c) Choroidal rupture. Always wait for the cryo ice ball to dissolve before taking it off the sclera.

(d) Freezing with cryoprobe shaft. This is uncommon but can result in inadvertent macular freezing. Always double-check that the retinal break is indented with the cryo tip (Video 8).

4. Inadvertent scleral perforation/SRF drainage

(a) It happens in about 5% of cases [14].

(b) Always use a spatulated needle and aim for a partial-thickness bite. Advance the needle carefully in the scleral lamellae. The base of the needle can also perforate the sclera as you pull the needle out so be careful not to "sink" that part in.

(c) Perforation may lead to abrupt severe hypotony, and rapid restoration of IOP by intravitreal injection of air or gas is necessary to prevent serious complications such as vitreous, choroidal, and subretinal hemorrhage.

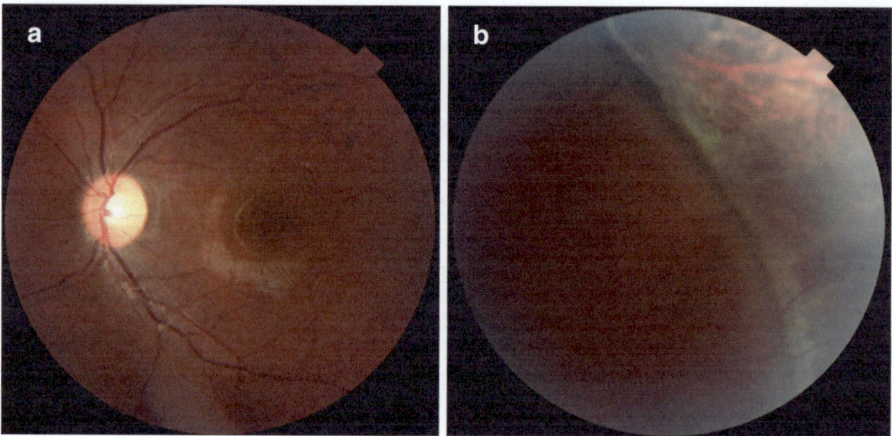

Fig. 7 Dispersion of retinal pigment epithelial cells that had settled along the upper temporal arcade (**a**) due to excessive cryopexy application to the peripheral retinal tear at the time of scleral buckle surgery (**b**)

Fig. 8 Retinal necrosis at the site of the primary break due to overtreatment with cryopexy. However, the retina remained attached as the area of necrosis was well supported by the buckle

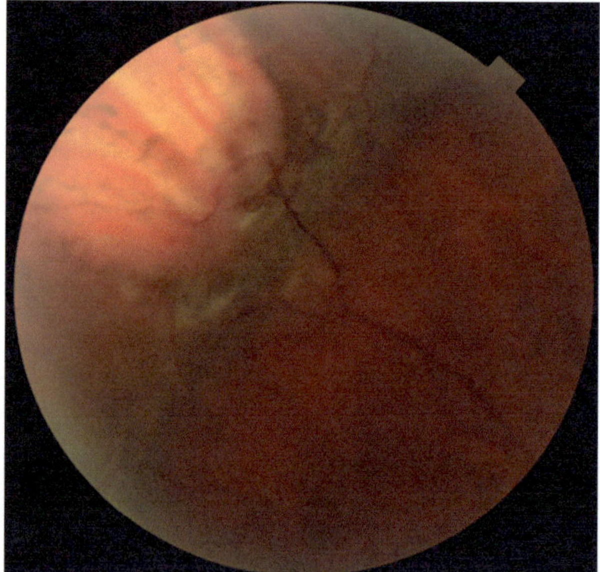

(d) If vitreous prolapse occurs at the perforation site, cut it with a scissor flush with the surface of the sclera.

(e) If there is a lot of SRF in the area where the perforation happens, no retinal injury will result. However, should a retinal injury be noted it is then impotant to revise the buckle sutures. This involves moving the posterior suture to a position behind the perforation site, ensuring that this area is included on the buckle.

5. Subretinal hemorrhage (Fig. 3a)

   (a) This is a dreadful complication of SRF drainage.
   (b) It happens in about 5% of cases [15].
   (c) Using a cut-down technique and preparing the choroid with diathermy or laser may decrease the risk.
   (d) It is crucial to avoid hypotony with drainage:

   - Keep the intraocular pressure high for 2 min directly after the drainage by pulling on the muscle sutures or pressing them with cotton buds.
   - Be ready with air to inject intravitreally after drainage and 1–2 min of pressure on the eye.
   - Note: Think of SRF drainage and injection of air as "one step," after which you examine the fundus.

   (e) If macular bleeding happens, position the eye to decrease gravitation to the macula by rotating it nasally. You could inject intravitreal tPA if bleeding has already reached the macula and inject gas to displace the blood [16]. We have tried converting to PPV and removing subretinal blood in this context [17]. This needs to happen very quickly to be effective before significant clotting of the blood takes place. In our experience, PPV and removing clotted blood, even though a large retinotomy, is challenging.

6. Retinal incarceration

   (a) The retina may get incarcerated in about 2–3% of cases at the drainage site [12, 18].
   (b) This complication should be avoidable. Always make a *small* opening in the choroid.
   (c) Peripheral incarceration can be treated by trying to reposition the retina and moving the buckle posteriorly, as in scleral perforation.
   (d) Alternatively, PPV and retinotomy will be required.

7. Vitreous hemorrhage

   (a) It usually happens in the context of scleral perforation.
   (b) If the hemorrhage is not dense enough to hinder surgery, we prefer to observe and operate later if it does not absorb.

8. Choroidal detachment

   (a) Observe as it usually settles on its own in about 2 weeks [19].

9. Ocular movement disorders

   (a) As a rule, avoid bulky and radial sponges under the muscles.
   (b) If movement disorders happen, observe as most cases resolve after 3–4 months.
   (c) Muscle surgery may be required if diplopia in primary and/or near position persists.

10. Explant exposure

   (a) It is more likely to occur with anterior and bulky sponges.
   (b) If the retina is attached, the buckle will need to be removed.
   (c) There is about a 5% risk of re-detachment after removal.

11. Refraction changes

   (a) Segmental buckle results in astigmatism that usually improves with time. Risk factors include the buckle height, radial buckle, and the anterior position of the buckle.
   (b) Encirclement results in permanent myopia, usually >2D. The myopic shift occurs due to increased axial length and is influenced by the degree of tightening of the buckle.

12. Buckle infection

   (a) It is a rare complication of modern sponge buckles necessitating removal and systemic/periocular antibiotics.

13. Vortex vein compression or injury during scleral buckle should be avoided as it could result in suprachoroidal effusion or hemorrhage, exudative retinal detachment, vitreous opacities, and anterior segment ischemia. These happen more with encirclement buckles [20].
14. Other complications encountered with tight encirclement buckles include high IOP, central retinal artery occlusion, and anterior segment ischemia.

   (a) With any buckle placed, one of the important points to assess after tightening the buckle is the central retinal artery patency. A patent or pulsating retinal artery is good. An attenuated artery and a pale disc are signs of a tight buckle and dangerously raised IOP. In this case, paracentesis, drainage of the SRF, or loosening of the buckle sutures is promptly needed.

9　Outcome of Scleral Buckle Surgery

– Overall, the success rate of scleral buckles is at least equivalent, if not higher, than PPV for primary retinal detachment. There is less retinal displacement. Cataract and PVR risks are lower.

   • According to the Primary Retinal Detachment Outcomes Study (PRO Study), single-surgery anatomic success was noted in line 155/169 scleral buckle cases (91.7%) vs. 207/249 PPV cases (83.1%). Scleral buckle has had significantly better visual outcomes for macula-on or split cases than PPV, even after accounting for decreased vision from post-PPV cataract [21].
   • The Royal College of Ophthalmologists national database study of vitreoretinal surgery reports higher single-surgery success was noted in 721,813 scleral buckle cases (89.6%) vs. 3549/4125 PPV cases (84%) [22].

- The ALIGN study showed a lower rate of retinal displacement with scleral buckle vs. PPV/ buckle, 16.7% vs. 38.8% (19 of 49) on fundus autofluorescence. Within the buckle group, displacement was less if there was no extenal drainage, 6.7% vs 22.5% [23].
- The success rate of scleral buckle with indirect ophthalmoscope vs. chandellier-assisted comparable [11].

– PVR risk after buckle surgery is ~10% compared to ~15% in PPV [24].

Key Points
- Identifying all retinal breaks is the key to successful retinal reattachment surgery.
- Scleral buckle is the best surgical option in young patients with no PVD RRD.
- It is best to use the smallest buckle needed.
- When considering SRF, remember two points—a small opening in the choroid and avoid hypotony.
- In the early postoperative period, the most important parameter is the tear-buckle relationship. Once the retina attaches, the important parameter to look for is optimum retinopexy around the tear.
- Using endoillumination simplifies scleral buckle surgery and is a great aid for teaching the surgery.

References

1. El Rayes EN, Elborgy E. Suprachoroidal buckling: technique and indications. J Ophthalmic Vis Res. 2013;8:393–9.
2. Lincoff H, Kreissig I. Results with a temporary balloon buckle for the repair of retinal detachment. Am J Ophthalmol. 1981;92:245–51.
3. Oge I, Birinci H, Havuz E, et al. Lincoff temporary balloon buckle in retinal detachment surgery. Eur J Ophthalmol. 2001;11:372–6.
4. Theodossiadis G, Chatzoulis D, Patelis J, et al. Extraocular observations in episcleral sponge implants. Ophthalmol J Int d'ophtalmologie Int J Ophthalmol Zeitschrift fur Augenheilkd. 1975;171:439–50.
5. Russo CE, Ruiz RS. Silicone sponge rejection. Early and late complications in retinal detachment surgery. Arch Ophthalmol (Chicago Ill 1960). 1971;85:647–50.
6. Hilton GF, Wallyn RH. The removal of scleral buckles. Arch Ophthalmol (Chicago Ill 1960). 1978;96:2061–3.
7. Tsui I. Scleral buckle removal: indications and outcomes. Surv Ophthalmol. 2012;57:253–63.
8. Shanmugam PM, Singh TP, Ramanjulu R, et al. Sutureless scleral buckle in the management of rhegmatogenous retinal detachment. Indian J Ophthalmol. 2015;63:645–8.
9. Landa G, Benevento J, Rosen R. Sutureless belt loops versus sutured buckle technique in combination with vitrectomy for retinal detachment repair: a comparative analysis. Ophthalmol J Int d'ophtalmologie Int J Ophthalmol Zeitschrift fur Augenheilkd. 2018;239:225–30.
10. Yorston D, Donachie PHJ, Laidlaw DA, Steel DH, Aylward GW, Williamson TH; BEAVRS database study group. Stratifying the risk of re-detachment: variables associated with outcome of vitrectomy for rhegmatogenous retinal detachment in a large UK cohort study. Eye (Lond). 2023 Jun;37(8):1527–1537.

11. Ahmed Saad, Albalkini Abdussalam M, Abdullatif Mohamed Saad, Albalkini Tamer A, Macky Ayman, Khattab Mohamed, Attya. CHANDELIER-ASSISTED VERSUS STANDARD SCLERAL BUCKLING FOR PRIMARY RHEGMATOGENOUS RETINAL DETACHMENT Retina 2022;42(9):1745–1755.
12. Chignell AH, Fison LG, Davies EW, et al. Failure in retinal detachment surgery. Br J Ophthalmol. 1973;57:525–30.
13. Paul Sullivan. Retina techniques of Scleral Buckling Elsevier 1669-1695.
14. Brown P, Chignell AH. Accidental drainage of subretinal fluid. Br J Ophthalmol. 1982;66:625–6.
15. Fallico M, Alosi P, Reibaldi M, et al. Scleral buckling: a review of clinical aspects and current concepts. J Clin Med. 2022;11:314.
16. Chen SN, Ho CL, Kuo YH, et al. Intravitreous tissue plasminogen activator injection and pneumatic displacement in the management of submacular hemorrhage complicating scleral buckling procedures. Retina. 2001;21:460–3.
17. Rubsamen PE, Flynn HWJ, Civantos JM, et al. Treatment of massive subretinal hemorrhage from complications of scleral buckling procedures. Am J Ophthalmol. 1994;118:299–303.
18. Wilkinson CP, Bradford RHJ. Complications of draining subretinal fluid. Retina. 1984;4:1–4.
19. Auriol S, Mahieu L, Arné J-L, et al. Risk factors for development of choroidal detachment after scleral buckling procedure. Am J Ophthalmol. 2011;152:428–432.e1.
20. Doi N, Uemura A, Nakao K. Complications associated with vortex vein damage in scleral buckling surgery for rhegmatogenous retinal detachment. Jpn J Ophthalmol. 1999;43(3):232–8.
21. Ryan EH, Ryan CM, Forbes NJ, et al. Primary retinal detachment outcomes study report number 2: phakic retinal detachment outcomes. Ophthalmology. 2020;127:1077–85.
22. Jackson TL, Donachie PHJ, Sallam A, et al. United Kingdom National Ophthalmology Database study of vitreoretinal surgery: report 3, retinal detachment. Ophthalmology. 2014;121:643–8.
23. Bansal A, Naidu SC, Marafon SB, Kohler JM, In S, Mahendrakar PA, Garima, Kashyap H, Susavar P, Bhende M, Ryan EH, Muni RH. Retinal Displacement after Scleral Buckle versus Combined Buckle and Vitrectomy for Rhegmatogenous Retinal Detachment: ALIGN Scleral Buckle versus Pars Plana Vitrectomy with Scleral Buckle. Ophthalmol Retina. 2023 Sep;7(9):788–793.
24. Patel SN, Salabati M, Mahmoudzadeh R, et al. Surgical failures after primary scleral buckling for rhegmatogenous retinal detachment: comparison of eyes with and without proliferative vitreoretinopathy. Retina. 2021;41:2288–95.

Giant Retinal Tears

Aman Chandra

1 Introduction and Etiology of Giant Retinal Tears

A giant retinal tear (GRT) is defined as a tear that extends more than 3 o'clock hours. GRT-related rhegmatogenous retinal detachment (RRD) comprises about 1.5% of all RRD. GRT may be associated with inherited vitreoretinopathies such as Stickler's syndrome, high myopia, and trauma, but most cases are idiopathic.

2 Challenges with GRTs

Giant retinal tear management poses significant challenges for several reasons:

1. The large size of the GRTs results in a higher risk of RRD.
2. The retina is very mobile with folding of the posterior edge of the GRT.
3. The progression of retinal detachment is fast, and there is a risk of proliferative vitreoretinopathy (PVR) due to a larger area of exposed retinal pigment epithelium (RPE).
4. In young patients, GRT RRD may happen without complete PVD. Posterior hyaloid separation during pars plana vitrectomy (PPV) in these eyes can be very difficult.

Supplementary Information The online version contains supplementary material available at https://doi.org/10.1007/978-3-031-47827-7_10.

A. Chandra (✉)
Ophthalmology Department, Mid and South Essex NHS Foundation Trust, Southend-on-Sea, Essex, UK
Vision & Eye Research Institute, Anglia Ruskin University, Cambridge, UK
e-mail: a.chandra@nhs.net

A. B. Sallam et al. (eds.), *Practical Manual of Vitreoretinal Surgery*,
https://doi.org/10.1007/978-3-031-47827-7_10

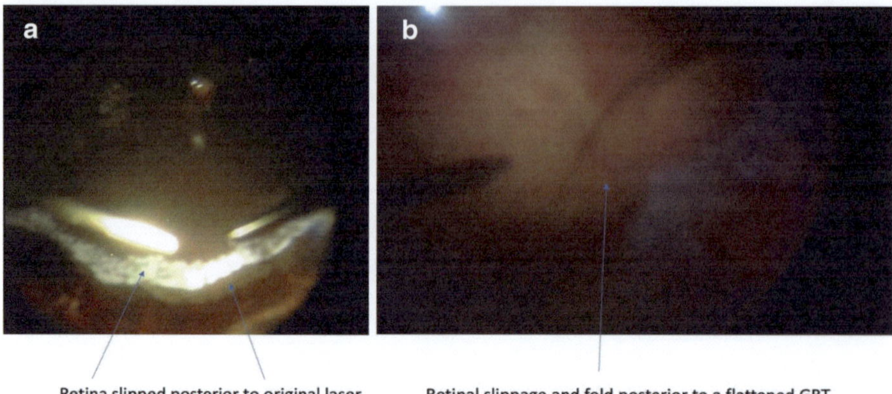

Fig. 1 Intraoperative posterior retinal slippage after air-perfluorocarbon liquid exchange in two different cases of giant retinal tear (GRT) detachment

5. A major challenge in PPV surgery for GRT is the risk of retinal slippage during the exchange of perfluorocarbon liquid (PFCL) for air or silicone oil (SO) (Fig. 1a, b). Slippage refers to the posterior displacement of the peripheral retinal edge of a giant retinal tear due to the posterior movement of the residual aqueous fluid under the retina caused by an incoming bubble of endotamponade. Slippage has been shown to occur much more frequently with PFCL-air exchange than PFCL-SO exchange. This is because air has a lower density which allows the residual subretinal fluid to be displaced posteriorly. Furthermore, the very anterior positioning of GRT provides rapid access for the aqueous to accumulate under the edge of the tear. On the other hand, the hydrophobic nature of both SO and PFCL results in good contact between the two fluids, to the relative exclusion of an aqueous or saline solution. This stabilizes the retina and shifts the aqueous layer above the SO layer rather than posteriorly. While a small degree of peripheral retinal slippage may not be problematic, large degrees can result in a wide area of exposed RPE and increase the risk of PVR, persistent or recurrent retinal detachment, and hypotony. It also can result in symptomatic posterior retinal folds. This latter issue is particularly relevant if the macula is involved with the RRD.

3 Preoperative Consideration

There is significant gender predilection toward men, and most cases of GRTs occur at a generally younger age than other forms of RRD, around 40–45 years.

Table 1 Differences between retinal dialysis and giant retinal tear (GRT)

	Retinal dialysis	GRT
Appearance	No anterior retinal flap present, only posterior flap	Anterior and posterior retinal flaps present
Vitreous status	Attached posterior hyaloid	PVD is usually present
Retinal mobility	Less mobile retina with usually no folding of the posterior tear flap	Very mobile retina and usually folding of the posterior flap
Treatment of choice	Segmental scleral buckle	PPV

Careful consideration must be given preoperatively for the following:

- Phakic status: As with all PPV surgery, the presence of a crystalline lens requires cautious maneuvers to avoid damage to the posterior aspect of the lens.
- As in other types of RRD, it is important to ascertain the status of the posterior hyaloid. GRTs often occur in the presence of a posterior vitreous detachment (PVD). However, this may not always be the case particularly in young myopic patients or eyes with inherited vitreoretinopathies and after trauma. This is important to note before the surgery as PVD induction in eyes of young patients with RRD can be technically challenging.
- Differentiating between GRT and retinal dialysis is important (Table 1).
- The extent of the GRT: Larger GRT (>180°) is likely to be associated with a more mobile retina.
- The location of the GRT: This will affect the consideration of which internal tamponade would be used.
- Foveal status: This will help inform the patient regarding visual prognosis. This is particularly relevant if the fovea is detached. Chronicity of foveal detachment will also be obviously important.
- Presence of PVR: As with most acute PVD-associated rhegmatogenous retinal detachment (RRD), the retina is often very mobile. If chronic, PVR may lead to reduced mobility of the retina with fixed retinal folds. PVR has important prognostic implications.

4 Management of GRT

4.1 *Retinopexy*

Giant retinal tear management poses significant challenges. However, if the retina is attached, laser photocoagulation may be performed posterior to the GRT [1]. This may be applied with indirect ophthalmoscopy, with two to three rows of laser being sufficient. However, if any neuroretinal detachment has occurred, more definitive surgical intervention is advisable, as RRD progression is likely to be too rapid to allow sufficient effect from retinopexy.

4.2   Explant Surgery

Although treating GRT-RRD externally with explant surgery, scleral buckle (SB) has been performed in the past, this is very challenging with the large break and very mobile RRD and a folded retinal flap. There may remain a role for external explant in cases with attached hyaloid without folding of the retina. These cases can be managed, similar to retinal dialysis management. Otherwise, it is generally regarded that PPV with modern techniques is a safer approach. Some surgeons recommend an additional placement of a buckle with PPV. This may be segmental in the area of the GRT or even an encircling element. This is generally not required with adequate PPV treatment in adults, and I do not endorse it.

A recent multicenter retrospective study showed that in children, 1-year SSAS rate was higher for PPV/SB (88.5%) than PPV (56.3%) ($P = 0.03$). In children, a supplemental SB may be beneficial as complete posterior hyaloid detachment, and vitreous shaving is difficult in this cohort [2].

4.3   PPV

Modern PPV is often elected for the management of GRT-RD. Small-gauge surgery with trocars is likely to reduce vitreous traction.

- As with all PPV in RD, it is important to ensure that the infusion is within the vitreous cavity. Small-gauge surgery with trocars and cannulas reduces the risk of the subretinal passage of instruments.
- If the patient is phakic, consideration needs to be given to avoiding contact with the posterior aspect of the lens. Some surgeons may elect to perform phacoemulsification with intraocular lens insertion at the same time as PPV for RD surgery. The author does not routinely perform this unless the cataract is too significant to allow adequate posterior segment view. Refractive outcome is likely to be better if biometry is performed with an attached retina, particularly the fovea. Furthermore, postoperative inflammation may be exacerbated with concomitant cataract surgery. The stability and final effective position of a freshly inserted intraocular lens may also be influenced by intraocular tamponade. With modern instrumentation, avoiding the posterior aspect of the crystalline lens is very manageable. Removing the anterior vitreous and the anterior lip of the GRT is possible with careful positioning of the cutter and diffuse lighting. An assistant performing scleral indentation may help with this, as can chandelier lighting if no assistant is available.
- A highly mobile retina is a frequent reality in GRT-RRD: do not underestimate the mobility of the retina. Keep the mouth of the vitrector facing anteriorly, and always be vigilant of its location (Video 1). As the vitreous is aspirated, the fluctuation of the retina may increase.

- We recommend ensuring that a posterior vitreous detachment is present. Although almost always present, in certain cases, such as trauma or Stickler's GRT, occasionally, a PVD may not be present (Video 1). A quick maneuver of aspiration over the disc will confirm the PVD.
- As with all RD-associated retinal tears, it is important to remove the vitreous and its traction from the lip of the GRT. With observation of the vitrector and tilting of the eye, this is very achievable. Scleral indentation either by an assistant or by the surgeon with the help of chandelier lighting makes this easier. The author recommends removing as much of the anterior lip of all retinal tears as can be safely completed, including a GRT. This helps ensure the removal of traction onto the tear and reduces any ischemia that the anterior lip may drive. Conversely, this may leave a large area of exposed RPE, stimulating hypotony and perhaps PVR. Thus, in very posterior GRT, the anterior flap can be preserved and lasered down.
- Once the vitrectomy has been completed, we recommend marking along the edge of the GRT with endodiathermy (Video 1). Once the retina is flattened, as with all retinal tears, visualization of the break becomes more challenging. Do not underestimate this phenomenon.
- Injecting PFCL: Before injecting the PFCL, reduce the infusion pressure to reduce the risk of rising IOP with the injection of PFCL. When inserting the PFCL cannula into the eye, direct the cannula away from the detached retina as soon as possible. This reduces the risk of drops of PFCL from the cannula migrating under the detached retina. The PFCL can be used to uncurl a folded edge of the GRT (Video 2). Subsequently, while injecting PFCL, it is important to ensure that this is not performed over the optic disc or the macula. It is possible for the jet of PFCL to penetrate the optic nerve and even an intact neuroretina (Video 3). Inject *slowly* away from the macula over the nasal retina. "Fish eggs" of multiple PFCL bubbles can be created on injection, which have a risk of these migrating subretinally or within the zonules. To reduce this, some advocate the use of dual-bore cannulas or simultaneously using an aspiration cannula in the second hand to aspirate while injecting. This latter technique, of course, would require a separate port for light or chandelier lighting. The author simply places the PFCL cannula into the formed bubble of PFCL and injects slowly to avoid "fish eggs."
- Once the retina is flattened with PFCL, further "interface vitrectomy" may be performed if there is any evidence of vitreous remaining peripherally. This may be aided with "staining" the vitreous (chromovitrectomy) with triamcinolone or vital dyes.
- Retinopexy must now be performed. If the GRT has been marked, identification of the location for this is straightforward. The options include diode laser, argon laser, and cryopexy. My most common tools are the latter two. The former has the advantage that it may be applied externally (Video 4). For the majority of the break, I would recommend laser retinopexy to minimize inflammation that would be present if extensive cryopexy is used. For argon laser application, I use a retractable/curved laser probe. This reduces the risk of damage to the posterior aspect of the crystalline lens while applying more peripheral laser from the contralateral side. I recommend a wide band of laser to be applied over the break, at

least three rows. Laser is applied to almost enclose the anterior "horns" of the break. If the horns are not completely covered, then I recommend applying cryopexy to these "horns." Cryopexy, being applied externally, allows retinopexy to be applied anteriorly to the ora serrata easier than with laser. The horns may be the most likely areas of accumulation of the subretinal fluid; thus, it is important to be sure of adequate retinopexy.

5 Tamponade

- The choice of tamponade should be considered preoperatively with the extent of the GRT in mind. As with all PPV, there are three choices: gas, short-term PFCL, and silicone oil. I reserve the latter only in cases of existing PVR. We have previously demonstrated that unexplained vision loss after silicone oil removal may be present in up to 49% of fovea-sparing GRT-RD [3].
- Choice of tamponade depends on the location of the GRT.

    - Inferior GRT can be managed with the PFCL. The PFCL, which had been inserted to flatten the neuroretina, may be left in place for up to 2-3 weeks while the retinopexy takes effect [4]. In practical terms, I would recommend suturing the ports (liquid tamponades have poorer wound contact angle than gas). It is recommendable to then prescribe intensive anti-inflammatory drops and if possible a short course of systemic anti-inflammatory medication. Within 3 weeks (in practice, within 10 days is sufficient), I would then perform a pars plana vitrectomy to aspirate the PFCL and exchange with air. When aspirating the PFCL, pay attention to washing the anterior chamber. In addition, I would perform repeated fluid-air exchanges to endeavor to encourage droplets of PFCL, which can collect in zonules and ciliary body, to present themselves.
    - Superior GRT would require considering gas tamponade. This poses a major challenge with GRT-RD, which is retinal slippage when exchanging PFCL with air. This is caused by the large size of the tear and its anterior location. Remaining saline and aqueous production easily migrate into the tear. This can lead to retinal slippage, with retinal redundancy draping more posteriorly, potentially leaving a fold, which can be visually significant, particularly if this fold is close to the fovea. Minimizing this risk requires reducing the saline in the eye and positioning the eye with the break dependent while aspirating at the edge of the break (Video 5).

        Fill the eye with PFCL till it flows into the infusion line. This should suggest that the eye is full of PFCL, though there will certainly be some saline remaining.
        Remove the infusion line, and turn the air on. Flush the saline out of the infusion line, and replace the infusion line onto the cannula.
        When ready, tilt the eye so that the GRT is dependent.

Keep your aspiration cannula at the edge of the break while air is entering the eye to try to aspirate the "wedge of saline" that will be present between PFCL and the air.

Keep aspirating at the edge of the PFCL; as the PFCL passes the GRT, dip to the GRT edge to remove any remnants of SRF. The end point is the edge of GRT being flat, stuck down, to the RPE.

Aspirate the PFCL bubble to the disc.

Drop a few droplets of saline onto the posterior pole. This allows any remnants of PFCL to form a bubble again within the saline bubble. This can then be visualized more easily to be aspirated (Video 6).

– If the GRT extends beyond inferior and superior meridians, I recommend leaving PFCL in situ and, once the ports are sutured, injecting a small volume, 0.1 mL, of 100% SF_6 gas as a top-up. This combination would allow tamponade support to a greater extent of the GRT.

- Silicone oil tamponade

  Traditional approaches have had a low threshold for the use of silicone oil (Fig. 2). This dates from old data, which suggests a low anatomical success rate for primary PPV for GRT-RD. Current data does not support the notion that acute GRT-RD has a poorer success rate [5]. With modern surgical techniques and early presentation, the risk of PVR and, thus, the need for SO tamponade are relatively low. In fact, there is growing evidence that SO tamponade may result in an unexplained visual loss in the macula on GRT-associated RRD [2]. However, in certain cases presenting with concurrent PVR, there may be a necessity for SO tamponade.

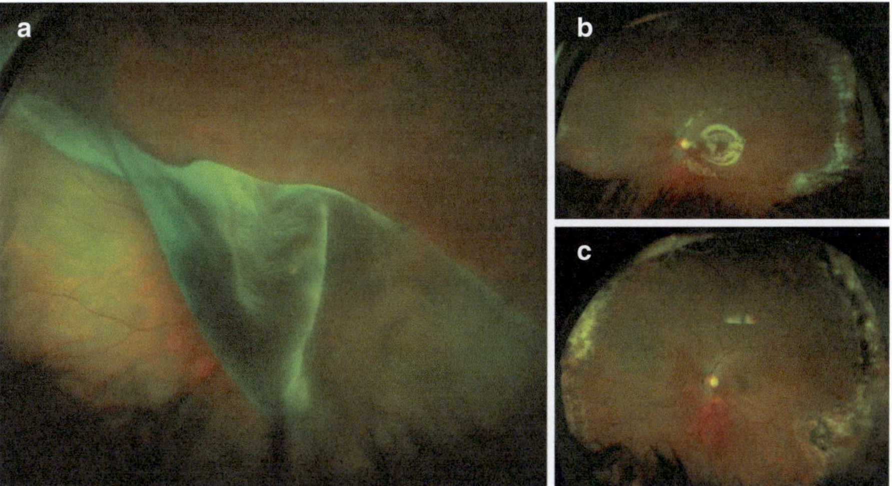

Fig. 2 Giant retinal tear of more than 180° with posterior flap folding (**a**) treated with silicone oil (SO) (**b**). Two years after SO removal (**c**)

- To exchange PFCL for SO, there are two approaches:

    - The PFCL can be exchanged for air (as described above) and then followed by SO exchange for the air (Video 7).
    - Alternatively, PFCL may be exchanged directly with silicone oil to help avoid retinal slippage [6]. This technique can be undertaken with a passive extrusion cannula, with the silicone oil injected via the third port. This may be via the infusion line or directly into the port with an assistant holding the injecting oil cannula. Simultaneously, the passive extrusion cannula may be placed posteriorly at the reducing pool of PFCL [7]. Passive aspiration is associated with a risk of high IOP since the aspiration of PFCL is less efficient than the active SO injection. Some vitreoretinal machines allow active injection of oil and active aspiration with one foot pedal control [8]. It is critical to have a low aspiration rate with this system to reduce the risk of hypotony with the slow injection rate of silicone oil. Further discussion on the techniques of direct PFCL-SO is found in chapter 5 "Vitreous Substitutes."

- When silicone oil or PFCL is left in situ, we would recommend suturing all the scleral ports.

6 Outcomes

The anatomical success of GRT-RRD surgery is encouraging and improving over time to approximately 85% with the first surgical intervention [4]. GRT-RRD most often presents acutely. However, if there is a proliferative vitreoretinopathy (PVR) already present, this will increase the risk of failure. Visual outcomes depend significantly on preoperative vision. To this extent, the status of the macula is critical. Where possible, it is wise to consider avoiding silicone oil in macula-sparing GRT-RRD. Post-surgical repair with PPV, cataract progression will limit visual recovery and can be managed when required. The presence of epimacular membranes or postoperative macular edema may also limit visual recovery, although comparisons of these complications to RRD not associated with GRT have not been undertaken.

Key Points
- Retinal detachment due to giant retinal tears poses significant challenges in their management.
- Preoperative considerations for GRTs include assessing phakic status, presence of posterior hyaloid detachment, differentiating GRT from retinal dialysis, and evaluating the extent and location of the tear and preexisting PVR.
- Vitrectomy with the use of PFCL is the current approach for GRT.
- The risk of retinal slippage during PFCL-air remains a major challenge.
- Short-term PFCL tamponade is suitable for inferior GRTs and gas tamponade for superior GRTs.
- Silicone oil is reserved for cases with existing proliferative vitreoretinopathy.

References

1. Ao J, Horo S, Farmer L, Chan WO, Gilhotra J. Primary laser photocoagulation for the treatment of giant retinal tears. Retinal Cases Brief Rep. 2018;12(4):371–4.
2. Ong SS, Ahmed I, Gonzales A, Al-Fakhri AS, Al-Subaie HF, Al-Qhatani FS, Alsulaiman SM, Mura M, Maia M, Kondo Kuroiwa DA, Maia NT, Berrocal MH, Wu L, Zas M, Francos JP, Cubero-Parra JM, Arsiwala LT, Handa JT, Arevalo JF. Vitrectomy versus vitrectomy with scleral buckling in the treatment of giant retinal tear related retinal detachments: an international multicenter study. Ophthalmol Retina. 2022;6(7):595–606.
3. Banerjee PJ, Chandra A, Petrou P, Charteris DG. Silicone oil versus gas tamponade for giant retinal tear-associated fovea-sparing retinal detachment: a comparison of outcome. Eye (Lond). 2017;31(9):1302–7.
4. Mikhail MA, Mangioris G, Best RM, McGimpsey S, Chan WC. Management of giant retinal tears with vitrectomy and perfluorocarbon liquid postoperatively as a short-term tamponade. Eye (Lond). 2017;31(9):1290–5.
5. Ting DSW, Foo VHX, Tan TE, et al. 25-years trends and risk factors related to surgical outcomes of giant retinal tear-rhegmatogenous retinal detachments. Sci Rep. 2020;10(1):5474. Published 2020 Mar 25.
6. Wong D, Williams RL, German MJ. Exchange of perfluorodecalin for gas or oil: a model for avoiding slippage. Graefes Arch Clin Exp Ophthalmol. 1998;236(3):234–7.
7. Madanagopalan VG. Sandwich technique with anterior silicone oil and posterior perfluorocarbon liquid for intraoperative retinal stabilization in eyes with large retinal breaks. J Ophthalmic Vis Res. 2019;14(2):232–5.
8. Ahmad KT, Sallam AB, Saad AA, Ellabban AA. Fully automated direct perfluorocarbon liquid-silicone oil exchange. Clin Ophthalmol. 2020;10(14):4355–8.

Proliferative Vitreoretinopathy Detachment: Surgical Management

Louisa Wickham and Ed Casswell

Proliferative vitreoretinopathy (PVR) is the most common cause of failure following retinal detachment surgery, with a reported incidence of 5.1%–11.7% [1]. Where there is a final failure of retinal detachment surgery, in over 75% of cases, PVR is responsible [1]. In this chapter, the surgical approach to patients presenting with PVR retinal detachments will be discussed.

1 Definition

PVR is defined as the growth and contraction of membranes within the vitreous cavity and on both surfaces of the retina following rhegmatogenous retinal detachment. These membranes can exert traction and reopen previously closed breaks, create new breaks and distort or obscure the macula [2] (Table 1) (Figs. 1 and 2).

Supplementary Information The online version contains supplementary material available at https://doi.org/10.1007/978-3-031-47827-7_11.

L. Wickham (✉)
Vitreoretinal Service, Moorfields Eye Hospital NHS Trust, London, UK
e-mail: louisa.wickham1@nhs.net

E. Casswell
Vitreoretinal, Moorfields Eye Hospital NHS Trust, London, UK
e-mail: edward.casswell@nhs.net

A. B. Sallam et al. (eds.), *Practical Manual of Vitreoretinal Surgery*,
https://doi.org/10.1007/978-3-031-47827-7_11

Table 1 The 1991 classification of proliferative vitreoretinopathy [3]

Grade	Features
A	Vitreous haze; pigment clumps; pigment clusters on the inferior retina
B	Wrinkling of inner retinal surface; retinal breaks with rolled or irregular edges; retinal stiffness; vessel tortuosity; decreased mobility of the vitreous
CP1–12	Posterior to the equator; focal, diffuse or circumferential full-thickness rigid retinal folds[a]; subretinal strands[a]
CA1–12	Anterior to the equator; focal, diffuse or circumferential full-thickness rigid retinal folds[a]; subretinal strands[a]; anterior displacement; condensed vitreous with strands

Sub-classification of grade C PVR (Machemer et al. 1991)

Type	Location (in relation to the equator)	Features
Focal	Posterior	Starfold posterior to the vitreous base
Diffuse	Posterior	Confluent starfolds posterior to the vitreous base. Optic disc may not be visible
Subretinal	Posterior/anterior	Proliferations under the retina: Annular strands near the disc; linear strands; moth-eaten-appearing sheets
Circumferential	Anterior	Contraction along the posterior edge of the vitreous base with central displacement of the retina; peripheral retina stretched; posterior retina in radial folds
Anterior displacement	Anterior	The vitreous base may be pulled anteriorly by the proliferative tissue; peripheral retinal trough; ciliary processes may be stretched and may be covered by membrane; the iris may be retracted

[a]Expressed in the number of clock hours involved

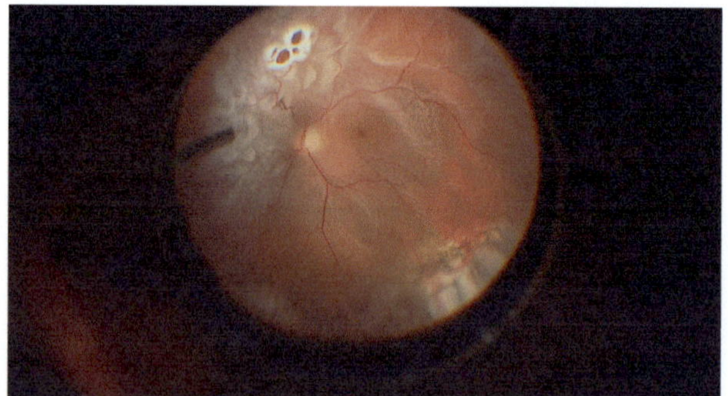

Fig. 1 Retinal photograph of proliferative vitreoretinopathy grade C showing anterior retinal traction and pre-retinal membranes. The causative breaks for the re-detachment are marked with diathermy

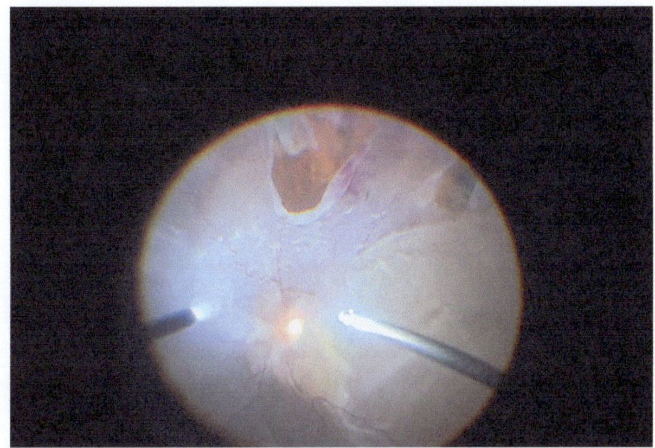

Fig. 2 Retinal photograph of proliferative vitreoretinopathy grade B showing rolled edges of the break

2 Can We Prevent PVR?

Although there has been a great deal of interest in the use of peri-operative and pre-operative adjuncts to prevent the formation of PVR, none are currently in widespread use, including methotrexate that has recently been investigated.

Given the limitations of surgical adjuncts at this stage, PVR is best prevented by identifying those at most risk of PVR and adjusting the surgical technique in response to this.

Risk algorithms have been developed to help identify at-risk patients, including the presence of PVR at the time of surgery, lens status and the presence of inflammatory stimulus such as vitreous hemorrhage or active uveitis [4–6]. Arguably the strongest determinant of the development of PVR is the presence of PVR at the time of presentation.

In cases thought to be at high risk of PVR development, the surgical approach should be tailored accordingly, with a low threshold for the use of long-acting tamponades.

3 Surgical Management of PVR

Treatment of retinal detachments with PVR can be distilled down to three basic principles:

1. Closure of all retinal breaks.
2. Release of traction.
3. Minimizing the recurrence of traction.

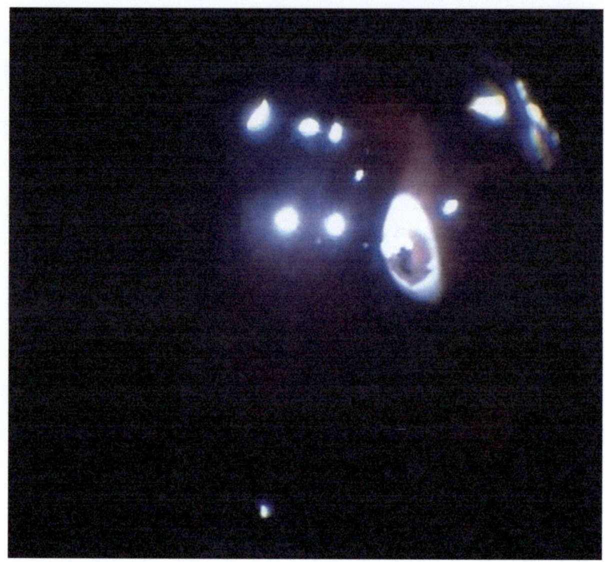

Fig. 3 Application of cryopexy to a retinal break in an air-filled eye. The cryopexy lights up the break. Where possible, one cryopexy application should be applied to cover the whole break to avoid overlapping cryo scars that have a greater risk of developing cryo-necrosis

3.1 Closure of Breaks

Closure of retinal breaks is achieved by stimulating chorioretinal adhesion and is usually achieved with cryopexy or retinopexy (Fig. 3).

4 Cryopexy

4.1 Advantages

- Broad band of adhesion.
- Will still work if residual SRF.
- Useful when view is poor.
- Good for anterior breaks.

4.2 Disadvantages

- Adhesion of the retina to RPE initially weaker post-application.
- Pro-inflammatory.
- Release of RPE cells with possible increased risk of PVR in large breaks.
- Potential for cryo machines to be unreliable in terms of uptake which can lead to undertreatment or cryo necrosis from overtreatment.

5   Laser Retinopexy

5.1   *Advantages*

- More immediate adhesion.
- Good for posterior breaks not accessible to cryopexy.
- Easier to titrate treatment in response to uptake.

5.2   *Disadvantages*

- Poor uptake if residual SRF is present.
- May increase time of surgery if frequent drying of the retina is required.
- Difficult to apply if view of the retina is poor.

In addition to chorioretinal adhesion, closure of retinal breaks may be aided by the use of a scleral buckle. Mild cases of PVR with a mobile retina may be treated by conventional, external buckling techniques without vitrectomy using a broad and moderately high encircling buckle to counteract tractional forces.

5.3   *Counteraction of Traction*

Contraction of epiretinal and subretinal membranes may cause new retinal breaks to form or prevent closure of those that have already been treated.

5.4   *How to Identify Traction*

- Areas of detachment associated with epiretinal and subretinal membranes.
- Persistent elevation after fluid-gas exchange.
- Areas of encapsulated subretinal fluid when using perfluorocarbon liquid (PFCL).

5.5   *How to Relieve Traction*

- Peeling epiretinal and subretinal membranes.
- Segmentation of epiretinal membranes.
- Retinectomy or retinotomy.
- Scleral buckling.

With the exception of scleral buckling, these techniques require an internal approach.

6 Membrane Peeling

6.1 Epiretinal Membranes

Peeling of epiretinal membranes relieves tangential traction that results in retinal folds. Identification of pre-retinal membranes may be aided with the use of adjuncts, for example, triamcinolone, trypan blue and brilliant blue (as a negative stain) [7]. Additional internal limiting membrane peeling in macula-off retinal detachment with PVR does not appear to confer additional anatomical or visual benefits [8].

6.2 Tips for Removing PVR Membranes

- Create an edge/flap by using a vitreoretinal pick, usually by gently moving the pick along the trough of a retinal fold.
- Using membrane forceps, commence peel at the posterior retina moving anteriorly as the retina is thicker posteriorly and provides stronger countertraction than the thinner anterior retina.
- Use slow movements as PVR membranes are often very adherent. A slow motion allows the membrane to disengage with less chance of tearing the underlying retina (Video 1).
- Membranes can only be peeled as far as the posterior border of the vitreous base. If anterior traction extends into the vitreous base, then additional surgical techniques such as retinectomy or buckle support are required (Video 2).
- If the underlying retina is atrophic, consider increasing countertraction by using a PFCL, for example, perfluorodecalin (Fig. 4).

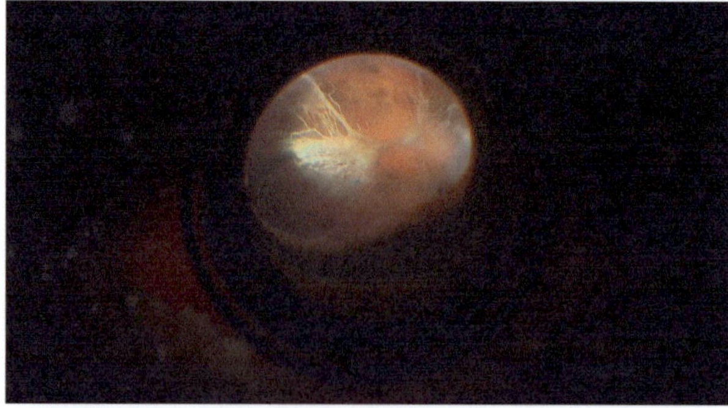

Fig. 4 Retinal photograph of a patient with proliferative vitreoretinopathy grade C with chronic inferior detachment leading to a very atrophic thin retina. Peeling adherent membranes on the surface is usually not possible due to the underlying weakness of the retina. Perfluorocarbon or a bimanual technique with a chandelier may be helpful, but in many cases, a retinectomy is required

Caution: PFCLs can be useful in the surgical management of PVR as they may reduce surgical time, decrease trauma from retinal manipulation, aid countertraction and be used to stabilise the macula. However, when used as an adjunct to the peeling of membranes, there is a risk of migration subretinally if a break occurs during peeling and residual traction remains. Similarly, if injected into an area of retinal traction, an open break may also act as a conduit for subretinal migration.

7 Subretinal Membranes

In many cases, subretinal bands do not exert significant traction and may coexist with attached retina. However, where they are contracted and causing elevation, they need to be removed (Fig. 5).

Depending on the location and the additional procedures being performed at the time, subretinal membranes can be removed either through an appropriately positioned retinotomy or by deflecting retina released during retinectomy.

7.1 Tips for Removing Subretinal Membranes

- Use forceps with a wide gripping surface (and where possible serrated).
- Where the membranes are long, countertraction may be exerted by using the light pipe as an additional point of countertraction (Video 3).

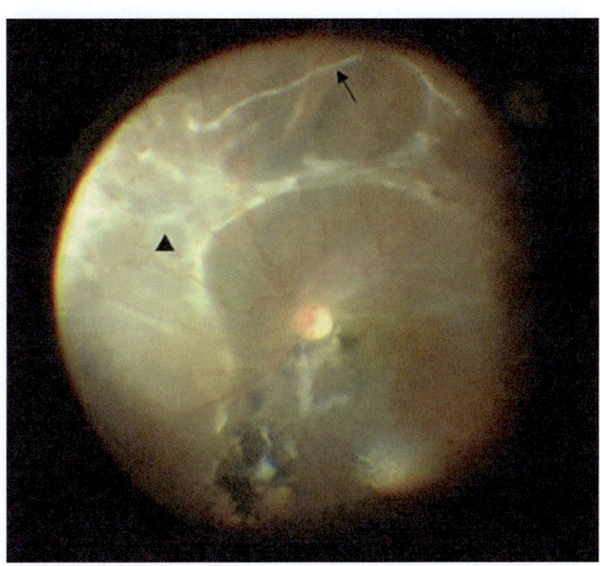

Fig. 5 Retinal photograph of extensive subretinal membranes, both sheets (arrowhead) and bands (arrow) which have contracted to cause a retinal detachment

8   Retinotomy and Retinectomy

This procedure involves cutting the retina in either a circumferential or radial manner to relieve traction, followed by retinopexy to attach the residual retina which is then supported by a long-acting intraocular tamponade. Following retinectomy, PFCL is usually injected to stabilise the retina and allows the application of laser retinopexy, after which a fluid-air exchange may be performed prior to injecting silicone oil (SO) or a direct PFCL/SO exchange may be used. When performing fluid-air exchange, active aspiration or passive aspiration may be used to equal effect.

8.1   Tips for Successful Retinectomy

- When removing PFCL (as part of either an air exchange or a direct SO exchange), start by aspirating at the edge of the PFCL bubble as anterior as possible to remove any residual irrigation fluid and reduce the risk of migration of fluid subretinally or retinal slippage.
- Residual fluid has been removed when the meniscus of the PFCL bubble can no longer be seen. Until that time, the aspiration cannula should straddle the edge of the meniscus bubble at the anterior margin. Once the PFCL meniscus is more posterior than the retinectomy edge, aspiration can be performed at the posterior pole.
- With direct SO exchange, always monitor the intraocular pressure by either visualization of arterial flow at the optic disc or manually checking the tone of the scleral wall.
- In cases where PVR is aggressive or still active, retinopexy of the retinectomy edge may be deferred until a later date prior to SO removal. This has the additional benefit of allowing some retinal movement or contraction without creating traction due to anchoring of the retinal edge with retinopexy [9].

Unfortunately, retinectomy is associated with poor anatomical and visual outcomes and an increased incidence of hypotony [10, 11]. In a retrospective study of 302 patients who underwent retinectomy, 51% achieved retinal reattachment following one procedure (72% final reattachment rate), but only 11.9% had a final visual acuity of greater than 6/24 [11].

Using SO as a tamponading agent in these cases appears to decrease the risk of post-operative hypotony [10]. Despite poor outcomes, this technique remains one of the most common approaches due to the lack of other surgical or adjunctive techniques to address retinal contraction.

9 Scleral Buckle

A circumferential buckle may be used as a way of relieving anterior traction caused by contraction of the vitreous base. A description of how to place a scleral buckle is given in Chap. 9 "Scleral Buckle Surgery".

In PVR buckling surgery, a high indent is desirable to relieve traction. In order to achieve sufficient height to the buckle, the eye needs to be softened. In a vitrectomised eye, drainage of aqueous fluid through a corneal paracentesis or vitreous cavity fluid via a pars plana needle is usually sufficient to create the space required. In a nonvitrectomised eye, an aqueous paracentesis may not create enough space, and additional procedures may be required, for example, drainage of the subretinal fluid, aspiration of the vitreous fluid or limited vitrectomy.

In a study of 95 eyes, a combined approach of vitrectomy and scleral buckling resulted in retinal reattachment in 75% of patients with severe PVR (grades D1–D3) compared to a much lower success rate of 19–23% using scleral buckling alone [12].

9.1 Minimizing Recurrence of Traction

Despite the best surgical techniques, PVR has a high risk of recurrence following surgery. To minimize the effects of recurrent traction whilst the PVR process burns itself out, long-acting endotamponades such as SO and C3F8 are used.

10 Should I Use Silicone Oil or Gas?

This was addressed in the Silicone Study. When the use of SO was compared with that of a longer-acting gas, C3F8 [13], there was no statistical difference in the anatomical success rate (73% vs. 64%) or in the number achieving a final visual acuity of greater than or equal to 5/200 (43% vs. 45%) at 18 months. More long-term follow-up (36 months) suggested an advantage favouring C3F8 in achieving complete posterior retinal reattachment (83% vs. 60%, $p = 0.045$). Use of SO was associated with a better visual outcome in patients with anterior PVR; however, the anatomical success rate was no better than that observed with C3F8 [14].

Despite this, many surgeons still prefer to use SO when managing patients with a high risk of PVR due to the degree of retinal stability with SO which aids monitoring patients in an outpatient setting. In cases where long-term oil is required or there is doubt as to whether it may ever be removed, some advocate the use of higher-viscosity oil which is thought to have a lower risk of emulsification and hence secondary glaucoma and retinal toxicity [15].

Heavy SO may also be used in circumstances when inferior tamponade is required. Studies have shown superior anatomical outcomes in eyes with inferior tears and PVR grade C compared to standard SO [16]. However, it is not avaialble in the USA and its use may be limited by observations of increased inflammation and the development of PVR in the superior retina [17, 18].

11 When Should Silicone Oil Be Removed?

The decision of when to remove SO is a difficult one. It is thought that a PVR cycle takes approximately 10–12 weeks to complete and that SO should remain in situ during this period. In cases where retinal detachment is seen prior to this period, then further surgery is warranted to address residual traction and the SO re-injected at the end of the procedure.

Even with full retinal reattachment, the rate of retinal detachment following SO removal is in the order of 15–25% [19–21]. If the retina re-detaches at this stage, an assessment of whether further SO tamponade (due to residual traction) or gas tamponade (untreated break without traction) is required is undertaken.

Staining the retina at the time of SO removal may have some benefit in identifying residual membrane and reducing the retinal re-detachment rate.

12 What Gauge Should I Use for PVR Surgery?

We mainly use 23-gauge PPV. However, the following should be considered when deciding on which gauge to use for PVR surgery.

13 Visualization and Access to the Anterior Retina

Most surgeons consider that removal of the peripheral vitreous is important and that indentation and visualization of the periphery are helpful in locating and treating retinal breaks. These steps can be more challenging to complete as the gauge becomes narrower due to differences in illumination and rigidity of instrumentation.

14 Potential Timing Implications

Removal of the vitreous takes longer as the gauge narrows and indentation is often required to remove the peripheral vitreous. In some instances, cataract extraction is performed at the same time to achieve sufficient vitreous clearance.

In cases where the use of SO (particularly high-viscosity oils) is planned, narrower-gauge systems can add significantly to the overall procedure time.

Some of these factors have been addressed by industry improvements in the instrumentation and fluid dynamics, and this is likely to positively impact on the future usability of smaller-gauge systems for complex retinal detachment.

15 Outcomes of PVR Surgery

The effects of PVR on visual function are well documented, with only 11–25% of patients achieving a visual acuity of 20/100 [13, 22].

Poor visual acuity has been associated with decreased performance of many activities of daily living, poor cognitive ability and ultimately poorer health-related quality of life (QOL). Further, in cases of PVR, multiple surgery can also lead to chronic pain and poor cosmesis that have an additional adverse impact on quality of life.

Key Points
- Despite advances in the treatment of primary retinal detachment, there are both lack of agreement and lack of an evidence base to make rational choices of technique when managing PVR.
- The current evidence base suggests that many surgical techniques can achieve similar success rates in specialist units and that perhaps familiarity and surgeon preference are the more compelling reasons for choosing a particular approach.
- Our most commonly used approach is to relieve traction wherever possible and proceed to retinectomy when attachment of the retina cannot be achieved by peeling alone. The use of SO as a tamponade is our preferred choice when PVR is still active or likely to recur; however, in cases where PVR is mild, a long-acting gas is preferable and associated with a lower risk of further ocular comorbidity.
- Use of pharmacotherapy to prevent PVR including methotrexate is still not widely used in clinical practice.

References

1. Charteris DG, Sethi CS, Lewis GP, Fisher SK. Proliferative vitreoretinopathy—developments in adjunctive treatment and retinal pathology. Eye. 2002;16:369–74.
2. The Retina Society Terminology Committee. The classification of retinal detachment with proliferative vitreoretinopathy. Ophthalmology. 1983;90:121–5.
3. Machemer R, Aaberg TM, Freeman HM, Irvine AR, Lean JS, Michels RM. An updated classification of retinal detachment with proliferative vitreoretinopathy. Am J Ophthalmol. 1991;112(2):159–65. PMID: 1867299.
4. Bonnet M, Guenoun S. Surgical risk factors for severe postoperative proliferative vitreoretinopathy (PVR) in retinal detachment with grade B PVR. Graefes Arch Clin Exp Ophthalmol. 1995;233:789–91.

5. Kon CH, Asaria RH, Occleston NL, Khaw PT, Aylward GW. Risk factors for proliferative vitreoretinopathy after primary vitrectomy: a prospective study. Br J Ophthalmol. 2000;84:506–11.

6. Wickham L, Bunce C, Wong D, Charteris DG. Retinal detachment repair by vitrectomy: simplified formulae to estimate the risk of failure. Br J Ophthalmol. 2011;95:1239.

7. Li K, Wong D, Hiscott P, Stanga P, Groenewald C, McGalliard J. Trypan blue staining of internal limiting membrane and epiretinal membrane during vitrectomy: visual results and histopathological findings. Br J Ophthalmol. 2003;87:216–9.

8. Obata S, Sawada O, Kakinoki M, Matsumoto R, Saishin Y, Ohji M; Japan-Retinal Detachment Registry Group. Effects of internal limiting membrane peeling on anatomical and functional outcomes in macula-off rhegmatogenous retinal detachment complicated by proliferative vitreoretinopathy: Japan-Retinal Detachment Registry. Japanese Journal of Ophthalmology. 2023;67(4):417–23.

9. Veckeneer M, Maaijwee K, Charteris DG, van Meurs JC. Deferred laser photocoagulation of relaxing retinotomies under silicone oil tamponade to reduce recurrent macular detachment in severe proliferative vitreoretinopathy. Graefes Arch Clin Exp Ophthalmol. 2014;252:1539–44.

10. Blumenkranz MS, Azen SP, Aaberg T, et al. Relaxing retinotomy with silicone oil or long-acting gas in eyes with severe proliferative vitreoretinopathy. Silicone study report 5. The silicone study group. Am J Ophthalmol. 1993;116:557–64.

11. Grigoropoulos VG, Benson S, Bunce C, Charteris D. Functional outcome and prognostic factors in 304 eyes managed by retinectomy. Graefes Arch Clin Exp Ophthalmol. 2007;245:641–9.

12. Hanneken AM, Michels RG. Vitrectomy and scleral buckling methods for proliferative vitreoretinopathy. Ophthalmology. 1988;95:865–9.

13. Silicone Study Group. Vitrectomy with silicone oil or perfluoropropane gas in eyes with severe proliferative vitreoretinopathy: results of a randomized clinical trial. Silicone study report 2. Arch Ophthalmol. 1992;110:780–92.

14. Diddie KR, Azen SP, Freeman HM, et al. Anterior proliferative vitreoretinopathy in the silicone study: silicone study report 10. Ophthalmology. 1996;103:1092–9.

15. Chan YK, Czanner G, Shum HC, Williams RL, Cheung N, Wong D. Towards better characterization and quantification of emulsification of silicone oil in vitro. Acta Ophthalmol. 2017;95:e385–92.

16. Tzoumas N, Yorston D, Laidlaw DAH, Williamson TH, Steel DH; British and Eire Association of Vitreoretinal Surgeons and European Society of Retina Specialists Retinal Detachment Outcomes Group. Improved Outcomes with Heavy Silicone Oil in Complex Primary Retinal Detachment: A Large Multicenter Matched Cohort Study. Ophthalmology. 2023;15:S0161–6420(23)00899–0.

17. Wickham L, Tranos P, Hiscott P, Charteris D. The use of silicone oil-RMN3 (Oxane HD) as heavier-than-water internal tamponade in complicated inferior retinal detachment surgery. Graefes Arch Clin Exp Ophthalmol. 2010;248:1225–31.

18. Rizzo S, Romagnoli MC, Genovesi-Ebert F, Belting C. Surgical results of heavy silicone oil HWS-45 3000 as internal tamponade for inferior retinal detachment with PVR: a pilot study. Graefes Arch Clin Exp Ophthalmol. 2011;249:361–7.

19. Laidlaw DA, Karia N, Bunce C, Aylward GW, Gregor ZJ. Is prophylactic 360-degree laser retinopexy protective? Risk factors for retinal redetachment after removal of silicone oil. Ophthalmology. 2002;109:153–8.

20. He Y, Zeng S, Zhang Y, Zhang J. Risk factors for retinal redetachment after silicone oil removal: a systematic review and meta-analysis. Ophthalmic Surg Lasers Imaging Retina. 2018;49:416–24.

21. Lam RF, Cheung BT, Yuen CY, Wong D, Lam DS, Lai WW. Retinal redetachment after silicone oil removal in proliferative vitreoretinopathy: a prognostic factor analysis. Am J Ophthalmol. 2008;145:527–33.

22. Wickham L, Ho-Yen GO, Bunce C, Wong D, Charteris DG. Surgical failure following primary retinal detachment surgery by vitrectomy: risk factors and functional outcomes. Br J Ophthalmol. 2010;95:1234.

Degenerative Retinoschisis and Related Retinal Detachments

Matthew R. Starr, Razieh Mahmoudzadeh, David Reed, and Sunir J. Garg

This chapter focuses on the natural history of degenerative retinoschisis as well as the surgical management of schisis detachments and progressive rhegmatogenous retinal detachments (RRD) associated with retinoschisis.

1 Retinoschisis

- Degenerative (previously known as senile) retinoschisis is a splitting of the retinal layers, typically in the peripheral retina. Retinoschisis occurs in approximately 1–4% of the adult population, and affected patients are typically asymptomatic. The area of retinoschisis is located inferotemporally in 75% and superotemporally in 25% of cases and is bilateral in 85% of patients. Most cases

Supplementary Information The online version contains supplementary material available at https://doi.org/10.1007/978-3-031-47827-7_12.

M. R. Starr
Mayo Clinic, Rochester, MN, USA
e-mail: starr.matthew2@mayo.edu

R. Mahmoudzadeh
Retina Service, Wills Eye Hospital, Philadelphia, PA, USA

D. Reed
Retina Department, Ophthalmic Consultants of Boston, Boston, MA, USA

S. J. Garg (✉)
Ophthalmology, Wills Eye Hospital/Thomas Jefferson University Hospital, Philadelphia, PA, USA
e-mail: sgarg@midatlanticretina.com

A. B. Sallam et al. (eds.), *Practical Manual of Vitreoretinal Surgery*, https://doi.org/10.1007/978-3-031-47827-7_12

of retinoschisis do not progress, and if they do, progression occurs over many years [1, 2].

- The etiology of retinoschisis is unknown. Some believe the cystic cavities develop due to vitreous traction; however, it is most commonly felt to be a degenerative disease affecting the inner retina as evidenced by the inability of posterior vitreous detachments to destabilize areas of retinoschisis.

- Over time, the support cells and neuronal interconnections between the inner nuclear and outer plexiform layers of degenerative retinoschisis fragment leaving a viscous fluid composed of mucopolysaccharide material. Additionally, the leftover footplates of Müller cells overlying the inner retinoschisis leave hyperreflective white dots or "snowflakes," a common clinical exam finding in patients with long-standing retinoschisis (Fig. 1—asterisk).

- Histologically, retinoschisis is divided into two subtypes, typical and reticular. Typical retinoschisis involves the splitting of the retinal layers at the level of the outer plexiform layer, while reticular retinoschisis develops at the level of the nerve fiber layer. While the two types are easily distinguished on histopathology, it is sometimes difficult to differentiate the two on clinical exam [1].

- Retinal detachments occur in approximately 0.04% of patients with degenerative retinoschisis. Given the similar appearance (Fig. 2a), it can be difficult to distinguish a retinal detachment from an area of retinoschisis. Table 1 highlights the major differences between degenerative retinoschisis and a retinal detachment.

- Recently, multimodal imaging has emerged as an adjunctive measure in differentiating retinoschisis from a retinal detachment. Perhaps the most reliable imaging modality used is optical coherence tomography (OCT) [3]. OCT is able to identify the splitting of the retinal layers with the outer retina remaining adherent to the underlying retinal pigment epithelium (RPE) in degenerative retinoschisis while detecting the subretinal fluid with retinal detachments (Fig. 2b). It may be difficult to obtain peripheral sweeps in some patients; however, with the advent of wide-field OCT, peripheral lesions are more easily captured. The infrared and

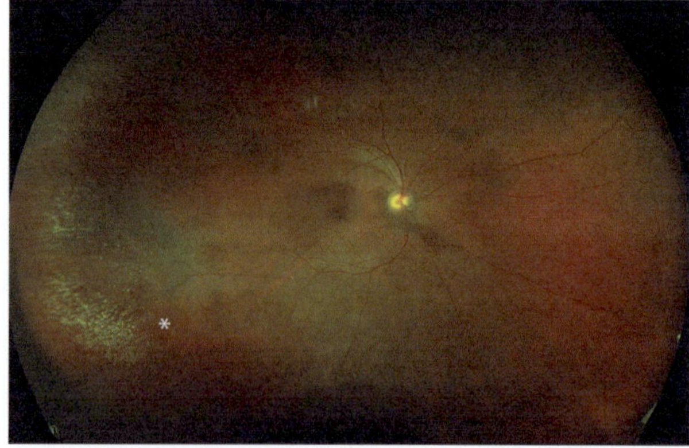

Fig. 1 Wide-field color image of a right eye in a patient with degenerative retinoschisis with extensive hyperreflective white dots or snowflakes (asterisk). These dots are commonly seen in patients with degenerative retinoschisis and are thought to be degenerative Müller footplates

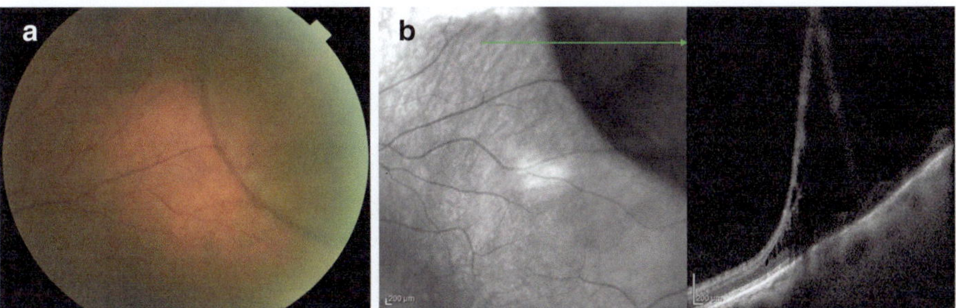

Fig. 2 Color image (**a**) of a patient with bullous degenerative retinoschisis. Corresponding optical coherence tomography (OCT, **b**) of the same patient exemplifying the splitting of the retinal layers between the inner nuclear layer and the outer plexiform layer, rather than a retinal detachment with the subretinal fluid

Table 1 Distinguishing degenerative retinoschisis from retinal detachment

	Degenerative retinoschisis	Retinal detachment
Symptoms	None	Symptoms if acute
Scotoma	Absolute	Relative
Appearance	Smooth, dome-shaped appearance, but can be shallow	Acute with corrugated retinal surface; however, chronic detachments may have a smooth retinal surface
White dots, Müller footplates	Common	Absent
Demarcation line	None	Present in chronic detachments
Laterality	Typically bilateral	Typically unilateral, but can be bilateral
Progression	Usually none. If it occurs, it is slow over years	Acute retinal detachments lead to vision loss within days
Effect of indirect laser	Due to the apposition of RPE with the outer retina, retinal whitening will occur	The retina will not blanch due to the subretinal fluid
Optical coherence tomography findings	Cavity between retinal layers with outer retina layers adherent to RPE	Complete split of the outer retina from RPE with the subretinal fluid

fundus autofluorescence to distinguish the two conditions are of varying utility with some reports identifying a hyperautofluorescent leading edge in retinal detachments, while others have not found either test to be sufficiently specific. Additionally, ultrasonography may be used to identify areas of retinoschisis. Retinoschisis can appear similar to a serous choroidal detachment on B-scan; however, retinoschisis is usually thinner with a single spike on A-scan compared to the double peak seen in choroidal detachments. With the introduction of newer imaging modalities, ultrasonography is not typically used to differentiate retinoschisis from retinal detachments.

2   Retinoschisis-Related Detachments

- Roughly one quarter of eyes with degenerative retinoschisis have outer retinal breaks. Outer retinal breaks are identifiable due to prominent rolled retinal edges with intact retinal vasculature coursing over the hole (Fig. 3). Outer retinal breaks may allow fluid from the schisis cavity to progress into the subretinal space. In combination with the inner retinal holes, the vitreous fluid may track through both the inner and outer retinal holes into the subretinal space. These holes can be typically observed given that the majority are stable over time; however, laser retinopexy may be performed to surround the area of the outer retinal hole to prevent any progression of the subretinal fluid beyond the borders of the break [1].
- There are two types of retinal detachments associated with degenerative retinoschisis, schisis detachments and progressive rhegmatogenous retinal detachments.

  - Schisis detachments occur when the subretinal fluid develops from an outer retinal break in the absence of an inner retinal hole and are difficult to detect. These detachments occur in 58% of patients with outer retinal breaks and overall in 6.4% of eyes with retinoschisis. These detachments can often remain stagnant with no progression over time and thus can be observed even if there is extension posteriorly as most patients are asymptomatic. Schisis detachments may be identified if a retinoschisis cavity develops an irregular contour or a demarcation line suggesting chronic subretinal fluid.
  - Progressive rhegmatogenous retinal detachments occur in the presence of both inner and outer retinal breaks. Breaks in both the inner and outer retina allow liquified vitreous entry to the subretinal space. These types of detachments are much rarer than schisis detachments. In a landmark paper examining 178 eyes with degenerative retinoschisis over a mean of 9 years by Byer, only 1 eye developed a progressive rhegmatogenous retinal detachment. These types of detachments are more easily identifiable due to acute, symptomatic changes in vision with a corrugated appearance of the retina [1].

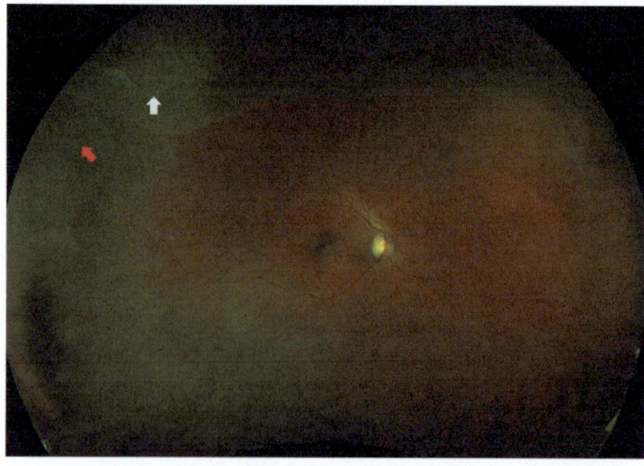

Fig. 3 Wide-field color image of a patient with far temporal degenerative retinoschisis. The red arrow highlights mild snowflakes, while the white arrow is pointing at an outer retinal hole which may develop underneath the schisis cavity

3 Pre-Operative Assessment

The most important pre-operative assessment is determining whether the area of concern is degenerative retinoschisis versus a retinal detachment. In cases of macula involving schisis detachments and progressive rhegmatogenous retinal detachments, surgical intervention is generally warranted.

- As with any rhegmatogenous retinal detachment, scleral-depressed peripheral retinal examination with scleral depression and identification of all retinal breaks remain critical. Careful examination with scleral depression of the contralateral eye is also to be performed given the typical bilateral nature of retinoschisis and to identify any full-thickness retinal breaks that should be treated in the peri-operative period of surgical eye.
- OCT to identify retinoschisis versus the subretinal fluid in new patients is a useful adjunct to the clinical exam and can help identify areas of subretinal fluid.
- Identification of a posterior vitreous detachment (PVD) on either OCT or direct fundus exam is also important to help determine the appropriate surgical technique.

4 Considerations for Surgery

Selecting the appropriate surgical technique depends on numerous pre-operative characteristics. A few important considerations are the location both of the outer retinal breaks and of the detachment, number of retinal breaks, PVD status, macular status, lens status, and type of retinoschisis detachment. Both schisis detachments and progressive RRDs related to retinoschisis have higher failure rates than typical RRDs.

- Schisis detachments.

    - Only, if there is noted progression of a schisis detachment toward the posterior pole, laser retinopexy may be applied to prevent further progression into the macula [4]; however, laser treatment of retinoschisis may be associated with retinal detachment due to the development of outer retinal layer defects [5].
    - When schisis detachments do involve the macula, they typically have outer retinal breaks that are located toward the posterior pole. Treating these breaks with cryoretinopexy is challenging due to the potential of macular extension; placing a radial element may lead to significant macular distortion and visual distortions post-operatively [6]. Some authors have proposed external drainage, cryoretinopexy, and long-acting gas tamponade with appropriate post-operative positioning without scleral buckling as a means to avoid very posterior radial elements in these schisis detachments [7].
    - When the outer retinal breaks are anterior to the equator, there are reports of encircling scleral buckles with cryoretinopexy and gas tamponade achieving

good anatomic success. There could be an increased schisis fluid soon after surgery (within 1–3 days), but this resolves over time.

- Pars plana vitrectomy (PPV) may be helpful in relieving any posterior vitreous traction followed by an internal drainage, air-fluid exchange, endolaser, and gas or oil tamponade.
- Often, the schisis cavity may re-open, while the previous area of retinal detachment may remain attached. Given the difficulty of schisis closure and nature of the absolute scotoma overlying the area of retinoschisis, some authors have proposed the complete removal of the inner retina in the area of retinoschisis. This enables the outer retina to remain attached without any cavities that may lead to intra-retinal traction and thus re-detachment. Additionally, some reports suggest placing endolaser to the entire area of retinoschisis as well as 2–3 mm posterior to leading edge of retinoschisis to promote adhesion of both the inner and outer retinal layers to the underlying RPE.
- There are case reports, though, of schisis detachments with absolute scotomas involving the macula regaining vision after successful retinal detachment surgery [8], and thus, these authors do not recommend removing the inner retina of the macula.
- Regardless of approach chosen by the surgeon, there are no large trials or series supporting one intervention over another. It is left to the surgeon's discretion to determine which approach is best for each specific schisis detachment. Vitreoretinal surgeons, though, should be aware of the higher single-surgery failure rates in schisis detachments and discuss them with patients pre-operatively.

- Progressive rhegmatogenous retinal detachments.

  - Compared to schisis detachments, progressive RRDs involve communication between the vitreous fluid and the subretinal space. Typically, the inner hole is extremely small, and often a small inner hole is not found on exam or intra-operatively. These detachments often present more acutely and behave more like typical RRDs, but still have a higher single-surgery (30%) and multiple-surgery (13%) failure rate than routine RRDs (15% and 5%) [2].
  - As with any RRD, the causative outer retinal break must be treated and either supported with a scleral buckle or the vitreoretinal traction relieved and subretinal fluid drained using PPV. In eyes with anterior retinal breaks and an absent PVD, typically, primary scleral buckles are favored, while eyes with a PVD or posterior retinal breaks may require a combination PPV and encircling scleral buckle or PPV alone to achieve anatomic success [2, 9].
  - Interestingly, treatment of the inner retinal hole and closure of the retinoschisis cavity may be optional in these cases. Similar to schisis detachments, though, the schisis cavity will likely re-open post-operatively if it closes during surgery. Thus, the same considerations can be made for treating the retinoschisis with endolaser applied to the area of retinoschisis as well as to the 2–3 mm posterior to the leading edge of the retinal detachment or removal of the inner retinal layers in the area of retinoschisis.

- Given the higher failure rates, surgeons often use longer-acting gas tamponade or silicone oil (Video 1) during the initial surgery in an attempt to achieve appropriate adhesions between the retinal layers as well as to the RPE [2, 10].
- There are also reports of in-office repair using cryoretinopexy and gas tamponade for select patients with appropriate RRDs who can position post-operatively [11].

5 Intra-Operative and Post-Operative Complications

There are risks to any surgery. Some particular to schisis-related detachments are as follows:

- As mentioned above, placing posterior radial elements may lead to macular distortion and subjective visual disturbances post-operatively despite re-attachment of the retina.
- Also unique to retinoschisis-related detachments compared to typical RRDs is the recurrent opening of the retinoschisis cavity.
- As with any chronic detachment, the subretinal fluid is extremely viscous, and attempts at external drainage with small bore needles may leave large amounts of retained subretinal fluid.

6 Case Scenario

A 62-year-old phakic female presented to the retina service for a formal evaluation of her retina at the request of her primary ophthalmologist. On examination, her visual acuity was 20/30 OD and 20/40 OS with an epiretinal membrane OU, posterior vitreous detachments OU, and superotemporal degenerative retinoschisis OU, more extensive in the right eye. The right eye had evidence of outer retinal holes with a prominent vessel coursing over the hole (Fig. 3 white arrow). There was also evidence of Müller footplates consistent with degenerative retinoschisis (Fig. 3 red arrow). She was observed with an exam every 6 months until she reported an acute change in her visual acuity OD 2 years after her initial retina evaluation. Her visual acuity worsened to count fingers OD, and she had evidence of a macula-off progressive RRD with fluid emanating from the area of superotemporal retinoschisis. The patient underwent a pars plana vitrectomy, encircling scleral buckle, peeling of the internal limiting membrane, internal drainage of the subretinal fluid through a drainage retinotomy, endolaser, and C3F8 gas tamponade with successful closure of the schisis cavity and repair of the retinal detachment.

Key Points
- It can often be difficult to distinguish degenerative retinoschisis from a rhegmatogenous retinal detachment on clinical examination.

- Areas of degenerative retinoschisis will have overlying white dots of Müller footplates, show retinal whitening when lasered, and rarely progress. OCT can be very useful in distinguishing the two entities.
- There are two types of retinal detachments associated with degenerative retinoschisis, schisis detachments and progressive rhegmatogenous retinal detachments.
- Schisis detachments occur when the subretinal fluid develops from an outer retinal break in the absence of an inner retinal hole, while rhegmatogenous detachments occur when both an inner and outer retinal hole are present.
- We will often consider performing a scleral buckle (with or without PPV) in these challenging cases.

References

1. Byer NE. Long-term natural history study of senile retinoschisis with implications for management. Ophthalmology. 1986;93(9):1127–37.
2. Xue K, Muqit MMK, Ezra E, et al. Incidence, mechanism and outcomes of schisis retinal detachments revealed through a prospective population-based study. Br J Ophthalmol. 2017;101(8):1022–6.
3. Jalalizadeh RA, Smith BT. Characterization and diagnosis of retinoschisis and schisis detachments using spectral domain optical coherence tomography. Graefes Arch Clin Exp Ophthalmol. 2023;261(2):375–80.
4. Okun E, Cibis PA. The role of photocoagulation in the management of retinoschisis. Arch Ophthalmol. 1964;72:309–14.
5. Johnson DL, Nieto JC, Ip MS. Retinal Detachment Due to an Outer Retinal Tear Following Laser Prophylaxis for Retinoschisis. Arch Ophthalmol. 2008;126(12):1775–1776.
6. Sulonen JM, Wells CG, Barricks ME, Verne AZ, Kalina RE, Hilton GF. Degenerative retinoschisis with giant outer layer breaks and retinal detachment. Am J Ophthalmol. 1985;99(2):114–21.
7. Ambler JS, Meyers SM, Zegarra H, Gutman FA. The management of retinal detachment complicating degenerative retinoschisis. Am J Ophthalmol. 1989;107:171–6.
8. Desjarlais EB, Garza PS, Johnson MW, Jayasundera T. Successful surgical treatment of maculainvolving degenerative retinoschisis by vitrectomy and drainage of the schisis cavity. Retin Cases Brief Rep. 2022;16(1):73–6.
9. Avitabile T, Ortisi E, Scott IU, Russo V, Gagliano C, Reibaldi A. Scleral buckle for progressive symptomatic retinal detachment complicating retinoschisis versus primary rhegmatogenous retinal detachment. Can J Ophthalmol. 2010;45(2):161–5.
10. Garneau J, Hébert M, You E, Lachance A, Bourgault S, Caissie M, Tourville É, Dirani A. Outcomes of surgical repair of Retinoschisis-associated retinal detachment compared to Rhegmatogenous retinal detachment. BMC Ophthalmol. 2022;22(1):10.
11. Lincoff H, Kreissig I, Uram D. Minor surgery for the repair of retinal detachment emanating from retinoschisis. Acta Ophthalmol. 2009;87(3):281–4.

Surgical Management of Epiretinal Membranes and Vitreomacular Traction

Ron A. Adelman and Marez Megalla

This chapter reviews the literature and discusses the surgical management of epiretinal membranes (ERM) and vitreomacular traction (VMT), which are disorders of the vitreoretinal interface.

1 Anomalous Posterior Vitreous Detachment

Posterior vitreous detachment (PVD) is defined as a separation between the posterior vitreous cortex and the inner limiting membrane (ILM) of the retina and is typically innocuous. Anomalous PVD with the incomplete separation of the posterior hyaloid from the retina may result in various vitreoretinal pathological signs due to static and dynamic tractional forces on the retina [1] (Fig. 1).

Supplementary Information The online version contains supplementary material available at https://doi.org/10.1007/978-3-031-47827-7_13.

R. A. Adelman (✉)
Department of Ophthalmology, Mayo Clinic, Jacksonville, FL, USA

Ophthalmology and Visual Science, Yale University School of Medicine, New Haven, CT, USA
e-mail: ron.adelman@yale.edu

M. Megalla
Ophthalmology, Yale School of Medicine, New Haven, CT, USA

A. B. Sallam et al. (eds.), *Practical Manual of Vitreoretinal Surgery*,
https://doi.org/10.1007/978-3-031-47827-7_13

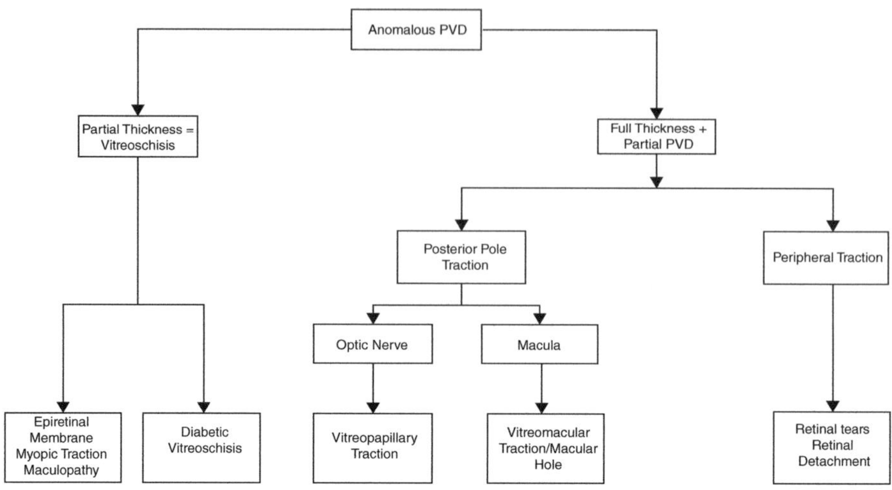

Fig. 1 Various vitreoretinal pathology that may arise from anomalous posterior vitreous detachment. (Courtesy of Ahmed Sallam, MD, PhD, USA)

2 Background, Causes, and Classifications

Vitreomacular traction describes the tenting of the retina due to the traction from the hyaloid face after partial vitreous detachment. The International Vitreomacular Traction Study Group developed a classification system to uniformly differentiate between vitreomacular adhesion, VMT, and macular holes [2]. Figure 2 shows the different patterns of VMT. ERM can be present in cases of VMT in about 20% of cases [3].

ERM consists of a layer of gliosis, cellular proliferation, and collagen fibrils forming on the inner retina. The etiology of ERM includes diabetic and vascular retinopathies, inflammation, trauma, retinal laser, cryopexy, intraocular surgery, or idiopathic epiretinal membrane (primary). The latter is more commonly encountered, with an incidence of about 5–18% in the general population. The development of ERM is thought to be related to the presence of residual cortical

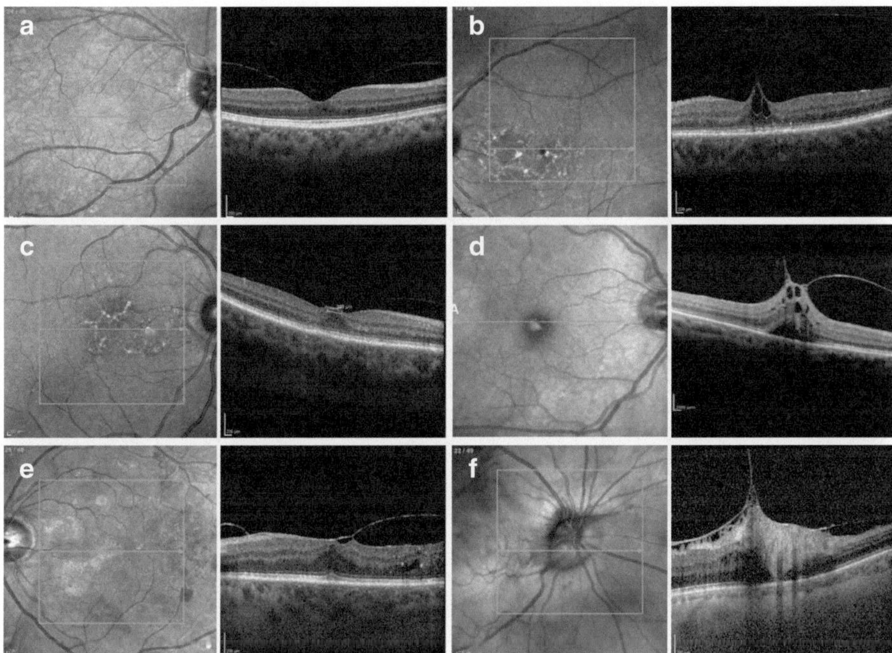

Fig. 2 Different patterns of vitreomacular traction (VMT), including vitreomacular adhesion (VMA), defined as perifoveal vitreous separation with remaining vitreomacular attachment and undisturbed foveal morphologic features (**a**), focal VMT (**b**), focal VMT with subretinal and intraretinal fluid (**c**), focal VMT with increased area of traction (**d**), broad VMT defined as more than 1500 μm area of adhesion (**e**), and vitreopapillary traction (VPT) (**f**)

vitreous on ILM surface secondary to a anomalous PVD or due to a break in the ILM that occurs with the separation of the posterior hyaloid, allowing the proliferation of glial cells on the retinal surface [4]. Inflammatory mediators also promote fibrocellular growth, especially in the setting of secondary ERM formation.

With the advancement and widespread use of optical coherence tomography (OCT), a classification of ERM based on whether the foveal pit is present and the definition of the retinal layers has been proposed [5], Fig. 3.

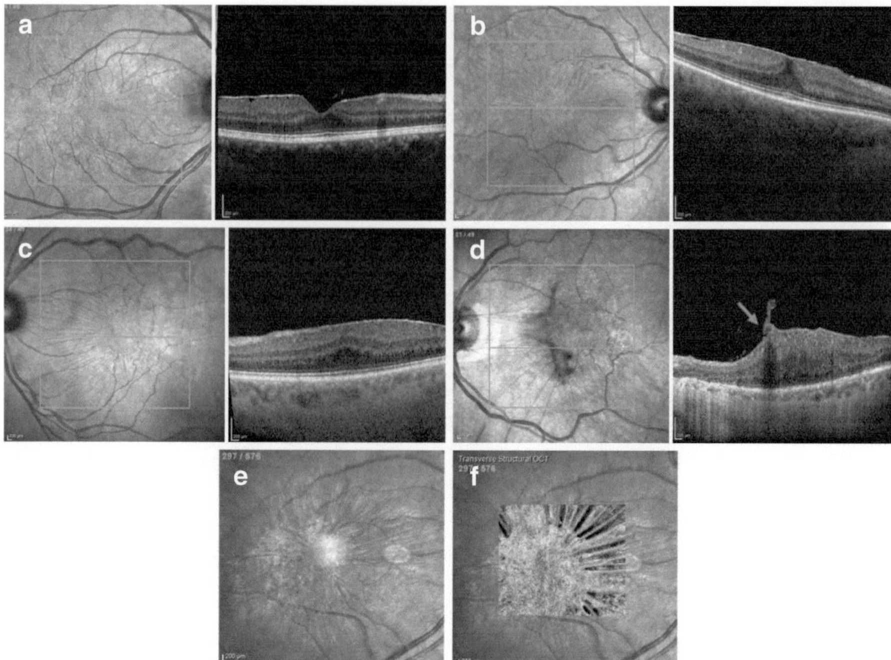

Fig. 3 Classification of epiretinal membrane (ERM) based on the status of the foveal pit and definition of the retinal layers. Stage 1, ERMs are mild and thin, and foveal depression is present (**a**). Stage 2, ERMs are associated with the widening of the outer nuclear layer and loss of the foveal depression (**b**). Stage 3, ERMs are associated with significant inner layer thickening and ectopic inner foveal layers crossing the entire foveal area (**c**). Stage 4, ERMs are thick, associated with continuous ectopic inner foveal layers, and retinal layers are disrupted (**d**). Also, note the schisis of the retinal nerve fiber layer in this case (arrow) (**d**). Enface optical coherence tomography photographs of a stage 3 ERM highlighting the extent of retinal traction (**e–f**)

3 Preoperative Assessment

- Primary ERM is more common in patients over the age of 60 years, while secondary ERM may occur at an earlier age.
- In VMT and ERM, patients often complain of decreased vision, photopsia, and metamorphopsia; however, patients with both entities could also be asymptomatic or have minimal non-disturbing symptoms.
- Assessing lens status preoperatively to determine the level of visualization intraoperatively as well as the possibility of performing combined or staged cataract extraction with intraocular lens implantation (CEIOL) and pars plana vitrectomy (PPV) should be discussed with the patient.
- ERM appears on ophthalmoscopic examination as a translucent, transparent, or pigmented membrane on the inner retinal surface with distortion of the outer and/or the inner retina.

- Do not presume that the ERM is primary until you exclude secondary causes. Examine the retina to diagnose/exclude retinal tears/RRD, posterior uveitis, or vascular occlusion.
- Primary ERM is usually associated with PVD.
- Preoperative OCT is crucial in assessing the extent of vitreoretinal traction and retinal distortion, as well as the presence of macular edema secondary to ERM or VMT (Fig. 3e–f). In addition, OCT allows the evaluation of external limiting membrane (ELM) and the ellipsoid zone (EZ), whose level of disruption is a prognostic factor for visual acuity post-surgical intervention [5]. Schisis of the retinal nerve fiber layer (sRNFL) (Fig. 3d) is a finding that is observed in up to 50% of ERM cases and has surgical implications [6]. Due to the vertical arrangement of Muller cells, the central region of the fovea is especially susceptible to traction. On OCT, this may manifest as a hyperreflective spot between the ellipsoid zone and the interdigitation zone (referred to as cotton ball sign) due to the upward elongation of the cone photoreceptors, foveal detachment, and hyperreflective subretinal material [7]. These signs, at times, may be mistaken for neovascular age-related macular degeneration.

4 Indications for Treatment

VMT and ERM with no symptoms or good vision should only be observed. Some cases of VMT may spontaneously resolve. In a single center study of 183 eyes, VMT resolved in 20% at about 15 months with improvement of symptoms, persisted in 60%, 10% developed a macular hole, and 10% had PPV because of their symptoms. Predictors of spontaneous resolution included better presenting VA, lower foveal thickness, and no associated ERM [3]. Common indications for surgery include visual acuity of 20/40 or worse or symptoms such as significant metamorphopsia or visual distortion interfering with daily activities. Symptoms are usually more troublesome when present under binocular conditions (with both eyes opened). Recent evidence supports earlier surgery in symptomatic patients, given that worse baseline visual acuity, increased glial proliferation, and total cellular density are important predictors of worse postoperative vision [4].

5 Non-surgical Treatment

Non-surgical management of VMT has been widely studied. Use of ocriplasmin, a recombinant protease targeting fibronectin which is involved in the adhesion between the vitreous face and internal limiting membrane, resolves VMT in 40–50% of patients. Positive prognostic factors of ocriplasmin success included female gender, age younger than 65, phakic status, and VMT area $\leq$ 1500 µm, as well as no ERM [8]. Adverse events included photopsia, vitreous floaters, and rarely retinal detachment [9]. Due to the high rate of adverse events and suboptimal efficacy, ocriplasmin is rarely used. While pneumatic vitreolysis has shown promise in releasing VMT in 70% of patients, including those who failed prior ocriplasmin, adverse events, including pupillary block, loculated subretinal fluid, and retinal detachments, did develop [10, 11].

5.1 Considerations for Surgery

1. Possible cataract extraction and lens implantation.
2. Vitrectomy.
3. Staining.
4. Membrane peeling with or without internal limiting membrane peeling.
5. Possible intravitreal gas.
6. Adjuvant therapies.

5.2 Surgical Order for Phakic Patients

- In phakic patients with visually significant cataract, consider performing CEIOL and PPV.
- For phakic patients with visually significant cataract and VMT, performing staged CEIOL and PPV may be beneficial as some VMT may spontaneously release after CEIOL.

5.3 Pars Plana Vitrectomy vs. Nonvitrectomizing Vitreous Surgery

- Often, 23- or 25-gauge (g) vitrectomy is utilized. Long-term visual outcomes were noted to be similar although 25-g were found to have faster visual recovery within the first postoperative week [12]. 27-g vitrectomy requires more time with no difference in outcomes to 23- and 25-g [13].
- First described in 1987 and rarely utilized nowadays, nonvitrectomizing vitreous surgery (NVS) has been employed with all available vitrectomy gauge systems for ERM [14]. The peeled epiretinal membranes were either left in the vitreous cavity or removed through the sclerotomy site with any attached vitreous separated with microscissors. While central retinal thickness outcomes were similar to groups receiving standard vitrectomy, NVS groups presented with preretinal hemorrhage, postoperative hypotony, and increased rates of ERM recurrence. NVS groups did, however, have significantly lower rates of postoperative cataract.

5.4 Staining

Type of Stains

- Most surgeons prefer to stain the ERM or ILM to facilitate visualization and peeling.
- Diluted ICG has been used for staining ILM. Care in concentration and length of retinal exposure to the stain, however, must be utilized as toxicity has been described. When using staining, we recommend low concentrations and minimal time exposure to the retina with a diffuse light source to limit phototoxicity [15].
- Brilliant blue G (BBG) in 0.25 mg/mL concentrations for ILM staining is reported to have lower light toxicity than ICG and is gaining increasing popularity [16].
- Although trypan blue (TB) has less reported retinal toxicity than ICG, TB does not stain the ILM well, requires air-fluid exchange before injection into the eye, and often needs to be mixed with glucose to increase its density compared to balanced salt solution (BSS), thereby increasing time of contact with the retina [16, 17].
- Diluted triamcinolone ($\leq$10 mg/mL), which integrates into the collagen fibers of the membrane surface, can help to identify the posterior hyaloid face but cannot differentiate residual ILM from the surrounding structures [18].

Technique of Staining

- After vitrectomy is performed, we inject the stain while the vitreous cavity is filled with fluid (termed wet technique) to identify and peel the ERM (Video 1). Sometimes to ensure adequate removal of the ERM and ILM, the stain is injected again (termed double stain technique).
- Some surgeons describe staining under air (termed dry technique) or using the double stain technique [16].

5.5 Peeling

Preoperative or Intraoperative Optical Coherence Tomography (OCT)

- Using the guidance of OCT, identify corrugations, the thickest part of the membrane, or where the membrane is most elevated above the retina [6]. If intraoperative OCT is available, it may preclude the need for staining for ERM peeling/VMT release identification of posterior hyaloid status, sRNFL (Fig. 4), and confirmation of complete ERM removal. Also, intraoperative OCT can be useful in identifying intraoperative events such unroofed cysts or macular hole formation. These occurrences may have implications for the surgical outcome, necessitating adjustments to the operative plan, which may include performing an ILM peel and utilizing intraocular gas [19].

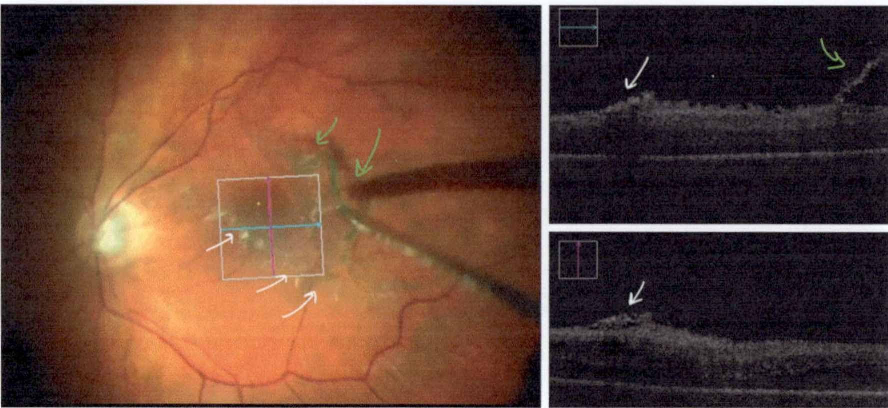

Fig. 4 Intraoperative view of the retina with corresponding intraoperative optical coherence tomography scans showing an area of schisis of the retinal nerve fiber layer (white arrows). The edge of the epiretinal membrane stained with indocyanin green dye is marked by green arrows

Instrumentation and Technique

- A macular lens is often used to magnify the fovea and membranes.
- If an edge is not already present, consider creating an edge inferotemporal to the fovea near the vascular arcades. Several instruments have been developed to initiate an edge and perpetuate the peel. We often use either vitreoretinal forceps to create a flap from traction or shearing in a rocking motion in the "pinch and grab technique" [20] or a thin membrane loop which has been shown to have less frequent inner retinal disruption on OCT [21]. A diamond-dusted membrane scraper, in which diamond fragments cover a silicone-tipped cannula to abrade the membrane creating an edge, can result in crescentic inner retinal defects and retinal diamond deposits using the scraper [22].
- We complete the peel with the vitreoretinal forceps circumferentially about two-disc diameters around the fovea.
- Recently, a micro-vacuum pick was developed as an all-in-one instrument to create a membrane edge, peel, and aspirate the membrane as well as perform fluid-air exchange; it has shown promising results in a preliminary study [23].

ILM Peel: "Double Peel"

- We routinely peel the internal limiting membrane (ILM) at the time of ERM surgery as although it does not improve the visual acuity, it may help reduce recurrences of ERM (Videos 2 and 3) [24, 25]. However, for VMT patients, removal of ILM is not necessary, and it was not found to result in significant visual outcomes (Video 4) [26]. Caution is needed when sRNFL is present, as due to axonal stasis, the area of nerve fiber schisis looks white and can be mistaken for ERM (Fig. 4). Also, dehiscence of the ILM is frequently present at the site of the schisis [6] (Video 5).

5.6 Intravitreal Gas Tamponade

- Generally, in the presence of retinal detachments or the development of total thickness macular holes, gas tamponade is employed. Without such complications, we do not use tamponade with gas but occasionally perform fluid-air exchange to decrease leakage through scleral ports. However, studies have shown it does not have an effect on visual outcomes [27].

5.7 Intravitreal Steroid vs. Nepafenac vs. No Adjuvant Therapy

- We do not routinely place intravitreal steroids or prescribe topical NSAIDs postoperatively as visual outcomes were not shown to be statistically different.

6 Surgery Outcomes

- Discussion with patients to manage their postoperative visual expectations is essential.
- About 80% of patients have visual improvement of about 2–3 Snellen lines with the improvement of distortion, but visual function rarely returns back to normal levels. In one study of primary ERM outcomes, average preoperative acuity was 20/80, and 43% of patients reached a postoperative visual acuity of 20/40 or better after 3–6 months [28].
- Improvement in visual functions after ERM surgery is slower than with cataract surgery. However, it is of note that distortion as compared to VA improves early on after ERM peel [29]. Most of the changes in VA and central macular thickness take place during the first 3 months and stabilize by 1-year post-surgery [4, 28].
- Improvement of outer retinal structure, ELM and EZ integrity on OCT, is a more important determinant for the long term visual acuity after ERM surgery then inner retinal paramaters such as improvement of foveal contour and CME resolution [30]. Histological biomarkers of poor visual prognosis after ERM surgery such as glial cell proliferation and increased total cellularity are usually present before vision significantly deteriorates and retinal structure changes are noted on OCT. These findings support early surgery for significantly symptomatic ERM.

- When compared to eyes with primary ERM, eyes with secondary ERM group usually had worse preoperative VA, slower visual recovery, and a twofold increase in postoperative CME [28].
- ERM may recur in up 10% of cases, and 5% may require reoperation [28, 31].

7 Intraoperative Complications

Focal intraretinal hemorrhages and retinal breaks occasionally occur in PPV for VMT surgery, with one meta-analysis reporting 5.6% and 1.6%, respectively [26]. Iatrogenic retinal breaks in ERM surgery were cited at 7% prevalence in one study [32]. that included cases operated with 20-, 23- and 25-g instruments with odds being higher with 20-g.

8 Postoperative Complications

As in other indications of vitrectomy, cataract is a common complication of surgery, and vitreous hemorrhage and retinal detachment are occasional complications. Postoperatively, the superficial and deep foveal avascular zone was noted to be significantly larger than in the preoperative setting; it has been suggested that recovery of the foveal avascular zone from the shearing of the ERM occurs slowly [33]. In addition, ILM peels and intravitreal gas tamponades were more associated with dissociated optic nerve fiber layer (DONFL) postoperatively (Fig. 5) [34]. Macular holes can develop following ILM peels, with one study citing an incidence of 2.6%. While most of the holes were eccentric and did not require surgery, there was a 0.5% incidence of central macular holes needing repair [35].

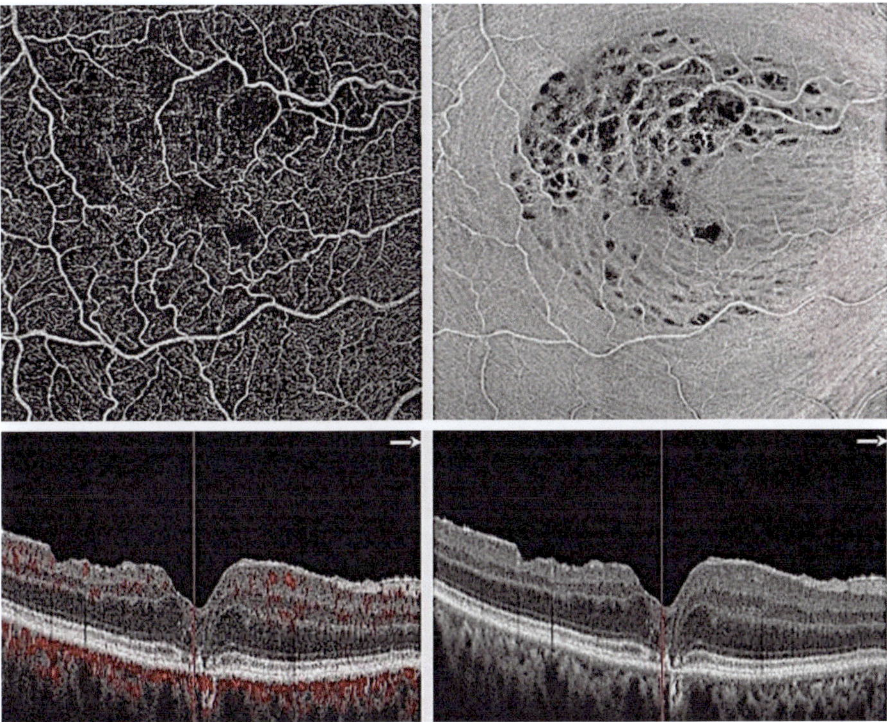

Fig. 5 Postoperative optical coherence tomography (OCT) of dissociated optic nerve fiber layer (DONFL) after combined epiretinal and internal limiting membrane peel. DONFL lesions are most obvious on the enface OCT scan (upper right image). (Courtesy of Mohamed Hassanein, MD, Egypt)

9 Case Scenario (Video 2)

A 70-year-old man complained of distortion and decreased vision OS. Visual acuity (VA) was 20/60. OCT macula showed a thickened epiretinal membrane with loss of the foveal pit but distinct retinal layers. After risks, benefits, and alternatives of combined cataract pars plana vitrectomy with epiretinal membrane were discussed, the patient desired to proceed with surgery. Intraoperatively, PVD was present. Epiretinal membrane was stained with trypan blue and removed with forceps. ILM peel was performed. Symptoms and visual acuity improved after the surgery.

Key Points
- ERM and VMT present with metamorphopsia and distorted vision though they could be asymptomatic in early cases.
- Surgery should only be considered for patients with significant symptoms.
- Preoperative planning is essential for determining prognostic factors of visual outcomes after surgical repair.

- Several stains and techniques have been employed for staining and peeling the membranes.
- ILM peeling has been associated with nerve fiber layer defect and may be best avoided in diabetics and in glaucoma patients.

References

1. Sebag J. Vitreous and vision degrading myodesopsia. Prog Retin Eye Res. 2020;79:100847.
2. Duker J, Kaiser P, Binder S, de Smet M, et al. The international vitreomacular traction study group classification of vitreomacular adhesion, traction, and macular holes. Ophthalmology. 2013;12(12):2611–9.
3. Errera MH, Liyanage SE, Petrou P, Keane PA, Moya R, Ezra E, Charteris DG, Wickham L. A Study of the Natural History of Vitreomacular Traction Syndrome by OCT Ophthalmology. 2018;125(5):701–707.
4. Wang LC, Lo WJ, Huang YY, Chou YB, Li AF, Chen SJ, Chou TY, Lin TC. Correlations between clinical and histopathologic characteristics in idiopathic epiretinal membrane. Ophthalmology. 2022;129(12):1421–8.
5. Govetto A, Lalane R, Sarraf D, Figueroa M, et al. Insights into epiretinal membranes: presence of ectopic inner foveal layers and a new optical coherence tomography staging scheme. Am J Ophthalmol. 2017;175:99–113.
6. Hussnain SA, Sharma T, Hood DC, Chang S. Schisis of the retinal nerve fiber layer in epiretinal membranes. Am J Ophthalmol. 2019;207:304–12.
7. Govetto A, Bhavsar KV, Virgili G, Gerber MJ, Freund KB, Curcio CA, et al. Tractional abnormalities of the central foveal bouquet in epiretinal membranes: clinical spectrum and pathophysiological perspectives. Am J Ophthalmol. 2017;184:167–80.
8. Varma R, Haller R, Kaiser P. Improvement in patient reported visual function after ocriplasmin for vitreomacular adhesion: results of the microplasmin for intravitreous injection traction release without surgical treatment (MINI-TRUST) trials. JAMA Ophthalmol. 2015;133(9):997–1004.
9. Tadayoni R, Holz F, Zech C, Liu X, et al. Assessment of anatomical and functional outcomes with ocriplasmin treatment in patients with. Vitreomacular traction with or without macular holes: results of OVIID-1 trial. Retina. 2019;39(12):2341–52.
10. Chan C, Mein C, Glassman A, Beaulieu W, et al. Pneumatic vitreolysis with C3F8 for vitreomacular traction with and without macular hole: DRCR retina network protocols AG and AH. Ophthalmology. 2021;S0161-6420(21):00353–5.
11. Crosson J, Thomley M, Chan C, Mein C. Loculated subretinal fluid after pneumatic vitreolysis. Am J Ophthalmol Case Rep. 2019;11:100462.
12. Sandali O, El Sanharawi M, Lecuen N, Barale P, et al. 25-, 23-, and 20- gauge vitrectomy in epiretinal membrane surgery: a comparative study of 553 cases. Graefes Arch Clin Exp Ophthalmol. 2011;249(12):1811–9.
13. Naruse S, Shimada H, Mori R. 27-gauge and 25-gauge vitrectomy day surgery for idiopathic epiretinal membrane. BMC Ophthalmol. 2017;17(1):188.
14. Reibaldi M, Longo A, Avitabile T, Bonfiglio V, et al. Transconjunctival nonvitrectomizing vitreous surgery versus 25-gauge vitrectomy in patients with epiretinal membrane: a prospective randomized study. Retina. 2015;35(5):873–9.
15. Rodrigues E, Meyer C, Farah M, et al. Intravitreal staining of the internal limiting membrane using indocyanine green in the treatment of macular holes. Ophthalmologica. 2005;219:251–62.
16. Bergamo V, Caiado R, Maia A, Magalhaes O Jr, et al. Role of vital dyes in chromovitrectomy. Asia Pac J Ophthalmol (Phila). 2021;10:26–8.

17. Haritoglou C, Eibl K, Schaumberger M, Mueller A, et al. Functional outcome after trypan blue assisted vitrectomy for macular pucker: a prospective, randomized comparative trial. Am J Ophthalmol. 2004;138(1):1–5.
18. Ashai M, Wallsh J, Gallemore R. Outcomes of epiretinal membrane removal utilizing triamcinolone acetonide visualization and internal limiting membrane forceps. Clin Ophthalmol. 2020;14:3913–21.
19. Heidi J, Huang D. Damla, Sevgi Sunil K, Srivastava Jamie, Reese Justis P, Ehlers. Vitreomacular Traction Surgery from the DISCOVER Study: Intraoperative OCT Utility Ellipsoid Zone Dynamics and Outcomes Ophthalmic Surgery Lasers and Imaging Retina. 2021;52(10):544–550.
20. Haug SJ, McDonald HR. Clinical pearls for performing ILM peeling in vitreoretinal surgery. Retin Physician. 2014;11:53–7.
21. Uchida A, Srivastava S, Ehlers J. Analysis of retinal architectural changes using intraoperative OCT following surgical manipulations with membrane flex loop in the DISCOVER study. Invest Ophthalmol Vis Sci. 2017;58(9):3440–4.
22. Lewis JM, Park I, Ohji M, Saito Y, Tano Y. Diamond-dusted silicone cannula for epiretinal membrane separation during vitreous surgery. Am J Ophthalmol. 1997;4:552–4.
23. Awh C, Bass E. A microsurgical vacuum pick for membrane peeling without forceps during vitreoretinal surgery. Ophthalmic Surg Lasers Imaging Retina. 2020;51(3):196–9.
24. Azuma K, Ueta T, Eguchi S, Aihara M. Effects of internal limiting membrane peeling combined with removal of idiopathic epiretinal membrane a systematic review of literature and meta-analysis. Retina. 2017;37(10):1813–9.
25. Sun Y, Zhou R, Zhang B. WITH OR WITHOUT INTERNAL LIMITING MEMBRANE PEELING FOR IDIOPATHIC EPIRETINAL MEMBRANE: a meta-analysis of randomized controlled trials. Retina. 2021;41(8):1644–51.
26. Jackson T, Nicod E, Angelis A, Grimaccia F, et al. Pars plana vitrectomy for vitreomacular traction. Syndrome a systematic review and metaanalysis of safety and efficacy. Retina. 2013;33(10):2012–7.
27. Emrani E, Matlach J, Guthoff R, Goebel W. Morphologic and functional outcome of epiretinal membrane surgery with and with-out gas tamponade—a pilot study. Invest Ophthalmol Vis Sci. 2014;55:3829.
28. Norton J, Soliman M, Yang Y, Kurup S, et al. Visual outcomes of primary versus secondary epiretinal membrane following vitrectomy and cataract surgery. Graefes Arch Clin Exp Ophthalmol. 2022;260:817–25.
29. Yoshikazu, Ichikawa Y, Imamura M, Ishida. METAMORPHOPSIA AND TANGENTIAL RETINAL DISPLACEMENT AFTER EPIRETINAL MEMBRANE SURGERY Retina. 2017;37(4):673–679.
30. Elhusseiny AM, Flynn HW Jr, Smiddy WE. Long-Term Outcomes After Idiopathic Epiretinal Membrane Surgery. Clin Ophthalmol. 2020;14:995–1002.
31. Grewing R, Mester U. Results of surgery for epiretinal membranes and their recurrences. Br J Ophthalmol. 1996;80:323–6.
32. Fajgenbaum M, Neffendorf J, Wong R, Laidlaw D, et al. Intraoperative and postoperative complications in phacovitrectomy for epiretinal membrane and macular hole: a clinical audit of 1000 consecutive eyes. Retina. 2018;38(9):1865–72.
33. Yoon Y, Woo J, Woo J, Min J. Superficial foveal avascular zone area changes before and after idiopathic epiretinal membrane surgery. Int J Ophthalmol. 2018;11(10):1711–5.
34. Park SM, Kim Y, Lee S. Incidence of and risk factors for dissociated optic nerve fiber layer after epiretinal membrane surgery. Retina. 2016;36(8):1469–73.
35. Rush R, Simunovic M, Aragon A, Ysasaga J. Postoperative macular hole formation after vitrectomy with internal limiting membrane peeling for the treatment of epiretinal membrane. Retina. 2014;34(5):890–6.

Surgical Management of Lamellar Macular Hole

Tarek Hammam, Hussain Ahmad Khaqan, and Mohamed Tawfik

Lamellar macular hole (LMH) is a partial-thickness macular change characterized by an irregular foveal contour, a break in the inner fovea, and a dehiscence of the inner foveal retina from the outer retina due to disruption of the Mullers cells in the foveal cone. There is no full-thickness foveal defect [1].

1   Causes and Pathogenesis

- The prevalence of LMH in the general population ranges from 1.1 to 3.6% [2].
- LMH is generally idiopathic. Other causes include ocular trauma, previous retinal surgery, uveitis, CME, and systemic diseases such as Alport syndrome.
- The pathogenesis of LMH has yet to be fully understood. However, there are three subtypes identified: [3]

  - Tractional LMH is usually associated with conventional thin hyperreflective ERM and is thought to be due to anomalous PVD with ERM.

Supplementary Information The online version contains supplementary material available at https://doi.org/10.1007/978-3-031-47827-7_14.

T. Hammam
Ophthalmology, Shrewsbury and Telford NHS Trust, Shrewsbury, UK
e-mail: Tarek.Hammam@nhs.net

H. A. Khaqan
Ophthalmology, PGMI, AMC, Lahore General Hospital, Lahore, Lahore, Punjab, Pakistan

M. Tawfik (✉)
Retina Department, Memorial Institute of Ophthalmic Research, Giza, Egypt

A. B. Sallam et al. (eds.), *Practical Manual of Vitreoretinal Surgery*,
https://doi.org/10.1007/978-3-031-47827-7_14

- Degenerative form with a thick iso-reflective ERM, schisis-like configuration often associated with outer retinal structure changes including external limiting membrane, and ellipsoid layer disruption.
- Mixed type.

2 Clinical Features

- Idiopathic cases of LMH are usually seen in older patients.
- LMHs can be asymptomatic in many cases. Patients may complain of metamorphopsia, decreased vision, and central scotoma when symptomatic.
- It is essential to correlate symptoms with macular changes. In many cases, symptoms such as central vision loss may be related to a pathology other than LMH, such as a coexisting cataract. The presence of metamorphopsia points out to a macular cause.
- Clinically, PVD is usually present, but may not be present in some cases. ERM coexists with LMH in up to 90% of cases.
- OCT is essential for diagnosing and identifying coexisting features such as vitreomacular traction, foveoschisis, and ERM. Two types of ERM have been identified based on OCT—thin, hyperreflective ERM and iso-reflective, thick epiretinal membrane, known as lamellar hole-associated epiretinal proliferation (LHEP) (Fig. 1) [3]. OCT also helps differentiate LMH from other non-surgical macular pathology with retinal thinning, such as macular telangiectasia.

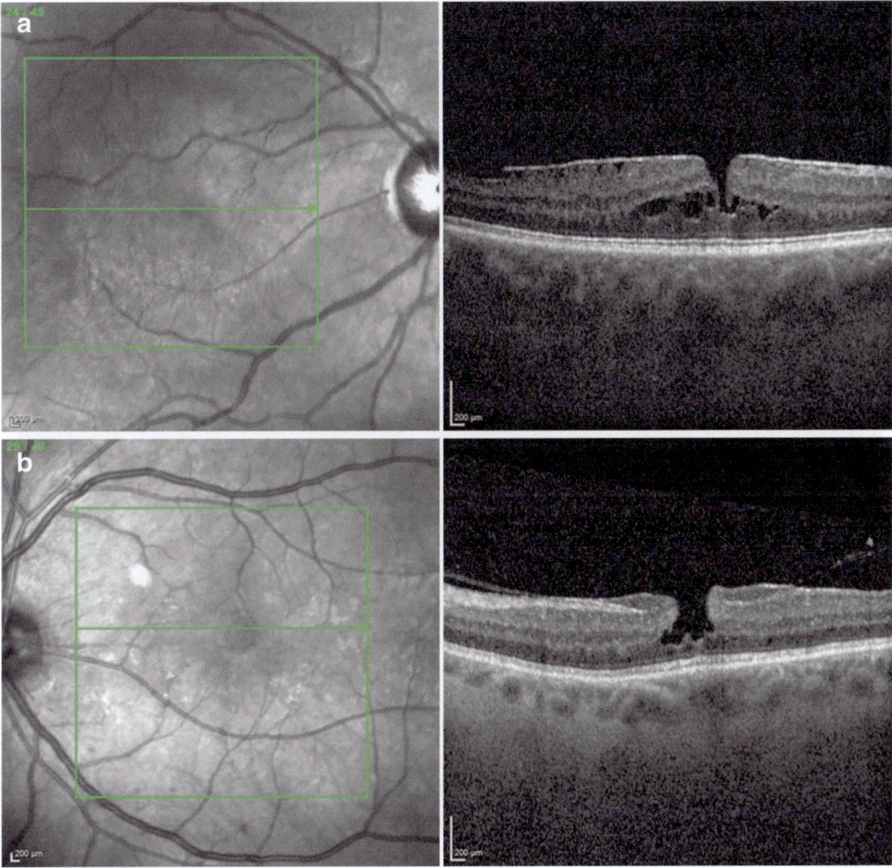

Fig. 1 Types of epiretinal membranes (ERM) associated with lamellar macular hole: thin hyper-reflective ERM (**a**) and (**b**) iso-reflective, thick epiretinal membrane, lamellar hole associated epiretinal proliferation (LHEP)

3   Natural Course and Treatment

- The natural course of LMH is benign with symptoms remaining stable over the years maintaining good vision (Fig. 2). Only a small number of cases exhibit progression or develop into full-thickness macular holes (FTMH) (Fig. 3) [1]. In a multicenter studies of approxiamtely 90 eyes, 10% of cases developed FTMH over 5 years and 15% lost ≥ 2 Snellens lines [4].
- Observation is, therefore, the main line of management. The indication for surgery in LMH is not well defined. Surgery in the form of PPV with induction of PVD if not present and ERM peel is offered mainly for cases with documented progressive visual symptoms (Video 1). Using air or gas tamponade was not shown to improve the outcome of LMH surgery [5].

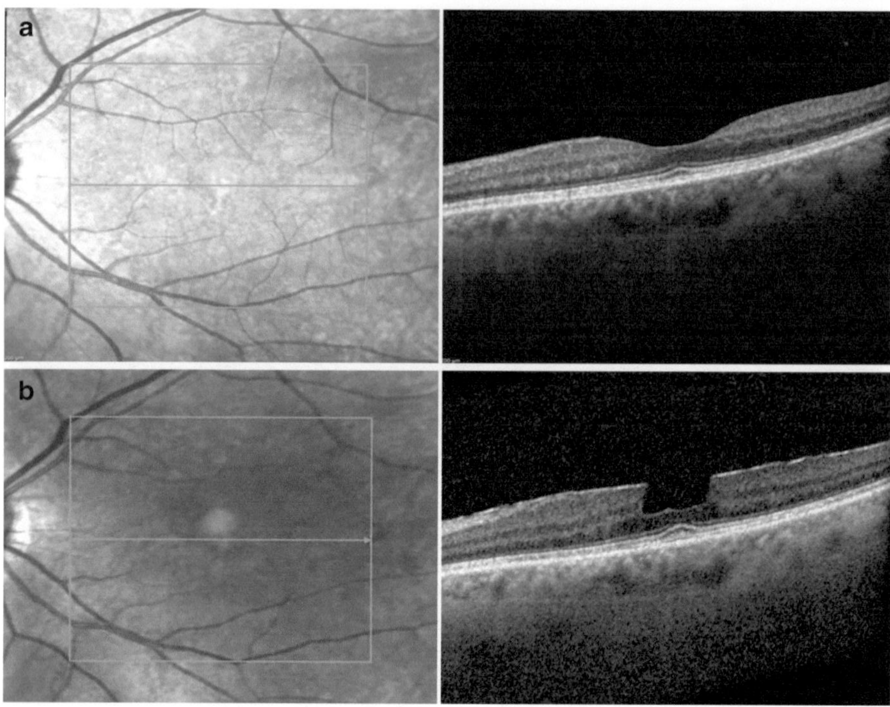

Fig. 2 A 64-year-old female with a normal left macula (**a**) developed lamellar macular hole (LMH) after 2 years of follow-up (**b**). The other eye had a small full thickness macular hole treated with pars plana vitrectomy SF6 gas without internal limiting membrane peel. The vision was 20/20 in the left eye, and LMH was therefore only observed

- The results of surgery for LMH in general are not as robust as for FTMH. Discordant outcomes have been reported regarding visual improvement ranging from no vision improvement to a 2–3 Snellen line gain [1, 2]. Generally, cases with conventional ERM achieve better vision gain than those with LHEP [6]. Eyes presenting with LHEP also have an increased risk of developing an FTMH after surgery of approximately 10% [1, 4]. To reduce this risk, several options have been proposed such as not peeling the internal limiting membrane (ILM) over the fovea, sparing the center part of the LHEP, leaving it attached to the macular center, and even using combined ERM and ILM flaps to cover the macular hole to restore the macular architecture [7].

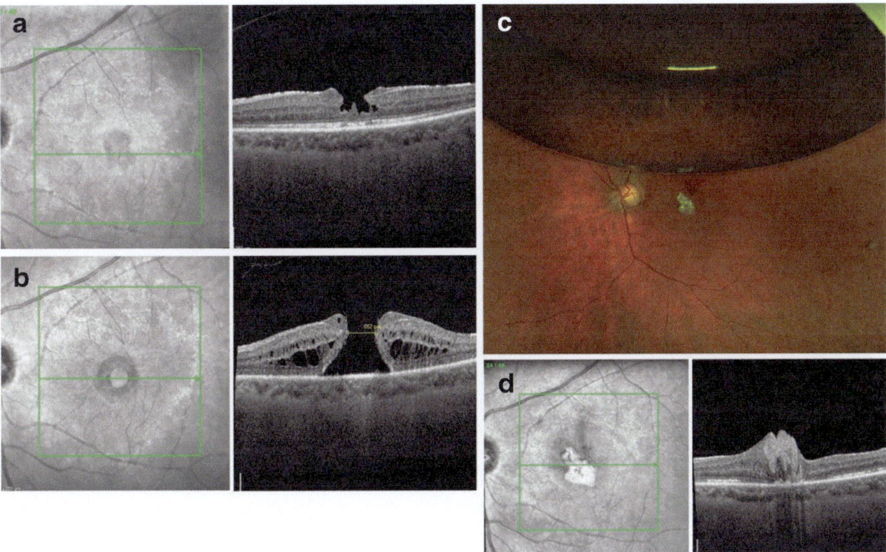

Fig. 3 Lamellar macular hole (LMH) with lamellar hole associated epiretinal proliferation (LHEP) and VA 20/30 (**a**). Progression after 4 years of follow-up to full thickness macular hole (FTMH) (**b**). FTMH was closed after vitrectomy, internal limiting membrane peel, amniotic membrane graft, and gas (**c** and **d**)

Key Points
- When reviewing patients with LMH, ascertain the reason for their symptoms, as LMH can be asymptomatic in the majority of cases.
- OCT helps determine the nature of LMH—tractional vs. degenerative.
- Observation is the main line of management of LMH.
- Be careful and conservative when undertaking ERM peel in the degnerative type of LMH due to the risk of FTMH.

References

1. Parisi G, Fallico M, Maugeri A, et al. Primary vitrectomy for degenerative and tractional lamellar macular holes: a systematic review and meta-analysis. PLoS One. 2021;16(3):e0246667.
2. Coassin M, Mori T, Di Zazzo A, Sgrulletta R, Varacalli G, Bonini S. Lamellar macular holes: monitoring and management strategies. Clin Ophthalmol. 2019;13:1173–82.
3. Witkin AJ, Ko TH, Fujimoto JG, et al. Redefining lamellar holes and the vitreomacular interface: an ultrahigh-resolution optical coherence tomography study. Ophthalmology. 2006;113(3):388–97.
4. Chehaibou I, Tadayoni R, Hubschman JP, et al. Natural history and surgical outcomes of lamellar macular holes. Ophthalmol Retina. 2024(3):210–22.
5. Sato T, Emi K, Bando H, Ikeda T. Retrospective comparisons of vitrectomy with and without air tamponade to repair lamellar macular hole. Ophthalmic Surg Lasers Imaging Retina. 2015;46(1):38–43.

6. Xu H, Qin L, Zhang Y, Xiao Y, Zhang M. Surgery outcomes of lamellar macular eyes with or without lamellar hole-associated epiretinal proliferation: a meta-analysis. BMC Ophthalmol. 2020;20(1):345.
7. Frisina R, Tozzi L, Gius I, Pilotto E, Midena E. Novel approaches to the assessment and treatment of lamellar macular hole. Acta Ophthalmol. 2021;100:e1287.

Surgical Management of Macular Holes

Kevin Eid, Ryan A. Shields, and Tamer H. Mahmoud

1   Introduction

Macular holes are an anatomical defect involving the fovea that typically arises from vitreomacular forces disrupting the foveal architecture and adhesion to the underlying retinal pigment epithelium (RPE). Macular holes can be classified as primary (idiopathic) or secondary, with primary idiopathic holes accounting for 87.1% of the total cases [1]. The most common secondary etiologies include high myopia, trauma, macular schisis, and age-related macular degeneration [2]. In the general adult population, macular holes are a relatively uncommon cause of decreased vision, represented by an annual incidence of 4–8.7 cases per 100,000 people; however, the prevalence of macular holes is threefold higher in women [3].

Supplementary Information The online version contains supplementary material available at https://doi.org/10.1007/978-3-031-47827-7_15.

K. Eid
Oakland University William Beaumont School of Medicine, Rochester, MI, USA

R. A. Shields
Associated Retinal Consultants, Royal Oak, MI, USA

T. H. Mahmoud (✉)
Oakland University William Beaumont School of Medicine, Rochester, MI, USA

Associated Retinal Consultants, Royal Oak, MI, USA

A. B. Sallam et al. (eds.), *Practical Manual of Vitreoretinal Surgery*, https://doi.org/10.1007/978-3-031-47827-7_15

2   Macular Hole Pathogenesis

The pathogenesis of idiopathic macular holes is highly contingent on the presence of vitreomacular adhesion in the fovea. The posterior hyaloid typically will detach from the posterior pole, including the optic nerve and fovea, leading to a posterior vitreous detachment (PVD). In instances where the posterior hyaloid remains attached to the fovea, anteroposterior contraction is the predominant force inducing a full-thickness macular hole (FTMH). The impact of vitreomacular traction (VMT) on macular hole development is evidenced by a significantly lower incidence of bilateral macular hole if the fellow eye has a complete PVD (11.7% in non-PVD vs. <2% in PVD) [4]. Additionally, tangential forces induced by the internal limiting membrane (ILM) are also involved in the development of a macular hole.

3   Classification of Macular Holes

Gass classified macular holes into four stages before the availability of optical coherence tomography (OCT). Stage 1 represents an impending macular hole. OCT will reveal VMT and abnormalities of the outer fovea without a full-thickness defect. Stage 2 represents a small hole <400 μm with persistent VMT. Stage 3 is a hole ≥400 μm with a small operculum covering the FTMH. Stage 4 has the same findings in stage 3 with a complete PVD [5]. Recently, FTMH have been reclassified based on three factors:

1. Size, as seen on OCT: small (<250 μm minimal linear diameter), medium (250–400 μm), and large (>400 μm).
2. Etiology: primary or secondary.
3. Presence of VMT [2].

4   Management Overview for Macular Holes

Prior to the use of pars plana vitrectomy (PPV), the standard of care for FTMH was observation; however, the results were less than satisfying with spontaneous closure occurring in 50% of stage 1 holes, 11.4% of stage 2 holes, and 3% of stage 3 holes [4]. In the 1990s, PPV alone improved the hole closure rate to 58% by removing anteroposterior vitreous traction from the fovea [6]. The surgical closure rate with PPV was further improved with the addition of the internal limiting membrane (ILM) peel [7]. There are multiple benefits of an ILM peel. First, any residual vitreous cortex is removed, ensuring negligible anteroposterior traction. Second, there is a reduction in the tangential traction circumferentially around the macula which improves the compliance to the retina. Third, there is a decreased risk for subsequent epiretinal tissue proliferation post-surgery. A greater success rate was achieved with ILM peeling once ICG (indocyanine green) was introduced in macular hole surgery to stain and identify the ILM to facilitate peeling [8]. In its current iteration, PPV with ILM peel has a single-surgery success rate of over 90% for idiopathic macular holes [9]. Despite this excellent single-surgery success rate, multiple features have been associated with surgical failure despite PPV with ILM peel.

- **Large Size**: Success decreases from 90% in holes with a minimal linear diameter of 400–649 μm to 76% in holes with a minimal linear diameter of 650–1419 μm [10]. Other studies have reported an even lower success rate of 50–60% in FTMH over 500 μm [11].
- **Chronicity**: Success decreases from 90% if surgical repair occurs within a year of symptom onset to <50% in those with delayed surgery beyond 1 year of symptom onset [12].
- **Myopia**: PPV with ILM peel success rate approaches 100% in eyes with normal axial length (AL <26 mm); however, the success rate drops to 91.7% in eyes with an AL of 26.0–29.9 mm and to 0% when AL is ≥30 mm [13].

5 Surgical Strategies

Once vitrectomy is initiated, confirmation of a PVD is paramount. If the posterior hyaloid is still attached to the posterior pole, a PVD must be induced. Multiple techniques can be employed in inducing a PVD including an aspirating cannula, microvitreoretinal (MVR) blade, or forceps; however, modern-day vitrectomy probe design is highly effective in aspirating and detaching the posterior hyaloid (Video 1). In cases of extremely difficult PVD induction, one can proceed with the ILM peel. This will create an opening in the posterior hyaloid, facilitating the induction of a PVD.

After PVD induction and vitrectomy, focus is then given to the ILM peel. Though not necessary, most surgeons prefer dyes (indocyanine green [ICG] or brilliant blue if available) to enhance ILM visualization. ICG is a highly selective stain for ILM but can be associated with RPE toxicity with high concentrations or long exposure time. It is strongly recommended that ICG be diluted to a concentration of 0.025% or less to minimize toxicity. Additionally, dilution with 5% dextrose solution is very helpful in increasing the osmolarity of the solution, allowing for excellent layering over the macula. Typically, ICG is left on the macula for less than 45 s.

The initiation of the ILM peel is often the most difficult step of the procedure, and thus, numerous techniques have been reported. ILM forceps can be used to gently pinch and then tear a flap of ILM with minimal damage to the underlying nerve fiber layer. Because of the risk of an aggressive (or deep) grasp of the retina with the "pinch and peel" technique, instruments including a diamond-dusted scraper or flex loop have been developed to atraumatically initiate and even complete the ILM peel (Video 1). A plethora of different techniques of utilizing the ILM for hole closure have been developed and will be covered subsequently.

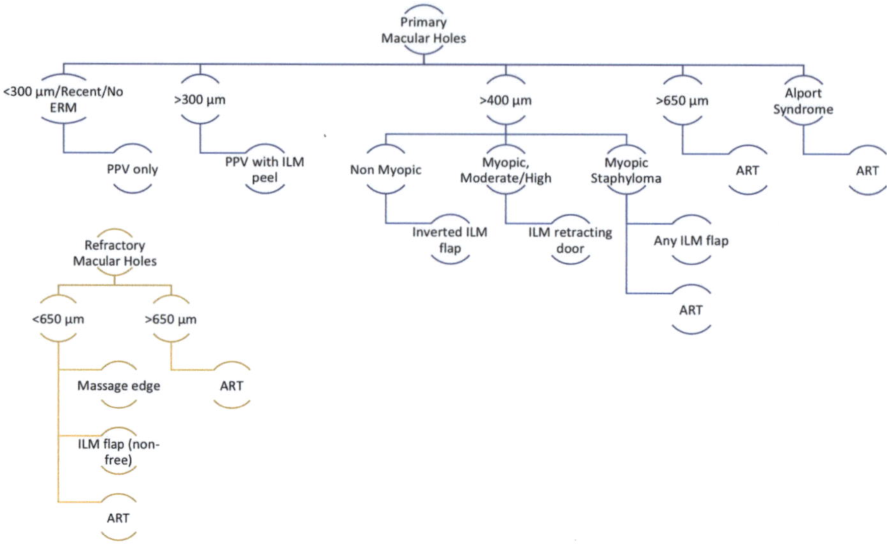

Fig. 1 Surgical preference flowchart based on etiology and minimal linear diameter

Figure 1 illustrates the current authors' algorithm in selecting the optimal procedure and/or modification in managing the range of macular holes and will serve as an outline for the rest of the chapter.

6 Small Holes

Small (<300 µm minimal linear diameter) primary stage 1 or 2 FTMH in the absence of other risk factors have a very high spontaneous closure rate and may benefit from observation for 4–6 weeks. If surgery is undertaken, either a PPV alone or a PPV with ILM peel is highly successful.

7 Medium Holes

Medium-sized (<400 µm minimal linear diameter) primary holes, or those with an associated epiretinal membrane (ERM), can be successfully treated with PPV and ILM peel. ILM peel width varies from 0.5 to 3 disc diameter (DD) around the fovea and is surgeon- and patient-dependent. Wide ILM peel does not affect the closure rate for holes of this size [9].

8   Large or Chronic Holes (Non-myopic)

Large primary (<650 μm minimal linear diameter) or chronic (>1 year) holes can be treated with a standard PPV with ILM peel, though ILM scaffold techniques may offer a greater primary closure rate. Of note, the Manchester study showed that over 90% of FTMH <650 μm closed with a wide ILM peel (arcade-to-arcade) and long-acting gas tamponade [10]. However, the ILM flap may provide more scaffold to facilitate closure and preserves more ILM for future use in case of a failed initial procedure. The ILM scaffold provides mechanical support for hole closure and a platform for proliferating Müller cells to grow on and release growth factors [14]. The most common ILM scaffolding techniques can be broadly categorized into two categories: inverted and non-inverted ILM flaps.

8.1   *Inverted Internal Limiting Membrane Flap*

In an inverted ILM flap, the ILM is peeled toward the macular hole edge and then inverted over the hole, completely covering it. What was originally the outer face of ILM is now directly facing the hole, no longer in direct contact with the vitreous cavity. This procedure provides the macular hole a structural scaffold to close and heal which has shown to be more effective than traditional ILM peel in large macular holes and macular holes in myopic eyes. A randomized controlled trial has shown that in FTMH sized 600–1500 μm, inverted ILM flap had a success rate of 90% compared to 70% in standard ILM peel [15]. In addition to an increased surgical success rate, a meta-analysis of multiple RCTs and retrospective studies shows that inverted ILM yielded a superior short-term visual acuity recovery than ILM peel in FTMH >400 μm [16].

The primary difficulty with the inverted ILM flap is maintaining the inverted positioning in the intraoperative and early postoperative periods. A temporal inverted flap allows suction forces at the disc during the fluid-air exchange to adequately position the flap over the macular hole and keep it in place.

9   Primary Myopic Holes

Multiple factors contribute to the high surgical failure in myopic holes including surgical difficulty from extreme axial length, the posterior staphylomatous contour exerting increased tangential traction, and high concurrence of retinal detachment with the macular hole [13, 17]. Due to these factors, additional support is needed to promote proper macular hole closure.

9.1   Inverted ILM Flap in High Myopic Macular Holes

Inverted ILM flap can be used to deflect anteroposterior traction while also increasing the closing force of the hole. In a large retrospective study of FTMH in high myopic eyes (>26 mm AL), it was shown that inverted ILM had a success rate of 88.4% vs. a success rate of 38.9% with traditional ILM peel [18]. For deep myopic staphyloma, it is very challenging to reach and design a flap. In such cases, any type of flap may help the closure including the perifoveal ILM tissue that can be folded 360° to cover the hole. Another challenge is that staining is usually very faint. A few tips can be incorporated to achieve successful myopic flaps including long forceps, perfluorocarbon liquid (PFCL) to stabilize the flap, and a flat contact lens for visualization since non-contact systems may be in the way of the forceps when perpendicularly oriented to reach the depth of the staphyloma.

9.2   Retracting Door

The retracting door flap is similar to the inverted ILM flap discussed earlier, in that the ILM is peeled and then draped over the macular hole (Video 2). The difference is that no inversion of the ILM flap occurs. The ILM is peeled from the nasal side of the macular hole, moving temporally as the peeled ILM goes around the hole [19]. The ILM is kept intact on the temporal side of the hole to act as a hinge for the peel. The peel is then draped back over the macular hole in a position where the hole is fully covered. Another benefit is that more ILM is preserved for future use in this procedure than in inverted flap or standard ILM peel.

OCT angiography (OCTA) shows that following PPV with ILM peel, there is nasal contraction of the macula [20]. In the retracting door technique, the tension of the taut flap counteracts this, allowing for a temporally directed tensile force of the ILM and a nasally directed contractile force of the retina, as visualized in Fig. 2. This technique can facilitate hole closure and retinal attachment in myopic macular holes while maintaining the proper orientation of ILM.

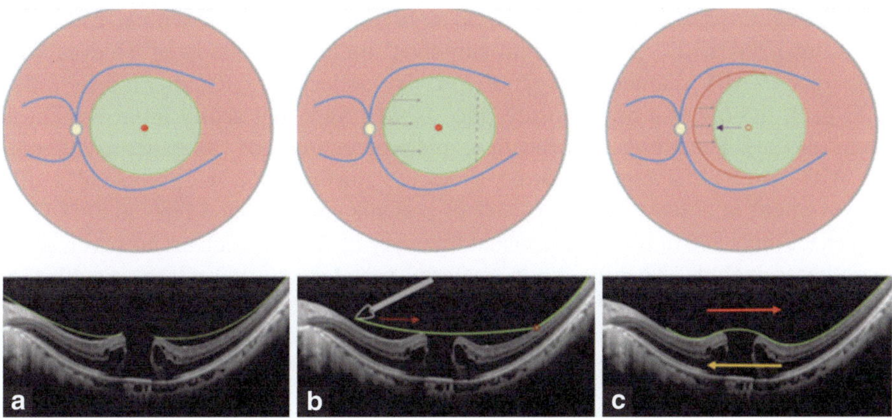

Fig. 2 Upper en face animation demonstrating nasal contraction of the retina and temporal contraction of the overlying internal limiting membrane (ILM) in the retracting door technique. Bottom panel (**a**) highlighting ILM in green before surgery, after the placement of the temporally hinged ILM flap back over the hole (**b**), and the direction of the retinal contraction (yellow arrow) and the ILM contraction (red arrow) after the retracting door technique (**c**). (Figure adapted from Finn AP, Mahmoud TH. Internal limiting membrane retracting door for myopic macular holes. Retina. 2019)

10　Very Large Holes

Macular holes larger than 650 μm (minimal linear dimension) pose a significant challenge not only for anatomical closure but also for visual recovery. Very large holes (if successfully closed) tend to heal with more gliosis and disruption of the normal retinal architecture [21]. One potential solution that may improve normal retinal architecture and physiology is an autologous retinal transplant.

10.1　Autologous Retinal Transplants (ART)

Autologous retinal transplant involves placing retinal tissue from the mid-periphery into the macular hole (Video 3). Visual recovery following ART depends on how well the graft tissue integrates into the surrounding macula. The grafted tissue requires tamponade agents to keep it in the correct position as it becomes grounded in place by glial cell proliferation. Successful graft integration can be visualized by OCT, and successful perfusion of graft blood vessels can be seen on OCTA. The initial description of this technique showed a 3-month postoperative visual acuity improvement from 20/200 to 20/80 in a highly myopic eye with a refractory 1100 μm FTMH [22]. In the initial surgeons' multicenter study of 41 eyes with refractory FTMH (diameter 621–2600 μm) that underwent ART after a prior failed ILM peel, there was a 88% closure rate, as well as visual acuity improvement in over half [23]. The global retrospective, multicenter study of 130 patients undergoing ART for FTMH repair showed a closure rate of 89% with a visual acuity improvement of at least 3 lines in 43% of patients and at least 5 lines in 29% [24]. The exact mechanism behind the visual recovery of ART is unclear; however, some hypotheses include synaptogenesis, material transfer, cell migration, growth factors, glucose transport, and the possibility of Müller cells acting as photoreceptor stem cells.

11 Refractory or Recurrent Holes

Historically, the standard of care for refractory or recurrent macular holes has been to repeat PPV and enlarge the ILM peel. Despite eliminating the key initiators of tractional forces that created the macular hole, removing the vitreous and ILM will sometimes not be enough to facilitate macular hole closure and healing. Additionally, because of the previous ILM peel, there is likely insufficient ILM to attempt an inverted ILM flap or retracting door ILM flap. The following are potential surgical options in managing recurrent macular holes.

11.1 Free Flap or Pedicle Flap

A free flap (Video 4), or pedicle flap, harvests ILM outside of the original ILM peel with either no continuity (free flap) or a small pedicle of connection to unpeeled ILM. This tissue can be either draped over the hole or folded in multiple layers as it fits over the hole. The free flap ILM transplantation successfully closes the hole in over 93% of refractory FTMH cases, in comparison to a closure rate of 64.2% when enlargement of the ILM peel is performed. Despite the improved hole closure rate when compared to additional ILM peel, free flap ILM transplantation can cause increased foveal fibrosis due to a proliferation of glial tissue seen in free flap repairs [25]. Furthermore, placement and retention of the free flap in its correct place pose an additional challenge, especially during the fluid-air exchange. This can be ameliorated with the use of PFCLs to help stabilize the flap before the fluid-air exchange. Alternatively, the flap can be tucked into the hole's edge, though this may damage underlying photoreceptors. We have not been satisfied with such outcomes, even with hole closure, since functional outcomes are limited.

11.2   Scaffold Tissue Alternatives

In situations where sufficient ILM is unable to be harvested, alternative scaffolding tissue may be used to help hole closure. These tissues include the lens capsule, amniotic membrane, and autologous retinal transplant (see earlier section on ART).

- *Lens capsule.*

  A lens capsule graft may be taken from the same or fellow eye. The anterior lens capsule is most frequently used as it is more rigid allowing for its placement over the macular hole without the use of stabilizing tamponades. The main limitation of this procedure is that it typically requires combined phacovitrectomy which is not available in all surgical centers.
- *Amniotic membrane.*

  A novel alternative to autologous ILM and lens capsule transplantation is the use of human amniotic membrane (hAM). The hAM itself secretes growth factors that could assist in the closure of the macular hole. The limited use of hAM subretinally has been promising so far. A prospective study of eight patients has shown neurosensory retinal tissue overfilling the hAM plug and closure of the hole within a week [26]. Similar success was replicated in highly myopic, recurrent macular holes (AL >30 μm) where >90% closure was achieved after repair with hAM [27]. Possible underlying concerns include the long-term persistence of the graft and effect on the overlying retina and mechanical damage to the RPE and surrounding macular tissue as the graft is being positioned.

12   Tamponades and Positioning

Following vitrectomy, endotamponades are used to stabilize the macular hole repair and help facilitate closure. The majority of macular holes close within 3–7 days, and thus, tamponade for that duration is theoretically acceptable. However, it is our experience that the more complicated the macular hole surgery is, the longer the tamponade should stay. Less complicated macular hole repairs usually use air or sulfur hexafluoride (SF6) as the tamponade. More complicated surgeries like refractory, large, or myopic macular holes may benefit from perfluoropropane (C3F8) or short-term PFCL.

One of the more debated and contentious issues following surgery is the necessity and the optimal amount of face-down positioning. Face-down positioning post-surgery may or may not be beneficial, as various studies have yielded conflicting results. One randomized controlled trial showed that there was no difference in outcome whether or not face-down positioning was practiced in macular holes <400 μm, while positioning did provide an advantage in holes >400 μm [28]. It is the authors' opinion that at least 1 day of chin-down positioning (still allowing the patient to be in an upright position) may best satisfy both the surgeon and patient. An almost complete fluid-air exchange to allow a dry macula in any position is key to closure without the need for positioning, especially in holes <400 μm.

13 Patient Counseling

Patients need to understand that improvements in visual acuity can take months to years. In successful patients, visual acuity usually improves continuously for 1–2 years at most before starting to stabilize. The strongest predictor of postoperative visual acuity improvement is anatomical closure of the hole and preoperative visual acuity [29]. That said, many patients who do have successful hole closure might not see any improvements in visual acuity postoperatively. Despite this, the prevention of further decreased visual acuity remains a primary goal in every macular hole repair. As discussed earlier, the chronicity of a hole represents an additional challenge to surgical success, so patients need to understand that early intervention yields the most favorable prognosis.

14 Case Scenario

A 69-year-old myopic (−1.5D) female underwent pars plana vitrectomy, internal limiting membrane peel, fluid-air exchange, and C3F8 gas-gas exchange for a stage 2, 300 μm, macular hole. Three months after the initial surgery, it was noted the macular hole was still open and was referred to our practice for a second opinion. The visual acuity was 20/200. She was phakic with 2+ nuclear sclerosis. The OCT demonstrated a large macular hole (~600 μm MLD and ~ 1600 μm at the base). She underwent a second surgery in which a free flap of ILM was peeled and placed into the macular hole under PFCL (Video 4). C3F8 gas was used as the tamponade, and she was instructed to remain face-down/chin-down during the day for 2 days. The macular hole closed nicely, and vision improved to 20/80 despite a progressive cataract.

Key Points
- VMT is the dominant force in the development of a primary/idiopathic macular hole.
- PPV with ILM peel has a high closure rate (>90%) in primary macular holes.
- Macular holes associated with high axial length, very large macular holes (> approximately 650 μm in MLD), and chronic macular holes (> 1 year of symptoms) have a lower closure rate with PPV/ILM peel alone.
- ILM flaps are broadly categorized into inverted and non-inverted flaps with advantages and disadvantages for each.

- Tissue scaffold including free ILM, lens capsule, amniotic membrane, or autologous retina is recommended for recurrent macular holes without sufficient ILM for an ILM flap.

References

1. Darian-Smith E, Howie AR, Allen PL, Vote BJ. Tasmanian macular hole study: whole population-based incidence of full thickness macular hole. Clin Exp Ophthalmol. 2016;44(9):812–6.
2. Duker JS, Kaiser PK, Binder S, et al. The International vitreomacular traction study group classification of vitreomacular adhesion, traction, and macular hole. Ophthalmology. 2013;120(12):2611–9.
3. McCannel CA, Ensminger JL, Diehl NN, Hodge DN. Population-based incidence of macular holes. Ophthalmology. 2009;116(7):1366–9.
4. la Cour M, Friis J. Macular holes: classification, epidemiology, natural history and treatment. Acta Ophthalmol Scand. 2002;80(6):579–87.
5. Johnson RN, Gass JD. Idiopathic macular holes. Observations, stages of formation, and implications for surgical intervention. Ophthalmology. 1988;95(7):917–24.
6. Kelly NE, Wendel RT. Vitreous surgery for idiopathic macular holes. Results of a pilot study. Arch Ophthalmol. 1991;109(5):654–9.
7. Eckardt C, Eckardt U, Groos S, Luciano L, Reale E. Removal of the internal limiting membrane in macular holes. Clinical and morphological findings. Ophthalmologe. 1997;94(8):545–51.
8. Da Mata AP, Burk SE, Riemann CD, et al. Indocyanine green-assisted peeling of the retinal internal limiting membrane during vitrectomy surgery for macular hole repair. Ophthalmology. 2001;108(7):1187–92.
9. Bae K, Kang SW, Kim JH, Kim SJ, Kim JM, Yoon JM. Extent of internal limiting membrane peeling and its impact on macular hole surgery outcomes: a randomized trial. Am J Ophthalmol. 2016;169:179–88.
10. Ch'ng SW, Patton N, Ahmed M, et al. The manchester large macular hole study: is it time to reclassify large macular holes? Am J Ophthalmol. 2018;195:36–42.
11. Susini A, Gastaud P. Macular holes that should not be operated. J Fr Ophtalmol. 2008;31(2):214–20.
12. Jaycock PD, Bunce C, Xing W, et al. Outcomes of macular hole surgery: implications for surgical management and clinical governance. Eye (Lond). 2005;19(8):879–84.
13. Suda K, Hangai M, Yoshimura N. Axial length and outcomes of macular hole surgery assessed by spectral-domain optical coherence tomography. Am J Ophthalmol. 2011;151(1):118–127.e1.
14. Kase S, Saito W, Mori S, et al. Clinical and histological evaluation of large macular hole surgery using the inverted internal limiting membrane flap technique. Clin Ophthalmol. 2016;11:9–14.
15. Kannan NB, Kohli P, Parida H, Adenuga OO, Ramasamy K. Comparative study of inverted internal limiting membrane (ILM) flap and ILM peeling technique in large macular holes: a randomized-control trial. BMC Ophthalmol. 2018;18:18.
16. Shen Y, Lin X, Zhang L, Wu M. Comparative efficacy evaluation of inverted internal limiting membrane flap technique and internal limiting membrane peeling in large macular holes: a systematic review and meta-analysis. BMC Ophthalmol. 2020;20(1):14.
17. Alkabes M, Pichi F, Nucci P, et al. Anatomical and visual outcomes in high myopic macular hole (HM-MH) without retinal detachment: a review. Graefes Arch Clin Exp Ophthalmol. 2014;252(2):191–9.
18. Rizzo S, Tartaro R, Barca F, Caporossi T, Bacherini D, Giansanti F. Internal limiting membrane peeling versus inverted flap technique for treatment of full-thickness macular holes: a COMPARATIVE study in a large series of patients. Retina. 2018;38(Suppl 1):S73–8.

19. Finn AP, Mahmoud TH. Internal limiting membrane retracting door for myopic macular holes. Retina. 2019;39(Suppl 1):S92–4.
20. Akahori T, Iwase T, Yamamoto K, et al. Macular displacement after vitrectomy in eyes with idiopathic macular hole determined by optical coherence tomography angiography. Am J Ophthalmol. 2018;189:111–21.
21. Liu Y, Wu C, Wang Y, et al. Risk factors for glial cell proliferation after idiopathic macular hole repair with internal limiting membrane flap. BMC Ophthalmol. 2019;19(1):264.
22. Grewal DS, Mahmoud TH. Autologous neurosensory retinal free flap for closure of refractory myopic macular holes. JAMA Ophthalmol. 2016;134(2):229–30.
23. Grewal DS, Charles S, Parolini B, Kadonosono K, Mahmoud TH. Autologous retinal transplant for refractory macular holes: multicenter international collaborative study group. Ophthalmology. 2019;126(10):1399–408.
24. Moysidis SN, Koulisis N, Adrean SD, et al. Autologous retinal transplantation for primary and refractory macular holes and macular hole retinal detachments: the global consortium. Ophthalmology. 2020;128:672.
25. Pires J, Nadal J, Gomes NL. Internal limiting membrane translocation for refractory macular holes. Br J Ophthalmol. 2017;101(3):377–82.
26. Rizzo S, Caporossi T, Tartaro R, et al. A human amniotic membrane plug to promote retinal breaks repair and recurrent macular hole closure. Retina. 2019;39(Suppl 1):S95–S103.
27. Caporossi T, Pacini B, De Angelis L, Barca F, Peiretti E, Rizzo S. HUMAN AMNIOTIC MEMBRANE TO CLOSE RECURRENT, HIGH MYOPIC MACULAR HOLES IN PATHOLOGIC MYOPIA WITH AXIAL LENGTH OF ≥30 mm. Retina. 2020;40(10):1946–54.
28. Guillaubey A, Malvitte L, Lafontaine PO, et al. Comparison of face-down and seated position after idiopathic macular hole surgery: a randomized clinical trial. Am J Ophthalmol. 2008;146(1):128–34.
29. Gupta B, Laidlaw DAH, Williamson TH, Shah SP, Wong R, Wren S. Predicting visual success in macular hole surgery. Br J Ophthalmol. 2009;93(11):1488–91.

Optic Disc Pit-Associated Maculopathy

Zofia Anna Nawrocka and Jerzy Nawrocki

1   Introduction

- An optic pit is a rare congenital colobomatous defect of the optic nerve head. The incidence is 1:10.000, and it most commonly occurs at the temporal side of the optic nerve.
- Optic disc pit is typically unilateral but may be bilateral in up to 15% of patients. It is usually sporadic, but autosomal inheritance has been suggested in some cases.
- In the absence of optic disc pit maculopathy (ODPM), optic disc pit is usually asymptomatic.
- ODPM occurs in up to 25–75% of optic nerve pits with the development of intra-retinal fluid (IRF) and subretinal fluid (SRF), causing visual deterioration [1, 2] (Fig. 1).

Supplementary Information The online version contains supplementary material available at https://doi.org/10.1007/978-3-031-47827-7_16.

Z. A. Nawrocka (✉) · J. Nawrocki
Ophthalmic Clinic Jasne Blonia, Lodz, Poland

A. B. Sallam et al. (eds.), *Practical Manual of Vitreoretinal Surgery*, https://doi.org/10.1007/978-3-031-47827-7_16

Fig. 1 Different morphological appearances of optic disc pit-associated maculopathy. (**a**) Subretinal fluid (star). (**b**) Intraretinal fluid (arrow). (**c**) Intraretinal (arrow) and subretinal fluid (star). (**d**) Outer lamellar macular hole with intraretinal fluid (arrow)

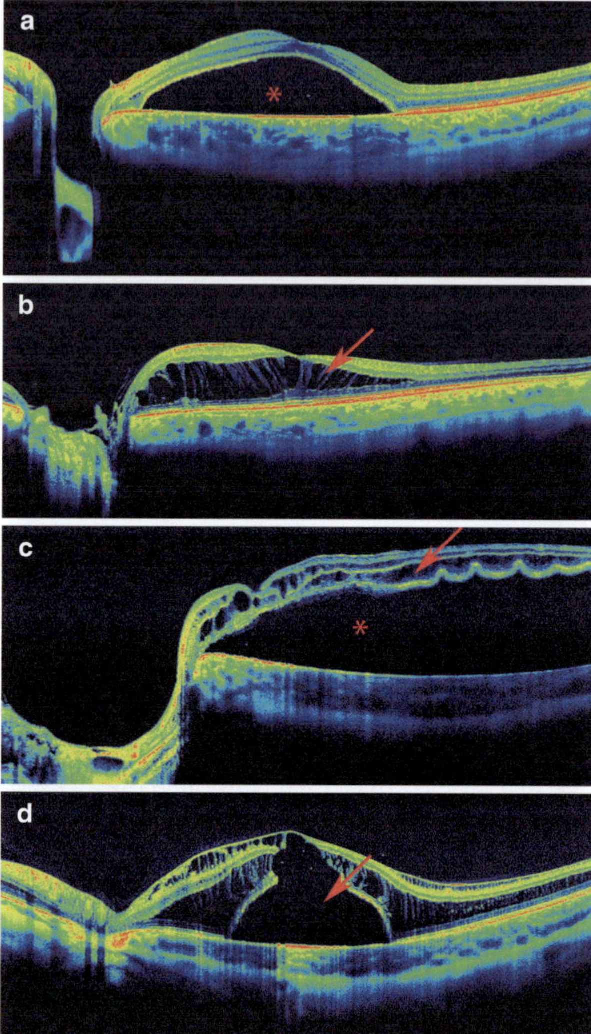

2 Pathogenesis

Optic disc pit results from the incomplete closure of the embryonic fissure. The origin of the fluid is unclear and is thought to occur from two potential sources, the cerebrospinal fluid and the vitreous. Theories supporting the vitreous source are based on the presence of adherent hyaloid and the difficulty in the induction of posterior hyaloid separation during surgery. Because there is a possibility that CSF may be a source of the fluid in optic disc pit maculopathy, it is best to avoid the use of silicone oil (SO) during surgery to avoid potential intracranial migration.

3 Disease Progression

ODPM can present with a combination of IRF and SRF [3, 4]. The fluid usually follows a pattern that first creates a schisis-like separation of the inner retina. Photoreceptor layer detachment may follow, resulting in an outer lamellar hole, and subsequently, the fluid reaches the subretinal space creating a macular neuro-epithelial detachment. Symptoms usually start in the third or fourth decade of life and include decreased central vision and visual distortion. Mild cases, particularly those with intraretinal fluid only, can be asymptomatic for many years [5] (Fig. 2, Video 1).

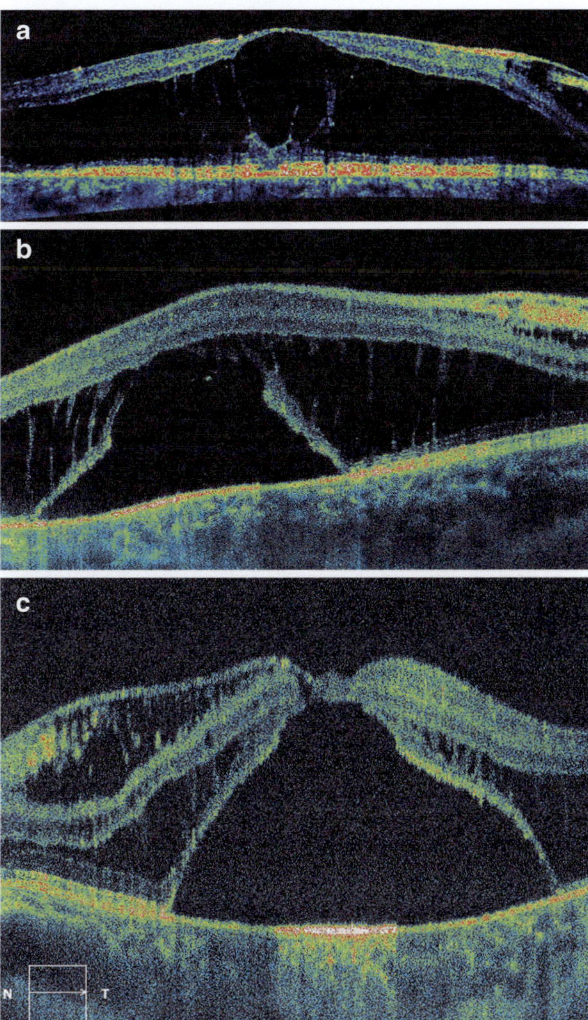

Fig. 2 Natural evolution of an untreated optic disc pit maculopathy in a 17-year-old girl. (**a**) Intraretinal fluid is visible. Striae between the outer plexiform layer and the outer nuclear layer are visible. Visual acuity was 0.8 Snellen fraction. (**b**) Two years later, visual acuity dropped to 0.3 Snellen, and an outer lamellar macular hole formed. Photoreceptors detached in the central fovea. (**c**) After 2 months, visual acuity spontaneously improved to 0.4 Snellen. New connections between the photoreceptor layer and the outer nuclear layer were observed. It was stable for another year

Fig. 3 Optical coherence tomography (**a**) and fundus photo (**b**) of a patient with optic disc pit-associated maculopathy. Elschnig's membrane is visible inside the optic nerve. It was earlier suggested that this membrane, if complete, might protect against the development of maculopathy

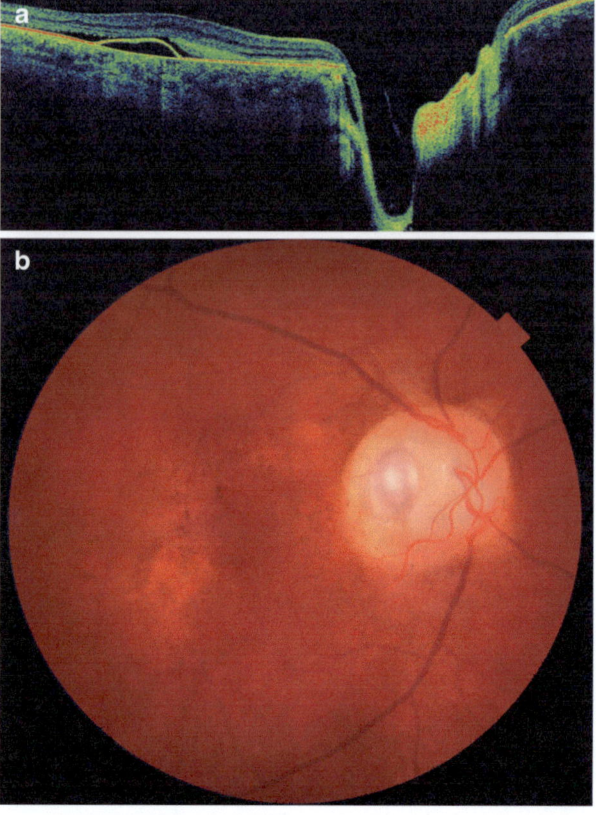

The diagnosis of ODPM is mainly based on the clinical appearance and optical coherence tomography (OCT) of the nerve and macula (Fig. 3). Optical coherence tomography angiography (OCTA) can also be helpful in diagnosis. In ODPM, similar to other diseases with IRF, artifacts can be found, especially in the deep fovea vascular layers. A novel finding in ODPM is an artifact resembling ice cracks on a frozen lake [6] (Fig. 4). We have also observed that elevated photoreceptors in outer lamellar macular holes correspond to a hyporeflective ring encircling a hyperreflective circle at the level of the choriocapillaris in swept-source OCTA (Fig. 5).

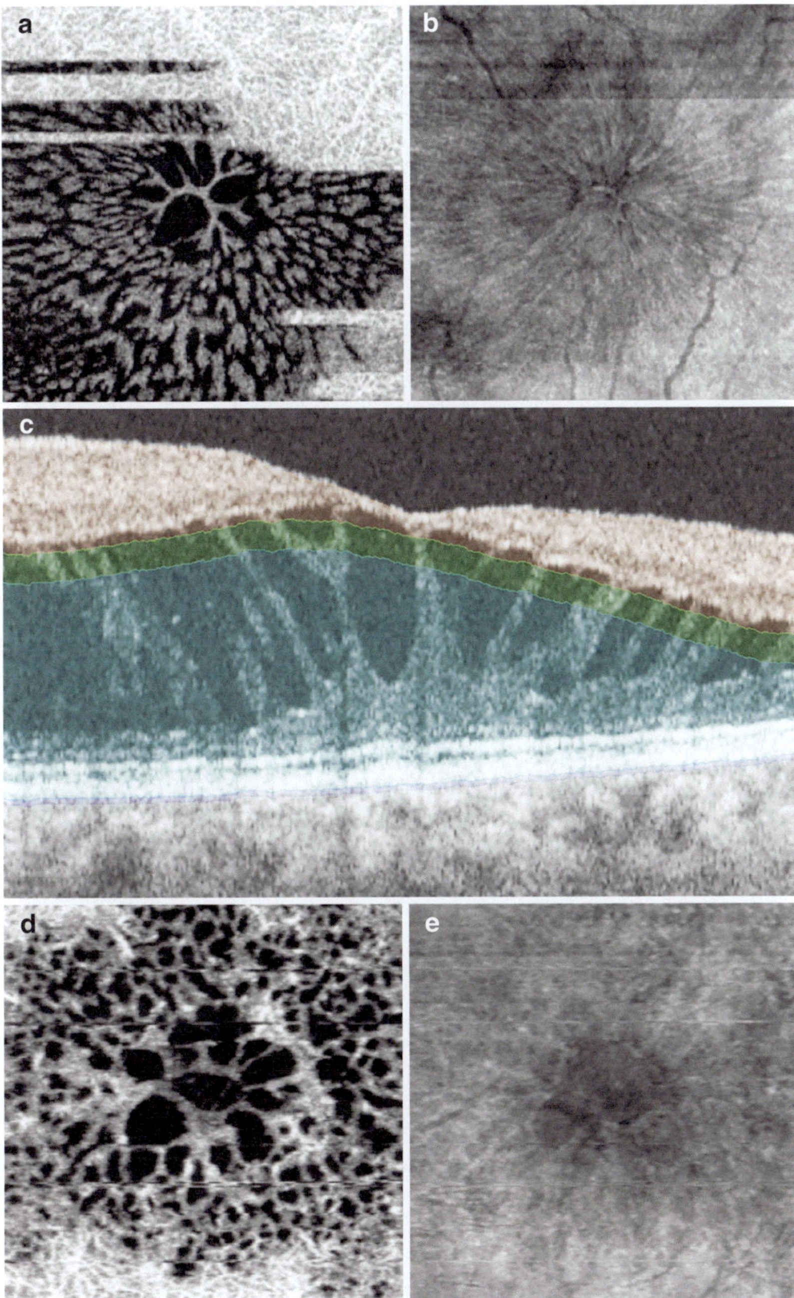

Fig. 4 Artifacts in swept-source optical coherence tomography angiography (OCTA) may occur in different retinal diseases due to the presence of intraretinal fluid and can result in misdiagnoses. (**a–c**) Optic disc pit-associated maculopathy. An artifact resembling ice cracks on a frozen lake is visible on OCTA. (**d–f**) Diabetic maculopathy images with artifacts. (**g–i**) Full-thickness macular hole images, with a medusa-like artifact. The images in (**a, d, g**) are at the level of the deep retina vessel layer on swept-source OCTA, (**b, e, h**) are en face images, (**c, f, i**) are swept-source OCT images

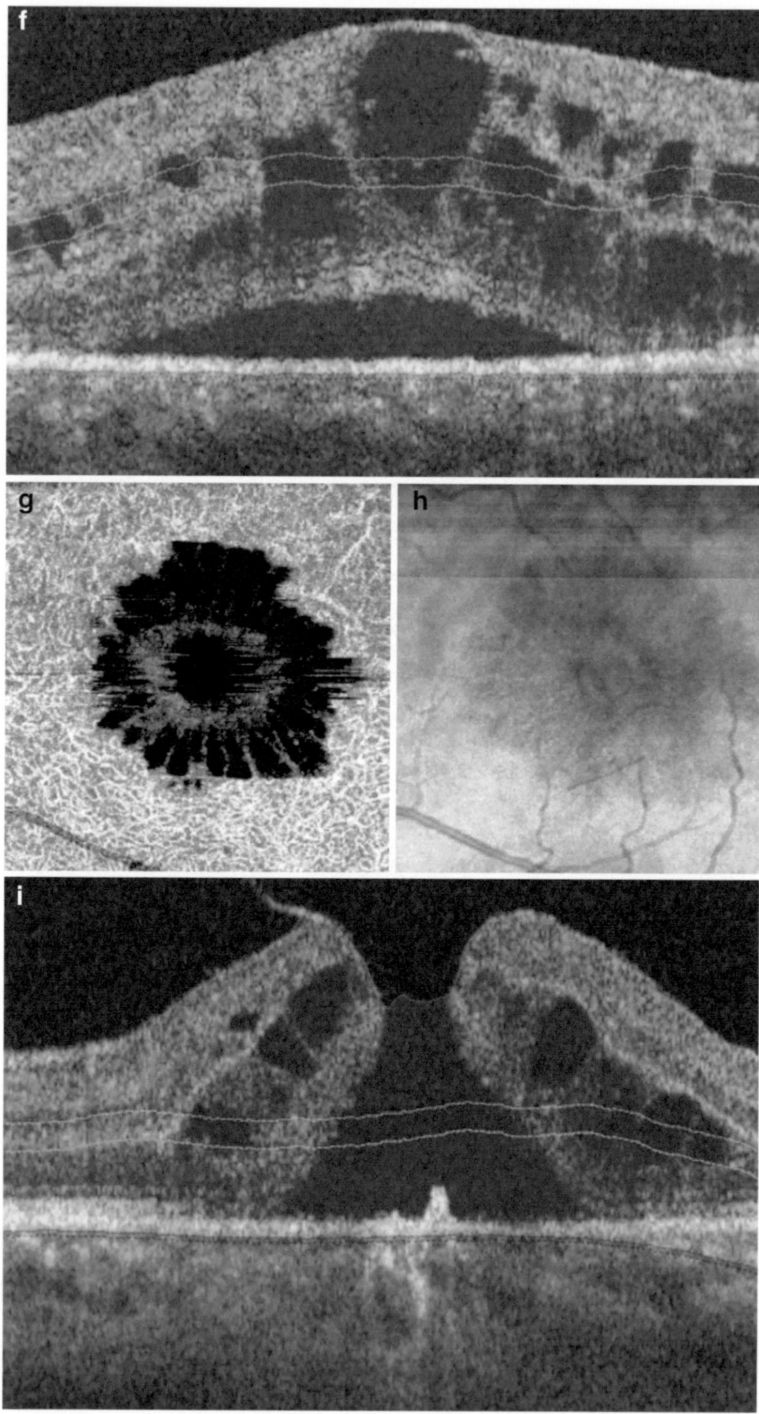

Fig. 4 (continued)

Fig. 5 (**a**) Swept-source optical coherence tomography of the fovea in an outer lamellar macular hole coexisting with optic disc pit maculopathy. (**b**) En face image. It is visible that elevated photoreceptors in outer lamellar macular hole corresponds to a hyporeflective ring encircling a hyperreflective circle at the level of the choriocapillaris on optical coherence tomography angiography

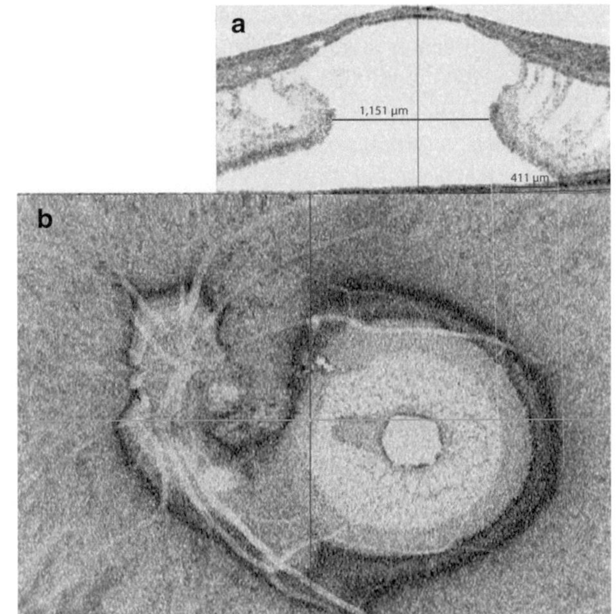

4 Differential Diagnosis

Due to the rarity of ODPM, misdiagnosis is not uncommon, especially in older patients. Important differential diagnoses include a choroidal neovascular membrane (> 90%), central serous chorioretinopathy, and macular edema. Most cases in a recently analyzed series were initially misdiagnosed as choroidal neovascular membrane (92.5%). Others were mistaken for central serous chorioretinopathy or macular edema. Most misdiagnosed cases exhibited SRF and outer retinoschisis resembling cystoid macular edema [7].

5 Treatment

- Asymptomatic cases of ODPM should only be observed.
- Laser treatment to the optic disc pit or the edge of the optic nerve is not effective.
- Pars plana vitrectomy with posterior vitreous detachment (PVD) induction is the method of choice, but there is ongoing discussion regarding the most optimal technique.
- The purpose of the surgical treatment of ODPM is to produce a permanent intra- and subretinal blockade of fluid migration.
- Due to the rarity of this disease, it is challenging to conduct a randomized controlled clinical trial.

- The role of laser photocoagulation as an adjunct to vitrectomy is controversial [8, 9]. A multicenter study analyzing the outcomes of 46 eyes with optic disc pit maculopathy concluded that laser photocoagulation does not influence the final outcome [10].
- The role of internal limiting membrane (ILM) peeling in the macular area is also controversial. In long-term follow-up, it has been associated with a reduction of macular thickness in spectral domain OCT. However, it may be associated with an increased risk of macular hole development [11].
- Regarding the type of tamponade, air might be sufficient, but most surgeons opt for short-acting SF6 gas. Because of possible intracranial migration, SO should be avoided [12].
- Because this is a congenital disease, recurrences of maculopathy after initial surgical success are not uncommon. Thus, different attempts to seal the pit have been proposed: radial optic neurotomy was reported as an effective treatment option in seven cases, but this technique was not widely used [13]. A case report of injecting autologous platelets over the optic disc pit also showed satisfactory results [14]. It was proposed to invert an ILM flap over the pit [15]. We previously used this technique but had the impression that long-term results were unstable, and eventually, the maculopathy reappeared. Travassos and colleagues introduced an autologous scleral transplant in three eyes [16].
- In 2016, we introduced the technique where an inverted internal limiting membrane (ILM) obtained by peeling the ILM from the temporal side of the disc and not the macula is manually introduced or, more colloquially, "stuffed" into the optic pit [6, 17] (Fig. 6, Video 2). The goal is to prevent the translaminar difference of pressure or blockade of the outflow of fluids. The advantage of the inverted ILM as a packing material is the simplicity of the technique making the use of allografts such as sclera or amniotic membrane unnecessary.

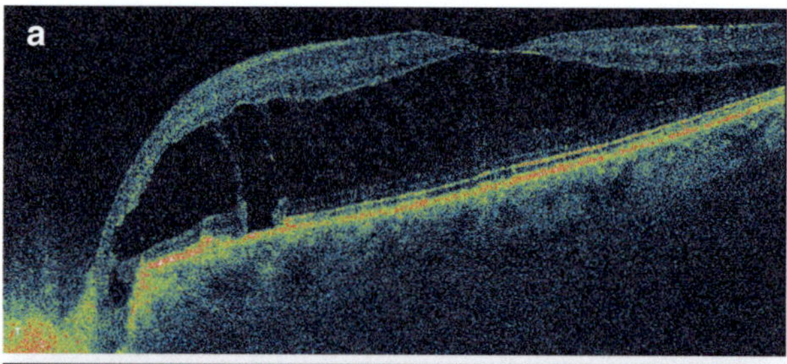
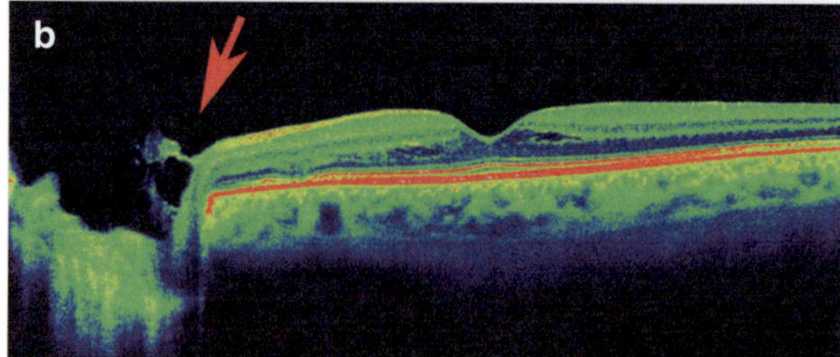

Fig. 6 Optical coherence tomography images before (**a**) and after (**b**) surgery. (**a**) Optic disc pit-associated maculopathy with intraretinal fluid. (**b**) Complete fluid reabsorption after vitrectomy by stuffing the internal limiting membrane into the pit (red arrow)

5.1 Surgery Outcome

- Most studies presenting standard vitrectomy results confirm an improvement of at least 1 Snellen line in more than 60% of cases [5, 18] correlating with resolving subretinal fluid, although this can take up to 30 months after surgery [18].
- When the optic nerve was "stuffed" with ILM, the resolution of SRF usually took approximately 1 week post-operatively. In some cases, it may take many months for IRF to disappear, which may be due to differences in pre-operative history. Final visual acuity in patients in whom the optic nerve was "stuffed" with ILM was 20/63 [6]. Thus, due to the natural history of eyes with SRF, these eyes likely had longer residual fluid when compared to eyes only with intraretinal fluid or eyes with intraretinal fluid and a lamellar macular hole. Even after creating a successful blockade with the ILM stuffing, photoreceptor defects might have been more severe, correlating with the lower visual recovery potential post-operatively.
- A recent multicenter study of 95 eyes with ODPM showed that vitrectomy with gas tamponade was associated with a higher likelihood of better anatomical and functional outcomes when compared to observation [19]. Additionally, juxtapapillary laser and ILM peeling during vitrectomy did not provide additional benefits [19].

Key Points
- ODPM can be misdiagnosed as choroidal neovascular membrane, especially when presenting later in older patients.
- IRF usually appears before SRF in ODPM.
- Vitrectomy and induction of PVD are the methods of choice. Inserting a plug from the ILM into the pit may enable stable and good long-term results.
- Gas tamponade should be used. SO should be avoided.

References

1. Brown GC, Shields JA, Goldberg RE. Congenital pits of the optic nerve head. II. Clinical studies in humans. Ophthalmology. 1980;87:51–e65.
2. Gordon R, Chatfield RK. Pits in the optic disc associated with macular degeneration. Br J Ophthalmol. 1969;53:481–e489.
3. Michalewski J, Michalewska Z, Nawrocki J. Spectral domain optical coherence tomography morphology in optic disc pit associated maculopathy. Indian J Ophthalmol. 2014;62:777–81.
4. Michalewska Z, Michalewski J, Nawrocki J. Natural course of macular detachment in relation to optic pit. Retina Today. 2010;9:60–1.
5. Steel DHW, Suleman J, Murphy DC, et al. Optic disc pit maculopathy: a two-year nationwide prospective population-based study. Ophthalmology. 2018;125:1757–e1764.
6. Michalewska Z, Nawrocka Z, Nawrocki J. Swept-source OCT and swept-source OCT angiography before and after vitrectomy with stuffing the optic pit. Ophthalmol Retina. 2020;4:927–37.
7. Iglicki M, Busch C, Loewenstein A, et al. Underdiagnosed optic disc pit maculopathy: spectral domain optical coherence tomography features for accurate diagnosis. Retina. 2019;39:2161–6.

8. Hirakata A, Inoue M, Hiraoka T, et al. Vitrectomy without laser treatment or gas tamponade for macular detachment. Ophthalmology. 2012;119:810–e818.
9. García-Arumí J, Guraya BC, Espax AB, et al. Optical coherence tomography in optic pit maculopathy managed with vitrectomy-laser-gas. Graefes Arch Clin Exp Ophthalmol. 2004;242:819–26.
10. Abouammoh MA, Alsulaiman SM, Gupta VS, et al. Pars plana vitrectomy with juxtapapillary laser photocoagulation versus vitrectomy without juxtapapillary laser photocoagulation for the treatment of optic disc pit maculopathy: the results of the KKESH international collaborative retina study group. Br J Ophthalmol. 2016;100:478–e483.
11. Chatziralli I, Theodossiadis G, Panagiotidis D, et al. Long-term changes of macular thickness after pars plana vitrectomy in optic disc pit maculopathy: a spectral-domain optical coherence tomography study. Semin Ophthalmol. 2015;26:1–7.
12. Kuhn F, Kover F, Szabo I, Mester V. Intracranial migration of silicone oil from an eye with optic pit. Graefes Arch Clin Exp Ophthalmol. 2006;244:1360–2.
13. Karacorlu M, Sayman Muslubas I, Hocaoglu M, et al. Long-term outcomes of radial optic neurotomy for management of optic disk pit maculopathy. Retina. 2016;36:2419–27.
14. Rosenthal G, Bartz-Schmidt KU, Walter P, Heimann K. Autologous platelet treatment for optic disc pit associated with persistent macular detachment. Graefes Arch Clin Exp Ophthalmol. 1998;236:151–3.
15. Mohammed OA, Pai A. Inverted autologous internal limiting membrane for management of optic disc pit with macular detachment. Middle East Afr J Ophthalmol. 2013;20:357–9.
16. Travassos AS, Regadas I, Alfaiate M, et al. Optic pit: novel surgical management of complicated cases. Retina. 2013;33:1708–14.
17. Nawrocki J, Bonińska K, Michalewska Z. Managing optic pit. The right stuff! Retina. 2016;36:2430–2.
18. Avci R, Yilmaz S, Inan UU, et al. Long-term outcomes of pars plana vitrectomy without internal limiting membrane peeling for optic disc pit maculopathy. Eye. 2013;27:1359–67.
19. Iros M, Parolini B, Ozdek S, Gini G, Nawrocka ZA, Ellabban AA, Faramawi MF, Adelman R, Sallam AB, EVRS Study Group. Management of optic disc pit maculopathy: the European VitreoRetinal society optic pit study. Acta Ophthalmol. 2022;100(6):e1264–71.

Myopic Traction Maculopathy

Barbara Parolini, Michele Palmieri, and Helena Dens

1 Introduction

This chapter covers myopic traction maculopathy (MTM), including the latest update in diagnosis and treatment. We aim to present a guide to inform management decisions.

1.1 Definition and Causes of Myopic Traction Maculopathy

High myopia is a refractive error above 6 diopters and/or axial length above 26.5 mm.

MTM is a pathology of high myopic eyes. It is reported in 9–34% of eyes with high myopia. It might manifest in different forms [1–3].

In high myopic eyes, different forces act on the retina and fovea as is shown in Fig. 1. Forces perpendicular to the retinal plane can cause maculoschisis or retinal detachment. Forces tangential to the retinal plane can cause lamellar macular holes (LMH) and full-thickness macular holes (FTMH).

Supplementary Information The online version contains supplementary material available at https://doi.org/10.1007/978-3-031-47827-7_17.

B. Parolini (✉) · M. Palmieri · H. Dens
Eyecare Clinic, Brescia, Italy

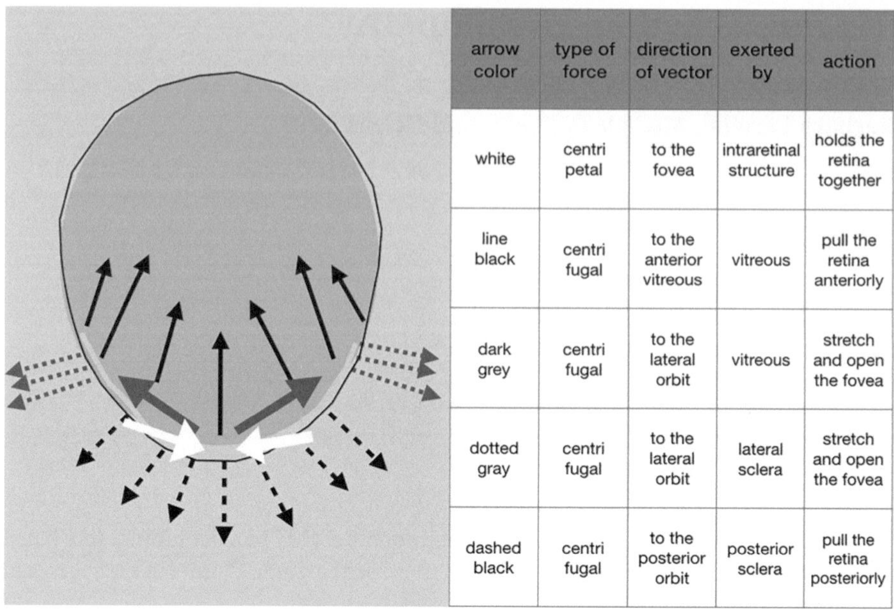

Fig. 1 Forces that are perpendicular and tangential to the retinal plane in high myopic eyes and their actions

1.2 Clinical Assessment of MTM

Color fundus examination can identify eyes with high myopia and the presence of a staphyloma. However, optical coherence tomography (OCT) is crucial for diagnosis and staging of MTM. Wide-scan imaging of the whole posterior pole, although still not widely available, is helpful to completely describe the clinical picture. The most critical OCT findings of MTM are inner or outer maculoschisis, macular detachment, inner and/or outer LMH, and FTMH. There is usually no need to request a fluorescein angiography test to diagnose MTM.

1.3 MTM Staging

MTM is a spectrum of different clinical pictures. The MTM Staging System (MSS) is based on OCT and describes the proposal of pathogenesis, the natural evolution, and the prognosis of MTM and offers potential guidelines for management [4].

The MSS is summarized in Fig. 2. The four rows represent the evolution of the disease in a direction perpendicular to the retina from inner/outer schisis (stage 1) to predominantly outer schisis (stage 2) to schisis detachment (stage 3) to complete

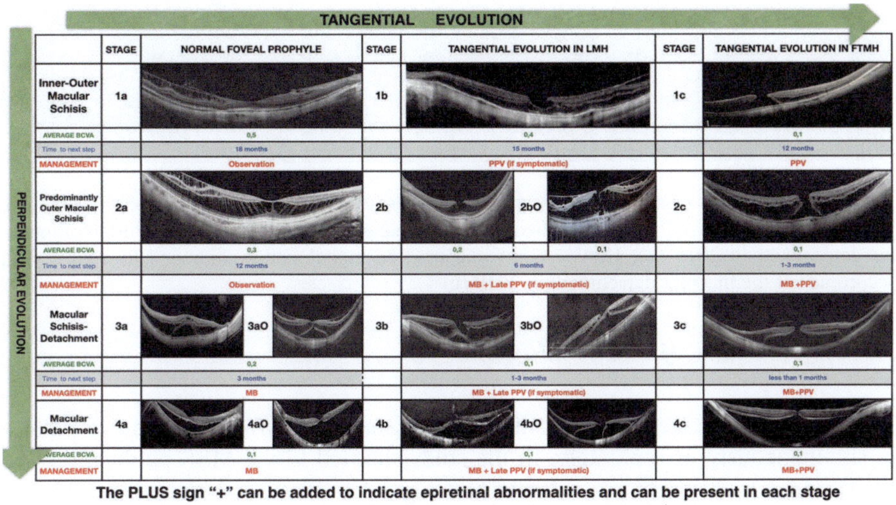

	STAGE	NORMAL FOVEAL PROPHYLE	STAGE	TANGENTIAL EVOLUTION IN LMH		STAGE	TANGENTIAL EVOLUTION IN FTMH
Inner-Outer Macular Schisis	1a		1b			1c	
AVERAGE BCVA		0,5		0,4			0,1
Time to next step		18 months		15 months			12 months
MANAGEMENT		Observation		PPV (if symptomatic)			PPV
Predominantly Outer Macular Schisis	2a		2b	2bO		2c	
AVERAGE BCVA		0,3		0,2	0,1		0,1
Time to next step		12 months		6 months			1-3 months
MANAGEMENT		Observation		MB + Late PPV (if symptomatic)			MB +PPV
Macular Schisis-Detachment	3a	3aO	3b	3bO		3c	
AVERAGE BCVA		0,2		0,1			0,1
Time to next step		3 months		1-3 months			less than 1 months
MANAGEMENT		MB		MB + Late PPV (if symptomatic)			MB+PPV
Macular Detachment	4a	4aO	4b	4bO		4c	
AVERAGE BCVA		0,1		0,1			0,1
MANAGEMENT		MB		MB + Late PPV (if symptomatic)			MB+PPV

The PLUS sign "+" can be added to indicate epiretinal abnormalities and can be present in each stage

Fig. 2 Tangenital evolution of myopic traction maculopathy

MD (stage 4). The three columns represent the evolution in a direction tangential to the retina and the fovea from the normal fovea (stage a) to inner lamellar macular hole (stage b) to full-thickness macular hole (stage c). The outer lamellar macular hole is marked as O and might occur in stages 2, 3, and 4. The presence of epiretinal abnormalities of any kind is marked as + (read as "plus") and might occur in every stage.

1.4 Definitions in MTM

- Maculoschisis refers to the increased thickness of the neurosensory retina which modifies with the layers of the retina separated and stretched in a column-like pattern. Maculoschisis can involve the inner retinal layers (inner nuclear layer to inner limiting membrane; inner maculoschisis) and outer retinal layers (outer plexiform layer to external limiting membrane; outer maculoschisis) or a combination of both.
- Macular detachment is the separation of the neurosensory retina from the retinal pigment epithelium (RPE) in the macula.
- LMH is a partial-thickness splitting of the macular layers. An inner LMH is confined to the inner retinal layers and does not compromise the photoreceptors. An outer LMH is an interruption in the photoreceptor layer.

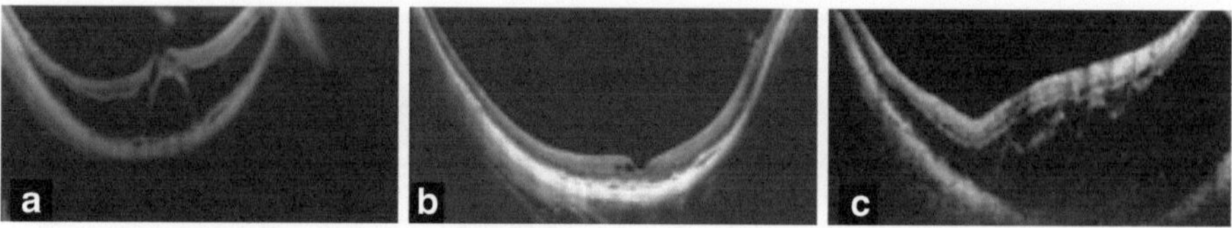

Fig. 3 The evolution of a high myopic eye that presented with macular detachment in 2014 (**a**). The patient was followed without any treatment and changed in a spontaneous resolution of macular detachment in 2015 (**b**). However, myopic traction maculopathy continued to evolve with recurrence of the macular detachment in 2018 (**c**)

1.5 Evolution of MTM Stages

The retina can change in time from stage 1 to stage 4 and from pattern a to pattern c, simultaneously or separately. In the study that led to the MSS publication, the mean time for evolution was 40 months (stages 1 to 2), 12 months (stages 2 to 3), and 3 months (stages 3 to 4).

There can also be a spontaneous improvement [5]. Figure 3 shows the evolution of a high myopic eye that presented with macular detachment in 2014 (a). The patient was followed without any treatment and changed in a spontaneous resolution of macular detachment in 2015 (b). However, MTM continued to evolve with recurrence of the macular detachment in 2018 (c) that was surgically treated.

1.6 Management of MTM

Early stages with intact fovea and good vision should be observed since progression is slow. For more advanced cases, treatment is required. Forces perpendicular to the retinal plane causing maculoschisis and detachment can be counteracted by placing a macular buckle (MB) which pushes the sclera toward the retina. Forces tangential to the retinal plane causing LMH or FTMH can be counteracted by pars plana vitrectomy (PPV) which creates a force pointing toward the center of the fovea. PPV can also counteract the forces perpendicular to the retinal plane exerted by the vitreous pulling the retina anteriorly.

In summary, the suggested management customized per stage is as follows [6]:

Stage 1a: observation on annual basis

Stage 1b: PPV in case of significant decrease in vision

Stage 1c: PPV

Stage 2a: observation every 6 months

Stage 2b: first MB and if necessary PPV afterward (when the inner LMH induces significant functional limitations or to treat residual epiretinal abnormalities)

Stage 2c: combined MB + PPV. Consider also MB then sequential PPV. It is easier to deal with a FTMH in an attached than a detached retina.

Stage 3a: MB

Stage 3b: MB and if necessary PPV afterward
Stage 3c: combined MB + PPV. Consider also MB then sequential PPV.
Stage 4a: MB
Stage 4b: MB and if necessary PPV afterward
Stage 4c: combined MB + PPV. Consider also MB then sequential PPV.

1.7   Prognosis for Vision After Surgery

Following the outlined treatment guidelines, visual acuity usually improves by an average of two lines. This is considered a good achievement as MTM surgery usually achieves anatomical success with no functional improvement [6]. Functional improvement is also influenced by the atrophic changes in the macula, the media opacity and possible amblyopia.

2   Surgical Techniques

2.1   Macular Buckle (Video 1)

The MB is placed behind the posterior pole to push the sclera anteriorly. The aim is to counteract the pulling effect exerted on the retina by the elongation of the sclera. The buckling side of the device is placed behind the posterior pole to push the sclera anteriorly.

Different models of MB have been proposed; we discuss our techniques below [7] focusing on our new design –NPB Buckle (New Parolini Buckle, AJL Spain). This is a one-piece MB that is made of polymethyl methacrylate (PMMA) and coated with silicone. It can be custom-made, based on the axial length of the eye. The buckle has two parts, one part is placed over the macular sclera, and it is called the "head of the buckle." The other part is for positioning the buckle, and is called the "arm of the buckle, Fig 4. The NPB can be more easily inserted with the use of the NPB loading device (Janach, Italy) Fig 4. The loading device has 3 main functions: 1. to allow a fluent buckle insertion; 2. to allow comfortable checking of the position by facilitating dynamic indentation movements; 3. to keep the NPB stable when placing sutures. Fig. 5 details the assembly steps of the protype of current buckle, off-label, made of titanium and silicone. This could be of benefit for surgeons who cannot obtain the NPB. Surgery may be performed under general or local anesthesia. For local anesthesia, we prefer sub-Tenon's anesthesia with a blunt cannula to avoid the potential risk of scleral perforation with retrobulbar injections in high myopic eyes.

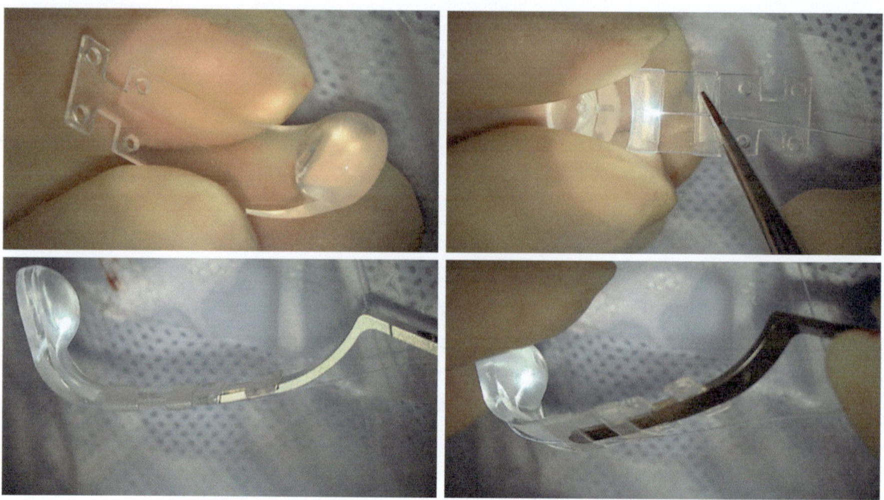

Fig. 4 NPB (New Parolini Buckle, AJL Spain) Top left: inner side of the NPB, which is supposed to face the sclera. The arm contains 4 holes for the sutures. The head buckles the macular sclera. Top right: outer side of the NPB surrounded by silicone sleeves to lodge the optical fiber and the loading device. Bottom left: lateral side of the NPB with the optical fiber illuminating the head and the loading device connected. Bottom right: NPB oblique view with the optical fiber illuminating the head and the loading device connected

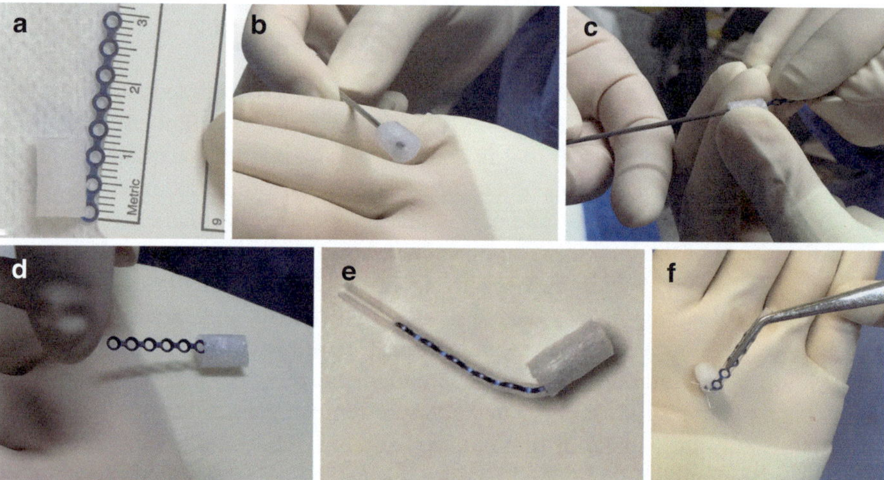

Fig. 5 (**a**) A protype of the current macular buckle made of titanium and silicone. The buckle is L shaped and has two parts, head and arm. (**b**) One part is placed behind the macular sclera and it is called "head of the buckle". (**c**) the second part is for positioning the buckle and it is called "arm of the buckle." (**d**) To create the head of the buckle, cut a 10 mm piece of 507 silicone sponge. (**e**) Use the 17-g needle to create a tunnel inside the sponge where to insert a 3 cm titanium stent. The tunnel should not be in the middle of the sponge but between one third and two thirds of the sponge thickness. (**f**) Cover the lateral titanium arm of the buckle with the 72 silicone sleeve in order to avoid direct contact of titanium to the sclera. Bend the titanium stent creating a 90° angle between the buckle head and the arm. Suture the silicone sponge to the titanium stent with a non- absorbable 7-0 suture.

Surgery Steps

1. *Superotemporal peritomy* is performed from 11 o'clock to 4 o'clock in the right eye and from 8 o'clock to 1 o'clock in the left.
2. *Two traction sutures* are placed around the lateral and superior rectus muscles.
3. *Insertion of the chandelier light.* This step is needed only if the surgeon selects to perform the surgery with a non-contact widefield viewing system. When using a flat contact lens, every step can be performed without any light. In alternative a 29,27 or 25 gauge light can be inserted into the head of the buckle (both the NPB and the titanium silicone one) to use the transillumination effect.
4. *Anterior chamber paracentesis*: Although lowering the IOP makes the insertion of the buckle easier, we now strongly recommend *not* to perform a paracentesis so as not to increase the risk of suprachoroidal hemorrhage during the surgery.
5. *Positioning of the NPB behind the posterior pole.* Grab the arm of the MB with the NPB loading device (or an alternative suitable forceps). With the other hand, gently pull the superior traction suture. It is helpful if a co-surgeon or a scrub nurse pulls the temporal traction suture. Slide the MB, head down, into the superotemporal quadrant between the superior and the lateral rectus muscle until a good indentation of the macula is induced.
6. *Assess the position of the MB.* Using a flat contact lens with direct view through the microscope (or as alternative a wide-field non-contact viewing system), check the position of the MB, and center it under the macula. The use of a flat contact lens allows a simultaneous view of the macula and the buckle under the microscope. The loading device (or a forceps) allows the surgeon to move the NPB to induce a visible indentation and confirm the correct position under the macula. It is not always easy to assess the correct position of the fovea intraoperatively, especially if the fovea is elevated. To further confirm the correct position it is useful to have information from the intraoperative OCT. If the intraoperative OCT is not available, it is advisable to have a color picture of the fundus with a marking on the fovea available and compare this preoperative image with the intraoperative view.
7. *Scleral marking of the sutures of the MB.* Once satisfied with the position of the MB, mark the position of the arm in order to suture it to the sclera. When using a non-contact wide field viewing system, this is probably the most crucial, difficult, and time-consuming part of the whole surgery. In fact, while the position of the buckle is assessed under the viewing system, the marks are done under the microscope, while the eye is necessarily moved nasally in order to expose the temporal side and the buckle arm. The surgeon needs to hold the arm of the buckle without moving the position in relation to the eye, and the assistant surgeon needs to clean the area from blood and peribulbar tissue and then mark the position of the arm of the buckle. To ease this step, we developed a nomogram that predict where to place the sutures based on the axial length of the eye. Our variable was the distance between the limbus in the middle of the superotemporal quadrant (at 2.30 o'clock for the left eye and at 10.30 o'clock for the right

eye) and the superior and temporal point of insertion of the needle. We called this variable "distance limbus-needle" (DLN). We collected data so far from 40 eyes with a range of axial lengths between 27.94 and 35.65 mm, using in every case an NPB with a total length of 23.6 mm, Table 1. Knowing the DLN also helps speed up the procedure.

Table 1 A nomogram that provides the distance limbus needle (DLN) in mm for the superior and temporal sutures for a given axial length in mm

AL pre (mm)	Superior DLN (mm)	Temporal DLN (mm)
27.94	8.50	7.00
28.06	11.00	9.00
28.61	10.00	9.00
29.02	11.50	9.00
29.23	12.00	8.00
29.37	9.50	9.00
29.60	9.50	9.00
29.78	10.00	10.00
30.03	12.00	9.00
30.09	11.50	10.00
30.36	12.00	11.00
30.62	13.50	13.50
30.62	11.50	9.00
30.78	11.50	9.00
30.85	11.50	10.50
31.03	11.00	10.50
31.17	12.00	10.00
31.52	11.50	11.50
31.55	12.50	12.00
31.59	12.50	11.00
31.62	11.50	11.50
31.90	13.00	12.50
32.18	13.50	12.00
32.45	16.50	15.00
32.81	13.00	13.00
32.91	13.50	12.00
33.74	17.00	15.50
33.89	14.50	14.00
34.31	14.00	14.00
34.49	15.00	14.00
34.51	14.00	14.50
34.85	13.50	12.50
35.65	16.50	15.00

8. *Apply the suture.* Use a T-Cron 6–0 suture to fix the arm of the NPB to the sclera. The NPB was designed with holes in the anterior side of the arm, to lodge the sutures. There are 2 holes close to the anterior edge of the arm and 2 other holes 3 mm more posteriorly. Placing the two anterior sutures provides sufficient indentation. Additional sutures may be placed through the posterior holes to provide more scleral indentation and enhance the buckle stability if needed.
9. *Check the position* of the buckle after suturing, and if the buckle is not in the perfect position, repeat steps 7, 8, and 9.
10. *Remove the chandelier lights. if applicable*
11. *Remove the traction sutures.*
12. *Close the Tenon and the conjunctiva*, with Vicryl 7–0.

Surgical Tips

- Avoid excessive indentation of the sclera. The final profile of the retina and the sclera should be as flat and horizontal as possible resembling a non-myopic macula.
- Intraoperative OCT can assist centering the buckle and setting the right amount of indentation.

2.2   *Pars Plana Vitrectomy for MTM*

The aim of PPV in MTM is to counteract the perpendicular MTM-inducing force exerted by the vitreous pulling the retina anteriorly. Epiretinal membrane (ERM) peeling or internal limiting membrane (ILM) manipulations counteract the tangential MTM-inducing force that leads to foveal splitting [4].

Our indication of PPV in MTM is aimed to:

(a) Remove ERM/traction after treatment with a MB, if residual distortion of the retina prevents vision improvement.
(b) Close an inner LMH after treating with a MB, if residual distortion of the retina prevents vision improvement.
(c) Close a full-thickness macular hole, simultaneously and sequentially to a MB insertion.

PPV in high myopic eyes can be challenging due to high axial length, posterior staphyloma, thinner and atrophic choroid, degenerated vitreous, and thinner sclera [8].

The first critical aspect of PPV in high myopic eyes is improved visualization. The presence of atrophic choroid reduces the contrast and the ability to identify the ILM, retinal holes, or ERM. Staining the vitreous, ERM, and ILM improves visualization and reduces the risk of iatrogenic tears.

Induction of posterior vitreous detachment (PVD) can be difficult due to vitreoschisis. Staining with dyes helps this step.

The increased axial length and the posterior staphyloma may make access difficult as standard-length instruments may not reach the posterior pole.

Surgery Steps

1. *23-g three-port system (25-g can be used, but in long eyes, stiffer 23-g instruments are more helpful)*
   Insert the trocars at 4 mm behind the limbus in phakic 3.5 mm behind the limbus in the pseudophakic eyes. Chandelier is rarely necessary.
2. *Core vitrectomy and posterior vitreous detachment.*
   Do a core vitrectomy, and identify the posterior hyaloid to verify if PVD is already present. Staining the vitreous with triamcinolone improves the posterior hyaloid visualization. Once the posterior hyaloid is free, extend the PVD to the mid-periphery, and complete the core vitrectomy. Shaving the vitreous base is usually unnecessary in MTM unless a peripheral detachment or break is present.
   At this point, the sequence of steps is different based on the clinical picture.
   If PPV is performed to:

   (a) *Remove ERM/traction.* We peel only the epiretinal membrane after trypan blue/brilliant blue (the dyes stains ERM and ILM).
   (b) *Close an inner lamellar macular.* We stain and peel the epiretinal membrane, if present, then peel and create a flap of ILM to stuff or cover the hole.
   (c) *To close a full-thickness macular hole.* similar to b.
   (d) *Close a full-thickness macular hole associated with a retinal detachment.* In this case, we use perfluorocarbon liquid (PFCL) to flatten the macula then stain and peel epiretinal membrane if persent folowed by an ILM flap and stuffing of the ILM over the hole. Then we exchange fluid/PFCL with air.

3. *Check the periphery* with scleral indentation, and perform peripheral laser coagulation if there are peripheral breaks or lattice degeneration lesions.
4. *Tamponade* we usually use air as tamponade of choice. Use gas SF6 at 20% concentration, whenever a tamponade longer than 1 week is necessary (if rhegmatogenous retinal detachment in the periphery or a full-thickness macular hole).
   Use silicone oil only in case of complicated retinal detachment with proliferative vitreoretinopathy (PVR).
5. *Removal of trocars*
   Despite the use of transconjunctival sutureless vitrectomy, the risk of sclerotomy leakage and postoperative hypotony is higher in high myopic eyes due to the thinner sclera and less vitreous plugging [9–11]. In case of leakage, we suggest suturing sclerotomies with 7–0 Vicryl or at least sealing the conjunctiva over it using diathermy.

Postoperative Posture

Posturing is needed in case of MH: we recommend a face-down position for 3 days in order to hold the flap over the MH.

Surgical Tips

- ILM manipulation is easier when performed on an attached retina. Consider a MB before PPV when a macular detachment is present.
- Intraoperative OCT can assist membrane peeling and positioning the MB and the ILM flap.

2.3   *Complications of Surgery*

- **Macular buckle:**

  - Temporary iatrogenic inner schisis, at 1 month after surgery and spontaneously resolving in 3 months, only if buckle is applied in stage 1 (which we do not recommend) (1%).
  - Temporary foveal detachment, at 1 month after surgery and spontaneously resolving in 3 months (1.9%).
  - Superficial extrusion of the lateral arm of the macular buckle (5%), which is not observed with the new model of macular buckle which is made from PMMA not metal.
  - Diplopia (5%).
  - Temporal choroidal hemorrhage (0.5%).

- **Pars plana vitrectomy:**

  - Temporary foveal detachment (2%).
  - Worsening of the retinal stage (20%).
  - Iatrogenic full-thickness macular hole (20%).
  - PVR (15%).
  - Other complications inherited to PPV including cataract, vitreous hemorrhage, retinal tears, and hypotony.

3   Case Scenario

Case 1
See (Fig. 6)

Case 2
See (Fig. 7)

Case 3
See (Fig. 8)

Case 4
See (Fig. 9)

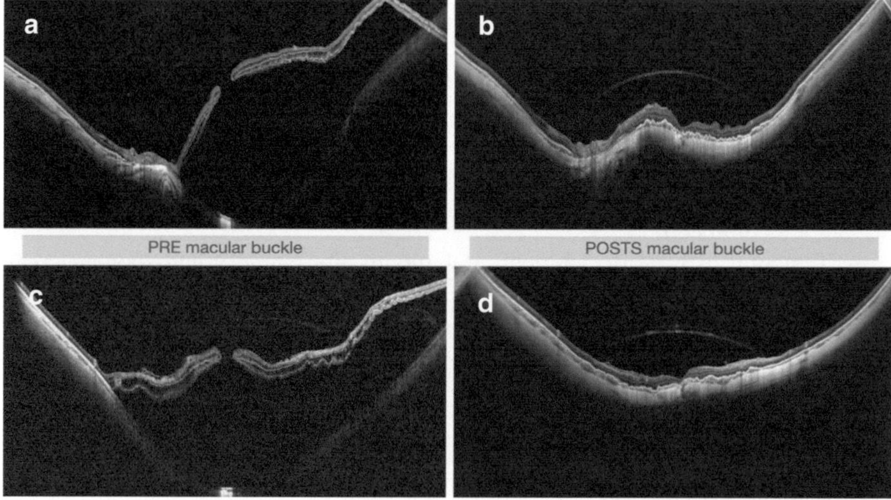

Fig. 6 A 62-year-old female presented with myopic traction maculopathy (MTM) stage 3a (**a**) in the right eye. Best corrected visual acuity (BCVA) was Snellen fraction 0.2. She was treated only with macular buckle with resolution of MTM (**b**). BCVA was 0.5 at 3 months

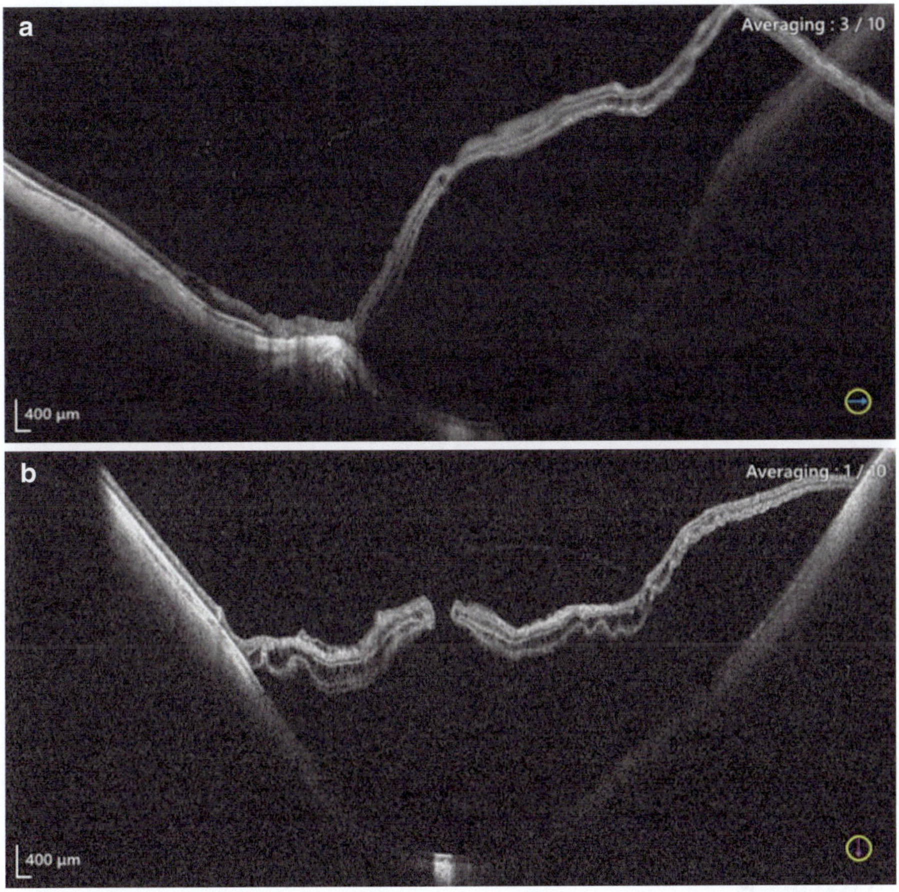

Fig. 7 A 57-year-old female, who presented with myopic traction maculopathy (MTM) stage 4c in the left eye (A horizontal and B vertical OCT scan. Scans are 23 mm by Canon Xephilio). She was treated with macular buckle and pars plana vitrectomy. Best corrected visual acuity was hand motion preoperatively and 0,1 postoperatively. The retina was attached, and the hole was closed (C horizontal and D vertical OCT scan)

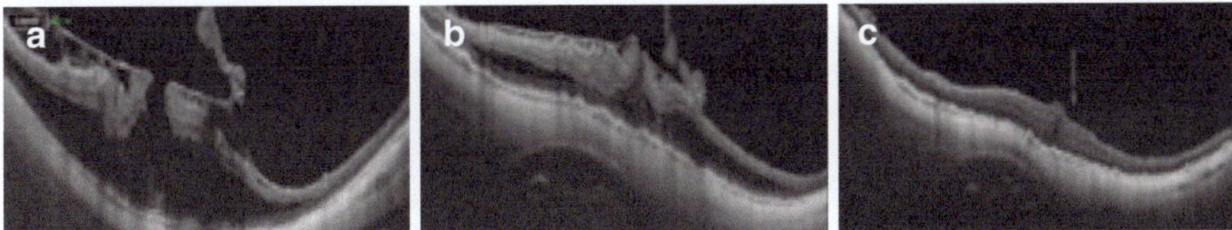

Fig. 8 A 60-year-old male presented with myopic traction maculopathy (MTM) stage 2b + (**a**) in the left eye. Best corrected visual acuity (BCVA) was 0.1. He was treated with a macular buckle to relieve the schisis. Pars plana vitrectomy (PPV) was initially avoided to lower the chance to induce an iatrogenic macular hole. BCVA improved to 0.2, but epiretinal abnormalities limited further vision improvement and induced metamorphopsia (**b**). PPV was performed which improved the inner retinal structure after 6 months (**c**). BCVA improved to 0.4 after an additional period of 9 months

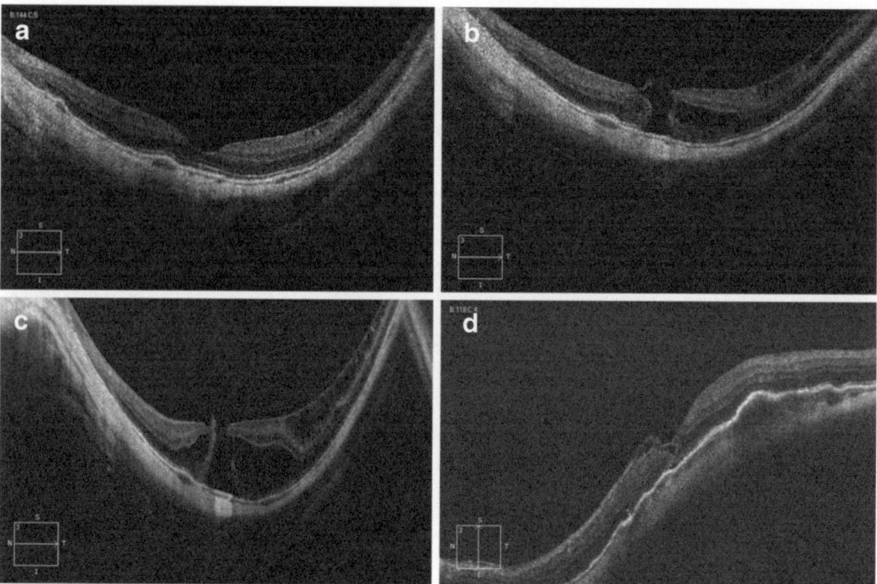

Fig. 9 A 64-year-old female presented in 2017 with myopic traction maculopathy stage 1a (**a**). Best corrected vison was 0.8. This evolved to stage 1C (**b**) in 2019 with a significant drop in vision to 0.1. Further progession to stage 2c with outer macular schisis and full thickness macular hole (**c**) happened in August 2020 and was operated with combined pars plana vitrectomy, macular buckle, ILM flap and gas in September 2020. Postoperatively, the retina was attached, and the hole was closed with an internal limiting membrane flap over the hole (**d**). Vision improved to 0.4 after 3 months

References

1. Panozzo G, Mercanti A. Optical coherence tomography findings in myopic traction maculopathy. Arch Ophthalmol. 2004;122(10):1455–60.
2. Baba T, Ohno-Matsui K, Futagami S, et al. Prevalence and characteristics of foveal retinal detachment without macular hole in high myopia. Am J Ophthalmol. 2003;135(3):338–42. Accessed 5 Apr 2015.
3. Benhamou N, Massin P, Haouchine B, Erginay A, Gaudric A. Macular retinoschisis in highly myopic eyes. Am J Ophthalmol. 2002;133(6):794–800. Accessed 21 Mar 2015.
4. Parolini B, Palmieri M, Finzi A, et al. The new myopic traction maculopathy staging system. Eur J Ophthalmol. 2020;31:1299.
5. Shimada N, Tanaka Y, Tokoro T, Ohno-Matsui K. Natural course of myopic traction maculopathy and factors associated with progression or resolution. Am J Ophthalmol. 2013;156(5):948–957.e1.
6. Parolini B, Parolini B, Palmieri M, Finzi A, Frisina R. Proposal for the management of myopic traction maculopathy based on the new MTM staging system. Eur J Ophthalmol. 2021;31:3265.
7. Parolini B, Frisina R, Pinackatt S, Mete M. A new L-shaped design of macular buckle to support a posterior staphyloma in high myopia. Retina. 2013;33(7):1466–70.

8. Arumi JG, Boixadera A, Martinez-Castillo V, Zapata MA, Macià C. Surgery for myopic macular hole without retinal detachment. Eur Ophthalmic Rev. 2012;06:204.
9. Woo SJ, Park KH, Hwang JM, Kim JH, Yu YS, Chung H. Risk factors associated with sclerotomy leakage and postoperative hypotony after 23-gauge transconjunctival sutureless vitrectomy. Retina. 2009;29:456.
10. Curtin BJ, Iwamoto T, Renaldo DP. Normal and Staphylomatous sclera of high myopia: an electron microscopic study. Arch Ophthalmol. 1979;97:912.
11. Coppola M, Rabiolo A, Cicinelli MV, Querques G, Bandello F. Vitrectomy in high myopia: a narrative review. Int J Retin Vitr. 2017;3:37.

Vitrectomy for Proliferative Diabetic Retinopathy

Riley Sanders, Hassan Al-Dhibi, and Ahmed B. Sallam

1   Introduction

- The hallmark of diabetic retinopathy is the loss of capillary pericytes, which distorts the blood-eye barrier, leading to incompetent vessels and eventual capillary dropout from long-term derangement in insulin regulation and glucose metabolism.
- The driving force of proliferative diabetic retinopathy (PDR) progression is thought to be the excess production of vascular endothelial growth factor (VEGF) from the resultant ischemic retina and retinal pigment epithelium (RPE).
- Histologically incomplete neovascular (NV) networks grow from native blood vessels onto the inner retinal surface and into the vitreous if posterior vitreous detachment (PVD) has not occurred. If PVD later occurs, the brittle vessels bleed into the subhyaloid space or vitreous gel. The NV can also fibrose and contract along the retinal surface, leading to traction retinal detachment (TRD) or combined traction/rhegmatogenous retinal detachment (CTRD). Neovascularization can also occur in the anterior segment, manifesting as pupillary abnormalities, hyphema, and neovascular glaucoma (NVG).

Supplementary Information The online version contains supplementary material available at https://doi.org/10.1007/978-3-031-47827-7_18.

R. Sanders
Ophthalmology/Retina, University of Arkansas for Medical Sciences, Little Rock, AR, USA

H. Al-Dhibi
King Khaled Eye Specialist Hospital, Riyadh, Saudi Arabia

A. B. Sallam (✉)
Jones Eye Institute, University of Arkansas for Medical Sciences, Little Rock, AR, USA

"

- Diagnosis of PDR can be made by clinical exam alone. However, wide-field fundus photography and wide-field fluorescein angiography are helpful to diagnose subtle cases and gauge the severity of retinal ischemia.

2 Diabetic Vitrectomy Challenges

- Eye surgery on diabetic patients presents several unique challenges and requires advanced fundamental knowledge and skills in anterior segment techniques and vitreoretinal surgery. Traction from an adherent posterior hyaloid makes complete pars plana vitrectomy (PPV) extremely difficult, with a considerable risk of iatrogenic breaks and intraoperative hemorrhage.
- Patients often have multiple coexisting surgical pathologies, including cataract, NVG, vitreous hemorrhage (VH), and TRD.
- The approach must therefore be carefully considered, with a balance between single- or multi-stage surgery and sometimes combined vitrectomy with cataract or glaucoma surgery. In this chapter, we cover the approach to diabetic vitreoretinal surgery.

2.1 Panretinal Photocoagulation

We do not intend to focus on panretinal photocoagulation (PRP) in this chapter, but we would like to highlight a few important remarks:

1. As ischemic retina producing VEGF is the reason behind PDR, the first "surgery" priority is typically PRP in clinic (outpatient), at the time of diagnosis of PDR. Patients are then followed for the regression or progression of their NV, as well as the progression of TRD or increasing VH.
2. VH does not indicate that PRP has failed, as the contraction of vessels may induce some bleeding. Changes in the caliber of vessels and density of NV networks are reliable indicators of response to PRP [1].
3. The temporal edge of the PRP should be 2.5-disc diameter (DD) temporal to the edge of the foveal avascular zone, and the nasal edge should be 1.5 DD nasal to the nerve for the preservation of the temporal visual field (Image 1a). Some physicians leave a large area of the temporal retina untreated posteriorly which should not be the case. Fundus autofluorescence (FAF) is an excellent way to visualize previous PRP spots and unlasered areas (Image 1b).
4. In general, we find slit lamp laser much easier to use than the laser indirect ophthalmoscope (LIO) in the clinic setting. It is less painful for the patient, especially using the short-duration laser, and ergonomically superior for the physician. You can reach peripheral enough with modern machines and viewing lenses. Short-duration laser is also less painful than conventional PRP using 100

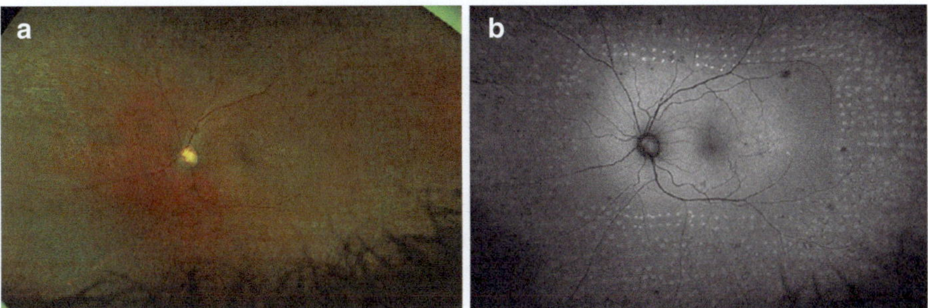

Image 1 (**a**) Optos™ wide-field multicolor image of panretinal photocoagulation (PRP) laser. Note 1.5–2 DD spared nasal to the nerve and 2.5–3 DD spared temporal to the FAZ. (**b**) Fundus autofluorescence (FAF) can aid in identifying laser marks

milliseconds (ms) laser but is less effective, and therefore, more shots are needed to have the same effect [2].The merit of LIO includes superior viewing in eyes with media opacity and better viewing of the extreme periphery.

5. The question is as follows: what should be done for eyes with persistent neovascularization of the disc (NVD)/iris (NVI)/elsewhere (NVE) despite adequate laser PRP? If these vessels are florid/active, we consider additional peripheral laser treatment with LIO and scleral depression usually followed by anti-VEGF treatment. We find laser treatment in this context painful, and we usually use sub-Tenon's anesthesia. If these vessels are fibrosed, we watch and consider PPV if there are repeat significant vitreous bleeds.

6. If media opacity (such as cataract or VH) is present which prevents the adequate delivery of PRP, and the disease is progressing to threaten vision, this constitutes an indication for surgery to complete the laser. After cataract extraction (CE), PRP may be completed with the laser indirect ophthalmoscope (LIO) in the same session or at a later date in clinic via slit lamp laser. Open surgical wounds need to be taken into consideration, and sterile technique should be used for LIO done in the OR immediately following CE. Likewise, time for adequate wound closure should be given before doing slit lamp laser with a contact lens. It is therefore helpful to place a corneal suture at the time of cataract surgery when early laser is planned postoperatively.

7. Intravitreal anti-VEGF agents are increasingly administered around the initiation of PRP to rapidly reduce VEGF levels and induce regression of neovascularization. Their effect is more potent and immediate than with laser, which has made them a cornerstone of PDR treatment [3]. This efficacy can sometimes induce an undesirable contractile response and worsen a TRD, in cases with large sheets of fibrosing NV membranes [4], though they are mostly safe for localized TRD when administered regularly for patients being closely observed [5]. However, currently available anti-VEGF treatment lasts only a matter of months, and unfortunately, there is a surprisingly high rate of loss-to-follow-up in patients with PDR [6]. Therefore, the durable effect of PRP is still critical to long-term success for most patients.

# 3	Indications for PPV Surgery

## 3.1	Vitreous Hemorrhage

One of the most common indications for diabetic vitrectomy is non-clearing vitreous or subhyaloid hemorrhage. Small pre-retinal hemorrhages may be observed if asymptomatic and good PRP can be done. Hemorrhages that obscure vision are more likely to require surgery. The Diabetic Retinopathy Vitrectomy study showed that early vitrectomy within 1–6 months of vitreous hemorrhage more than 1 month duration was associated with a better outcome, particularly type 1 DM [7]. Nowadays, with the advancement in vitrectomy surgery, most surgeons would only wait between 1 and 2 months before surgery. In an eye with VH and adequate PRP, waiting up to several months may be reasonable. Still, early surgery within weeks may be considered in certain situations including (a) eyes with no/little PRP before bleeding, (b) poor seeing fellow eye, and (c) eyes with NVI/NVG and ghost cell glaucoma. In the latter scenario, we usually operate within days. If an observation period is agreed upon, and the VH is dense enough to obscure fundoscopic details, regular B-scan ultrasonography must be performed to ensure that tractional membranes are not progressing to TRD.

## 3.2	Retinal Detachment

(a) TRD is another indication of PPV, especially when it involves the macula inside the arcades. TRD progressing on serial exams may also be an indication for surgery, especially if the patient has symptomatic changes in their visual field. Extramacular TRD may be observed if stable, and the patient has good vision and minimal symptoms. In fact, it is usually better to wait on these patients, due to the risk/benefit profile of diabetic PPV.

   In cases with localized extramacular TRD and good vision, it is better to start with PRP and observe progression. Keep away from areas of fibrovascular membranes, and be aware that some patients have dramatic contracture after laser (Image 2). If significant traction is already present, consider proceeding with surgery before laser. The vitreous may be easier to remove before PRP has been applied, tractional membranes will be less contracted, and surgeons can do endolaser PRP. The caveat is that overzealous endo-PRP can lead to worse post-operative inflammation, up to post-vitrectomy fibrinoid syndrome. Intravitreal steroid injections at the surgery's closing may help mitigate this [8].

(b) Combined TRD/RRD (CTRD) (Image 3) is an indication for surgery even if the detachment is non-macular. Because of the presence of a retinal break, the detachment will inevitably progress, and rapid interventions are needed.

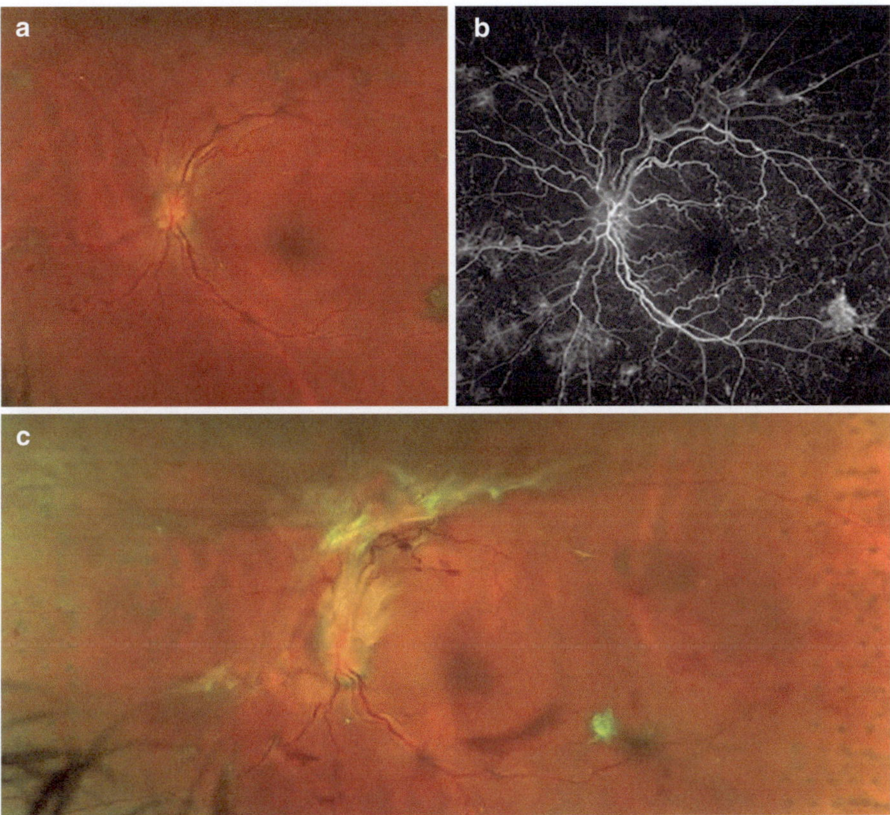

Image 2 (**a**) Fundus image demonstrating proliferative diabetic retinopathy of a patient's left eye. The extent of neovascular membranes is better seen on FA (Panel **b**). One month after PRP, the neovascular membranes have contracted, leading to traction retinal detachment of the superior peripapillary retina and superior macula (**c**)

3.3 Macular Edema

(a) Vitreoretinal traction and taut posterior hyaloid/epiretinal membrane can also contribute to persistent intraretinal fluid or macular edema, which is best seen on OCT (Image 4). PPV may be considered in these cases as well.

(b) The role of PPV and internal limiting membrane (ILM) peel in chronic macular edema with no traction is unclear. There is no consensus whether the improvement in macular thickness that is sometimes observed post-surgery is a factor of retinal thinning post-ILM peel or represents actual improvement in vision. It is also hard to comment on VA as many of the studies on this topic included combined cataract PPV surgery and some had a vitreous hemorrhage that was removed. In general, we do not endorse PPV for non-tractional macular edema.

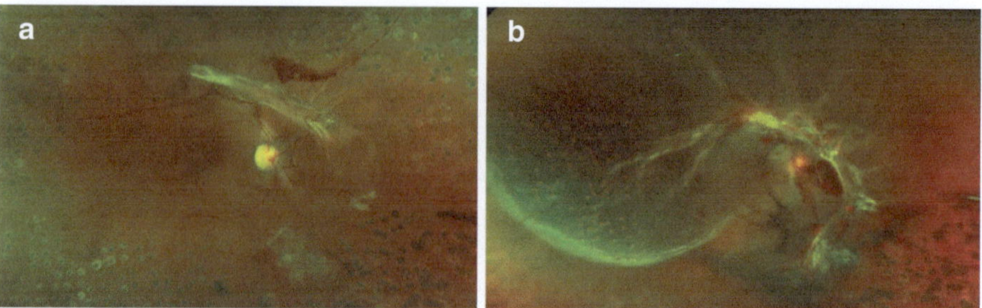

Image 3 Progression of tractional retinal detachment (TRD) to combined combined rhegmatogenous tractional detachment. In panel **a**, there are fibrovascular membranes and associated TRD around the nerves and arcades. In panel **b**, the retinal detachment is more bullous temporally, indicative of rhegmatogenous component. The retinal break is not seen, but likely small and located at the base of a band of traction

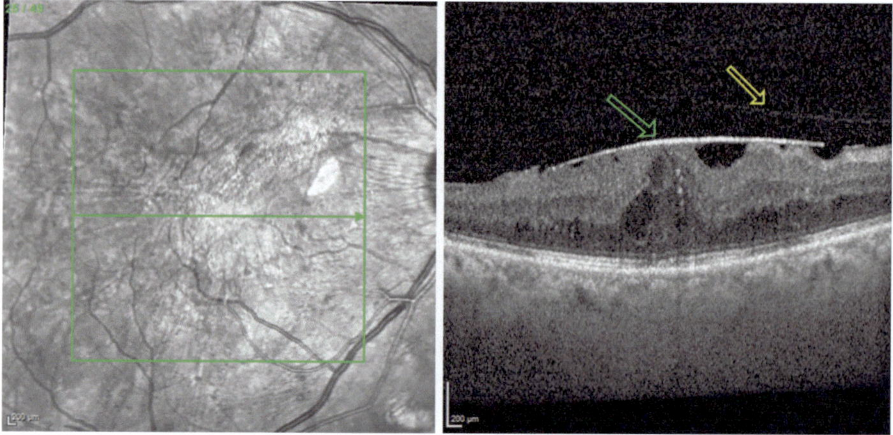

Image 4 Diabetic macular edema with significant tractional component. This edema was poorly responsive to multiple anti-vascular endothelial growth factors injections. Note the adherent hyaloid (yellow arrow) and the epiretinal membrane (ERM) (green arrow)

3.4 Anterior Segment Neovascularization

Neovascularization of the iris (NVI) or NVG, without an adequate view to complete PRP, is an indication for surgery. CE may be adequate, but if significant VH or traction is present as well, combined CE/PPV should be considered. If severe NVG has already occurred, the intraocular pressure (IOP) is unlikely to normalize with these measures alone due to synechial angle closure, and in selected cases, combining PPV and glaucoma drainage implant may be appropriate.

Other surgical indications to consider: Persistent NV despite good laser, particularly if associated with repeat vitreous hemorrhage.

4 Preoperative Considerations

4.1 Status of the Crystalline Lens

In general, if a patient is young enough to have accommodative faculty of the crystalline lens, effort should be taken to preserve it during vitrectomy. However, priority is given to complete treatment of the retinal pathology. Dextrose 50% infusion has been suggested to reduce intraoperative cataract formation [9], but evidence on its efficacy is mixed, and we usually do not use it. In cases where lens removal is not inevitable but may become necessary due to intraoperative opacity or lens damage during hemorrhage removal, it is advisable to do preoperative measurements and calculations for an intraocular lens (IOL) prosthesis. For more information, refer to the chapter on diabetic cataract surgery.

4.2 Pupillary Dilation

Although poor pharmacological pupillary dilation is common in diabetics likely due to a combination of iris muscle ischemia and neuropathy, topical mydriatics (phenylephrine 2.5% and tropicamide 1%, beginning 1–2 h preoperatively) usually provide adequate visualization using modern wide-field viewing systems. Intracameral epi-Shugarcaine (epinephrine 0.025%/lidocaine 0.75%) often works well to pharmacologically dilate the pupil, but its effect diminishes with repeated intraoperative dosing. Therefore, we recommend holding it until necessary (e.g., the pupil comes down after cataract surgery or starts to constrict during the PPV), since the first administration seems to give the greatest effect.

In cases where good pupil dilation is not achieved, mechanical pupil dilation using rings or hooks may be necessary. This is mostly in cases needing combined CE/vitrectomy or in eyes with NVI.

4.3 Pre-Existing PRP

Some surgeons advocate for doing as much PRP as possible prior to surgery. Endolaser is inflammatory, and there is a concern for worse postoperative inflammation. However, if surgery is already indicated and can be done promptly, consideration can be given for deferred laser, with endo-PRP at the time of surgery. Fibrovascular vitreous membranes will be less contracted, and the peripheral hyaloid is easier to remove prior to laser.

4.4 Anti-VEGF Treatment

In eyes with active diabetic neovessels undergoing PPV, injection of intravitreal anti-VEGF prior to PPV is helpful in decreasing intraoperative bleeding and therefore shortening surgery time and reducing iatrogenic breaks during surgery [10]. It can be given from 1 week up until several hours before surgery. While it first decreases vascular elements, it is important to note that between 10 and 20 days, there is an increase in fibrous and contractile elements, which may make traction become worse [11]. The clinical significance of this angiofibrotic switch is arguable. In general, we use anti-VEGF before delamination surgery, injecting 2–3 days preoperatively.

4.5 Anti-Coagulant Therapy

We do not recommend stopping or changing anti-coagulant agents if the patient has significant cardiovascular morbidity indicating their use. Liaising with prescribing physicians is usually too complex, and stopping these medicines may have systemic severe implications. Although there may be an increase in the risk of bleeding on these agents during PPV, several studies have shown no significant bleeding risk when anti-coagulants were not stopped [12].

4.6 Glaucoma

Consideration should be given to combined PPV and tube placement in patients with NVG. The tube may be placed through the pars plana once a complete vitrectomy has been done. In this approach, the tube of the valve may be placed in the pars plana rather than in the anterior chamber (AC), which may be advantageous to prevent iris chafing or corneal endothelial damage. Understandably, peripheral vitrectomy must be thorough if a pars plana tube is placed, due to risk of vitreous blockage.

Additionally, patients with open-angle glaucoma can also develop PDR. These patients should continue their glaucoma medications up until surgery and be followed closely for high pressure following vitrectomy.

4.7 Anesthesia Choice

For short cases (90 min or less), we prefer monitored (local) anesthesia, with minimal to no sedation. Even longer cases can be done under local anesthesia in select patients. However, general anesthesia is often a better choice when prolonged surgery is expected, in young or anxious patients, and in those with claustrophobia or trouble lying flat.

4.8 Other Patient Factors

PDR is a disease of the unwell. Patients often have significant cardiac comorbidity and renal failure and may have had concomitant strokes and subsequent devices such as tracheostomy or gastric tube placement. Localized or systemic infection is also common. Diabetic retinopathy of any severity is associated with increased incidence of stroke, heart attack, and all-cause mortality [13]. The average survival from time of TRD diagnosis is <5 years with a nearly 50% mortality rate at 10 years [14].

The ophthalmologist must be proactive in the co-management with the primary care physician, cardiologist, nephrologist, neurologist, and other surgeons to be sure patients are optimized for eye surgery when possible. Only so much optimization is possible. Many times, it is in the patient's best interest to undergo eye surgery despite being otherwise ill, especially when rapid deterioration of the visual potential is expected. That said, anesthesiologists and surgeons must work together in determining which cases should wait until better control of a given comorbidity. A question that always arises is as follows: what is the blood glucose level above which PPV or cataract surgery must be canceled? The answer is that there is none, and we advise not postponing surgery if the patient is hemodynamically stable and not in ketoacidosis. You could even argue that patients can help themselves more and take their medicine if they get surgery and their vision improves [15].

4.9 Surgical Consent

Diabetic vitrectomy is among the most challenging retina surgeries, and sight-threatening intraoperative and postoperative complications are common. The disease, surgical plan, risks, benefits, and alternatives should be discussed first in the clinic. Showing the patient their own images helps explain the severity of their condition. It is helpful to involve the patient's family/caregivers. On the day of surgery, the surgery and post-op care plan should be again reviewed, but it should not be the first time the patient hears about surgery risks!

As a rule, it is best to "underpromise and overdeliver" in diabetic patients. In some cases, the retina is very ischemic, and vision may not improve significantly even after removing traction and media opacities.

5   Surgical Procedure

This section will focus mainly on managing diabetic traction detachment and diabetic fibrovascular delamination. Diabetic vitreous hemorrhage was covered under the vitreous hemorrhage chapter and cataract surgery in the diabetic cataract surgery chapter.

5.1   Surgical Setup

The surgeon's microscope must be equipped for both wide-angle viewing and high-magnification work. Non-contact systems with diagonal image inversion are most used today. At a minimum, a three-port pars plana vitrectomy is usually needed. Additional ports may be necessary for chandelier lighting when bimanual surgery is performed.

If cataract surgery is to be done simultaneously, it is best to pre-place the pars plana trocar ports at the start of the case.

Using the Resight viewing system, we like to start with the green (60D) lens which provides an excellent view of the whole posterior pole to the arcade and beyond, with reasonable magnification. If we are not using 3D surgery, we usually utilize a contact plano-convex lens for macular work such as macular ERM peel or ILM peel. With 3D, the non-contact green lens suffices. For peripheral vitreous removal and laser, we use the wide-field yellow (128D) lens.

5.2   Choice of Gauge Size

25-gauge (g) is usually our gauge of choice for most vitrectomy cases including diabetic delamination. At this gauge, the instruments are reasonably sturdy, endoillumination is wide and bright, and the vitrector size allows appropriate access to diabetic membranes. For some cases, where the spaces between the diabetic membranes and the retina are very tight, we may combine this with an additional 27-g cutter. 27-g vitrector probes provide the smallest possible sphere of influence around the cutter port and allow precise delamination and segmentation of membranes near the retina. We prefer the high cutting probes (20,000 cuts per minute/CPM) with beveled tips that make the port opening closer to the retina for better access (Image 5). For this reason, a hybrid 25/27-g system offers all the advantages of both systems. In cases of traction/rhegmatogenous detachments with a highly mobile detached retina, bimanual surgery is likely required. In these instances, consideration is given to starting with 23-g ports, for the best availability of forceps and scissors for bimanual surgery.

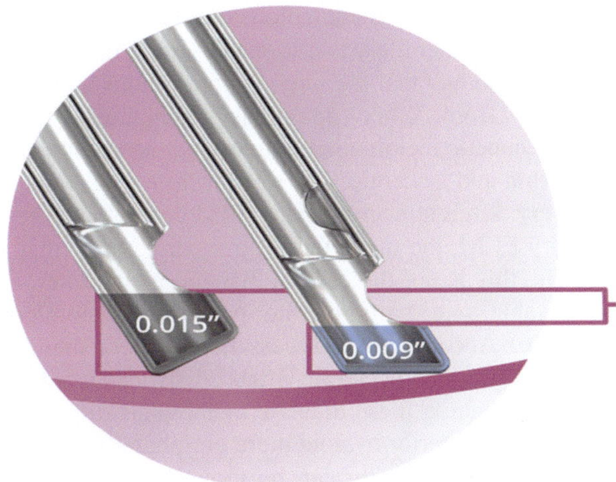

Image 5 Comparison of Alcon™ 27-gauge cutters, with a standard tip cutter on the left. The beveled tip allows the port opening to be 40% closer to the retinal surface

5.3 *Diabetic Vitreous Anatomy*

Separation of the posterior hyaloid is the cornerstone of a good vitrectomy. Without separating the hyaloid, vitrectomy will seem redundant: the surgeon circles around the vitreous cavity, each time finding more vitreous! This is because only layers of central vitreous are being removed, and there is always more underneath.

The diabetic posterior hyaloid is notoriously difficult to separate from the retina, due to two main factors: (1) growth of NV into the posterior vitreous face and (2) vitreoschisis, in which one or more "false" posterior hyaloid faces may be encountered and separated from the retina.

NV roots itself into the vitreous if there is no PVD and creates areas of vitreous adhesion. Neovascular ingrowth will be most prominent in the areas of firm vitreous attachment; thus, the location varies with patient age and vitreous status. In patients under 50 and with no previous surgery, the posterior hyaloid is usually completely attached. Accordingly, the majority of NV and traction is found at the posterior pole. In patients with partial PVD, NV may have grown into the vitreous more peripherally, with traction in these areas. Pre-retinal hemorrhage indicates partial separation of the vitreous from the retina. Pre-retinal hemorrhage can appear very localized if no spontaneous PVD is present or appear "boat-shaped" when it is pulled by gravity and settles along the edge of the PVD. The appearance of hemorrhage can give valuable clues for finding a plane of separation between the retina and posterior hyaloid during surgery.

The posterior vitreous face/hyaloid is a multi-layered or laminate structure [16]. In non-diabetics, these layers are fused and can be surgically separated all at once from the retina. However, in diabetics with TRD, there is usually schisis between these layers in most cases, and it is possible that the inner layers may be lifted separately from the outer layers. Surgeons must therefore be wary of "false"

PVD. Staining with triamcinolone or vital dyes such as brilliant blue or ICG is helpful to tell whether there is true separation of the hyaloid over the retina.

It is important that the surgeon understands that diabetic membranes in TRD are different from other epiretinal membranes such as primary (idiopathic) ERM. Diabetic membranes are more adherent to the retina, and the underlying retina is thin and ischemic. The relationship of diabetic membranes to the vitreous is also very different from primary ERM due to the presence of vitreoschisis. While in primary ERM, the membrane is a separate layer that is found under the posterior hyaloid, this is not the case in diabetic membranes, which are best thought of as inseparable and parts of the posterior hyaloid/posterior vitreoschisis leaflet (Image 6). Accordingly, to access these diabetic membranes, the surgeon must identify and lift up the posterior vitreoschisis leaflet from the retina, outside the membrane. Dissecting these diabetic membranes off, the retina will open the plane to remove the posterior hyaloid more peripherally (Video 1).

Vitreoretinal traction can be thought of in three main types: (1) anterior-to-posterior (AP), (2) tangential, and (3) bridging (Image 7). Often, all three are present. AP traction extends from the anterior vitreous face to the posterior pole, forming adhesions to the posterior hyaloid. Tangential traction occurs when a fibrovascular hyaloid contracts along the retinal surface. At the epicenters of the NV, it is often inseparable from the retina. Bridging traction occurs when contraction of tangential membranes creates folds within the retina, with tightly stretched hyaloid between the peaks of these folds.

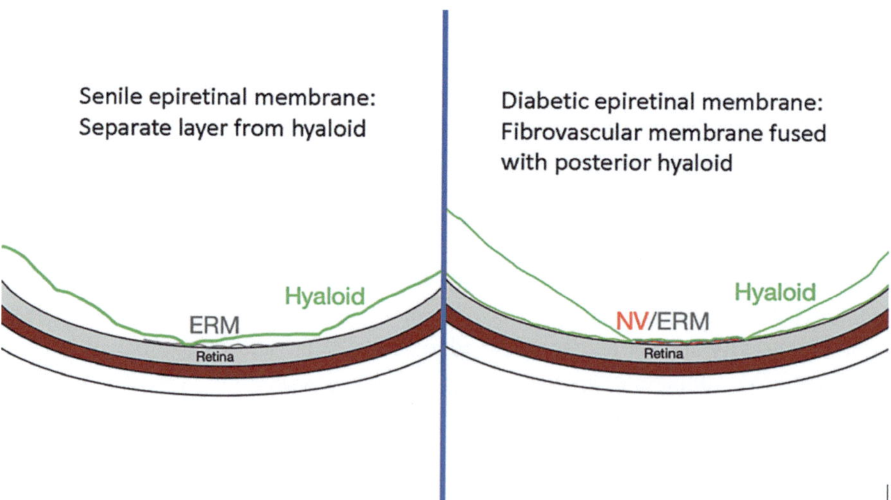

Image 6 Comparison of senile and diabetic epiretinal membranes

Image 7 Schematic showing different types of diabetic vitreous traction and vitreoschisis

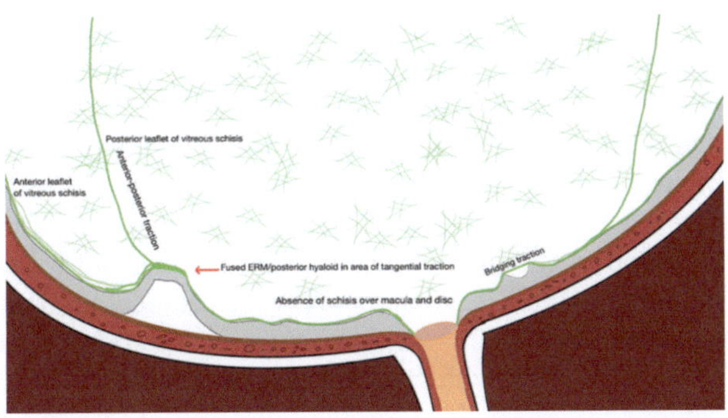

5.4 Posterior Hyaloid and Fibrovascular Membrane Dissection Plan

With the principles of vitreoretinal traction and vitreoschisis in mind, the surgeon can begin to approach diabetic vitrectomy. The process should proceed as such:

1. Clearing a window of the vitreous around the trocar entry sites.
2. Severing obvious sheets of AP traction as you move toward the posterior hyaloid. AP traction may be seen extending from the vitreous base down to the edge of posterior tangential tractional membranes. Additional AP layers can be found and addressed later.
3. Clearing vitreous hemorrhage if present over the macula and optic nerve to get an adequate view of the hyaloid and tractional membranes.
4. Attention is then turned to the posterior hyaloid and any tractional membranes that are present. This will comprise the bulk of the surgery. As the posterior hyaloid is typically fused with fibrovascular membranes in PDR, the following discussion applies to both the hyaloid and these membranes.
5. Peripheral vitreous removal, often with indentation to clear more hemorrhage.
6. Further surgical steps (e.g., endolaser, iridotomy, steroid implants, etc.).

Dissection of posterior hyaloid/membranes in our view should usually begin in an "in-out" direction, i.e., starting near the optic nerve and moving peripherally. When one can achieve a dissection plane in the peripapillary area, it is usually full thickness through the entire hyaloid, and it will be easier to continue moving peripherally under the hyaloid (Video 2). Starting elsewhere is not only less systematic, but it carries a greater risk of creating "false" PVD. It is sometimes appropriate to do an "out-in" dissection moving more toward the nerve. For example, a pre-retinal hemorrhage or an area of bridging traction close to the disc may provide a safe area to open the hyaloid, due to the pre-existing separation plane. One can then move back to the disc to continue separation. If no obvious plane is evident, it is best to just pick an area at the disc border away from the papillomacular bundle and start there.

A sharp instrument, such as a retinal pick, is useful in starting the dissection plane. End-grasping forceps can also be considered to start the dissection, but caution should be exercised as pulling too hard over the nerve can create retinal breaks and shear blood vessels in the surrounding retina. Once a plane is started, the membrane is pulled up little by little and then cut and removed. This comprises membrane *delamination*. Delamination can be accomplished with either a vitrectomy probe or a combination of bimanual forceps and scissors. As dissection proceeds, the surgeon must watch not only his instrument tip but the surrounding vitreous and retina. One must be aware of areas of vitreoretinal adhesion "epicenters" as the hyaloid is lifted with blunt pulling force. These areas often represent NV pegs, where new vessels have grown out of retinal vessels and into the vitreous. When these areas are identified, the surgeon should shift attention to sharp dissection around these areas. Pegs should be cut short, rather than being entirely pulled out. Blunt pulling on epicenters can create retinal breaks or shear the walls of native vessels and lead to more bleeding. When broad-based centers of tangential traction are too adherent to delaminate safely, membranes can be cut along bridging traction and be *segmented*, which is another effective way to relieve tractional forces acting along the plane of the retina (Image 8).

With the ability of the vitrectomy probe for both vacuuming and cutting, small-gauge vitrectomy probes (especially beveled 27-gauge) are an ideal first choice for single-handed delamination in many membranes today. Once an opening in the posterior hyaloid has been made, the probe's port can be placed on the edge of the membrane to dissect it along the plane of the membrane. This is called *conformational* delamination and is employed when the membrane is tightly adherent. With a beveled 27-gauge cutter, the port is within 0.09 in. (2.3 mm) from the retina,

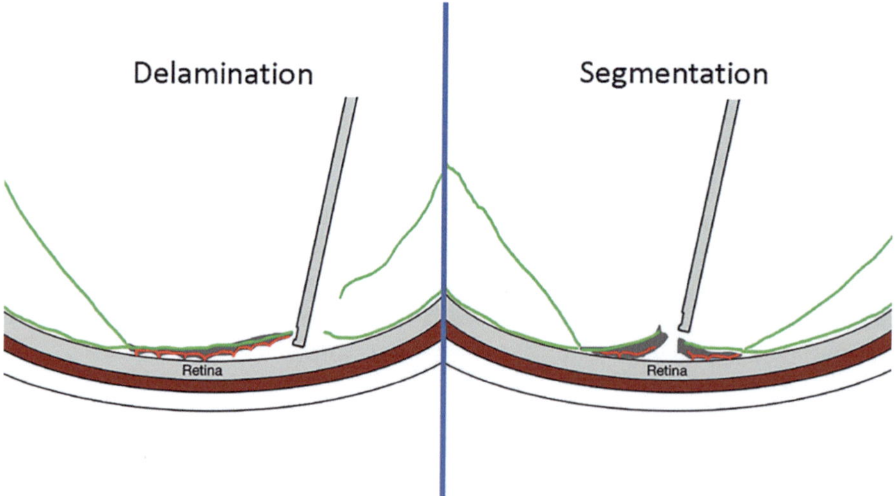

Image 8 Schematic of delamination (lifting the whole membrane as a sheet) versus segmentation (separating firmly adherent membranes along bridging areas between broad-based adhesions)

allowing membrane trimming very close to the retina without significant retinal touch occurring (Image 5). Once more of the membrane edge has been freed, the cutter can be held anterior to the membrane while the cutter and vacuum are activated. This causes the free edges of the membrane to lift up, or *fold back*, into the port for rapid consumption (Video 3).

Bimanual delamination with forceps and horizontal scissors, combined with segmentation using vertical scissors, is another option (Video 4). We use it when adhesions are too firm to create a plane using the vitrector. Another situation that calls for a switch to bimanual technique is CTRD, where the retina is too mobile to safely delaminate membranes with the vacuum of the vitrectomy probe. A variety of horizontal scissors and forceps are available in 23- and 25-gauge size for this purpose. When extensive bimanual dissection is anticipated, starting with 23-gauge ports allows a wider variety of instruments to be used. The 23-gauge DORC® Ovali™ spatula scissor (Image 9a) has a blunt outer side which can be used for gentle blunt dissection under the membrane, followed by the cutting of fine adhesions. Sharp dissection under the membrane is preferable to blunt dissection to avoid shearing of vascular pegs, but the surgeon should be wary of cutting into the retina in folded areas. Other horizontal scissors may be straight or curved. Use of a curved scissors, such as the Alcon® Grieshaber DSP™ (available in 23- and 25-gauge), can be helpful for both segmenting and delaminating (Image 9b).

Vertical scissors with a pick-like tip can be used to wedge under the edge of a tightly adherent membrane and make small cuts for segmentation (Image 9c) [6].

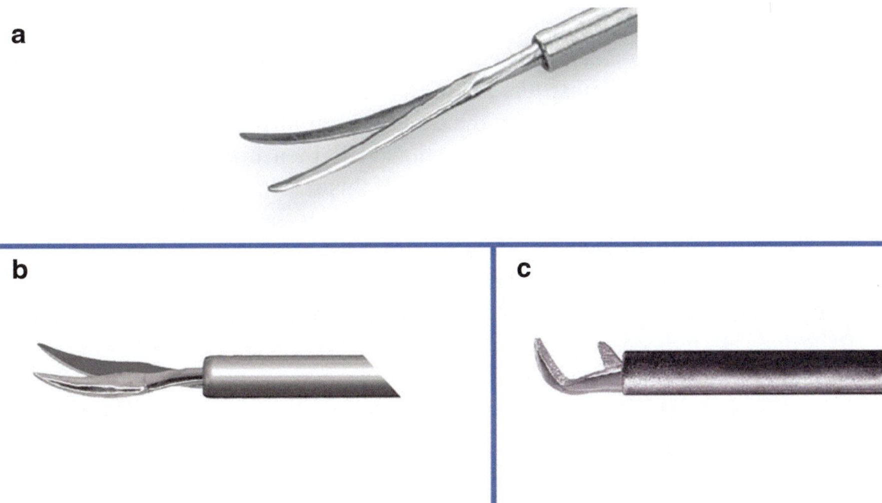

Image 9 (**a**) Tip of 23-gauge DORC Ovali™ spatula scissors. When closed, it has a relatively flat and blunt shape, which can be used for gentle blunt dissection, and then be opened to use for sharp cutting. (Image courtesy of DORC). (**b**) Alcon Grieshaber™ curved scissors instrument tip. (Image courtesy of Alcon). (**c**) Alcon Grieshaber™ vertical scissors (Image courtesy of Alcon)

A technique of injecting viscoelastic underneath a membrane for *viscodissection*, to aid in creating a plane of separation from the membrane and retina is used by some surgeons. We have rarely found this to be necessary. It also exerts hydraulic force on the retina, can create tears, and is difficult to remove.

Once the posterior vitreous face and tractional membranes have been adequately dissected, the surgeon can move on to complete the peripheral vitreous removal.

We try to avoid using PFCL in general during surgery unless it is really required. One scenario is in combined TRD/RRD (CTRD), where the retina is very mobile and membrane dissection is needed. We use PFCL in this situation to support the posterior retina after dissecting posterior membranes and work our way peripheral to the PFCL bubble, very similar to PVR surgery.

For completion, we want to mention a technique called trimanual dissection for delamination where bimanual surgery is performed under PFCL for controlling bleeding and providing support to the retina during dissection [17] (Video 5). We have limited experience with this technique, and we worry that if a break happens, PFCL may go under the retina during dissection.

5.5 Extent of Posterior Hyaloid and Fibrovascular Membrane Dissection

- Ideally, one wants to dissect all fibrovascular membranes/posterior hyaloid off the retina to relieve retinal traction and decrease the risk of POVCH. This is a perfect scenario, but it is difficult to achieve in many cases.
- With extensive dissection, the risk of creating retinal tears should be considered.
- A good rule to remember in diabetic delamination is to avoid/minimize creating iatrogenic retinal tears (just like in ROP surgery). Retinal tears may affect the visual outcome and may result in the development of RRD and PVR. However, if retinal tears do occur during dissection, it is then important to continue to remove all traction around the tear(s) even if this results in creating other retinal tears. This may include limited focal retinectomy if there is a plaque around the tear that cannot be dissected.
- When only a few tears and traction on these tears have been relieved, the retina usually settles down well under gas, and rhegmatogenous retinal detachment/PVR does not happen.
- Difficulties and problems arise when numerous tears occur, and traction remains around these tears. This is a situation you do want not to get in. The key is to learn to stop before creating retinal tears particularly if the macula and the arcade area have already been cleared, which is the main goal of diabetic delamination surgery.
- Table 1 provides some guidance on our rating of surgery goals and expected anatomical outcome. The main point here is to try to avoid breaks in areas of extensive traction, where it will be difficult to relieve traction on these breaks.

Table 1 Our rating of surgery goals during membrane dissection and the expected anatomical outcomes

Residual fibrovascular membranes	Iatrogenic retinal tears	Intraocular tamponade	Our rating for expected outcome
No	No	BSS/air	Excellent
Yes (outside arcade)	No	BSS/air	Good/very good
No	Yes, only a few	Gas	Good/very good
Yes, but no traction around retinal tears	Yes, only a few but no traction around them	Gas	Good/very good
Yes	Yes	Silicone oil	Unfavorable
Yes/no	Large retinectomy	Silicone oil	Unfavorable

5.6 Vitreous Base Shaving

- In the absence of peripheral PVR retinal detachment, we usually do not perform vitreous base shaving. We believe that this is an unnecessary step that does not improve the visual result and is associated with increased surgery time as well as the risk of creating retinal tears or touching the crystalline lens.
- The only exception is in eyes with inferior vitreous base hemorrhage, where "leaching" of blood from this area may cause early postoperative bleeding, and cautious shaving of the vitreous base inferiorly could therefore be of benefit.

5.7 SRF Management

- In TRD, we advise leaving the fluid, and it will self-absorb. There is no need to convert a TRD to a CTRD and add risks of PVR. A scenario where we may do a drainage retinotomy is where a large area of the retina that was not lasered before is detached from traction. We may in this situation perform a posterior drainage retinotomy, AFX to flatten the retina, and laser under air. Alternatively, you could use PFCL to push the subretinal fluid peripherally to a clean retinal area with no membranes, laser under PFCL, and then perform a drainage retinotomy, AFX, and laser around the retinotomy site.
- In CTRD, at least some subretinal fluid needs to be drained to be able to laser around the tears. Several options are available as in RRD including drainage from the break, drainage retinotomy, external drainage, or using PFCL. An important point is that in order to safely make a drainage retinotomy in the presence of TRD, one has to do it in a clean retinal area with no surrounding membranes or traction. We prefer not to use PFCL as much as possible.

5.8 *Eyes with Advanced Traction or Coexisting PVR*

- We encounter eyes with very severe TRD and extensive membranes. For better or worse, the outcome of these eyes is very guarded, and the presenting vision is usually poor that surgery risk is relatively low.
- Extensive dissection in these cases will eventually end up with lots of iatrogenic retinal breaks and unrelieved traction. Therefore, we think the best way to approach these eyes is similar to what we do in ROP: clear the center, make no breaks, and do not use SO, i.e., a very conservative approach.
- If the abovementioned complication occurs and in cases where there are large fibrovascular plaques around retinal breaks combined with PVR, large retinectomies of 180° or more may be needed to release traction. In general, the outcome of retinectomies in TRD is poor due to a combination of reasons including exaggerated PVR, hypotony, and SO use. An encircling buckle may be also an alternative in cases with less extensive peripheral pathology.

5.9 *Internal Limiting Membrane Peeling*

- Some advocate peeling of the internal limiting membrane (ILM) as well as removing the diabetic ERMs to reduce the risk of reproliferation [18].
- ILM peeling is a difficult step, especially when the diabetic retina is thin and ischemic. Caution needs to be exercised in eyes with marked diabetic macular edema so as not to deroof macular cysts and cause a macular hole.
- Vital dyes (indocyanin green, tissue blue, etc.) are helpful in staining the internal limiting membrane. Use of a vital dye can also be helpful to tell if there is still ERM or vitreous present over the ILM. Be aware of the staining properties of the dyes you have available.
- In general, unless significant traction is present post-ERM dissection, we like to leave the ILM in place. Let alone the risk of ILM peels, it is there for a reason, and the ganglion cell layer is already thin in diabetics compared to non-diabetics! [19].

5.10 *Management of Intraoperative Bleeding*

- Some amount of oozing is unavoidable when removing fibrovascular membranes.
- When a more significant bleed occurs, the first step should be to momentarily raise the infusion pressure. We use 60 mmHg pressure for 1–2 min, which often is enough of a tamponade to slow the bleeding enough for a small clot to form.
- When this fails, various other strategies can be employed, including physical tamponade of the vessel with the head of the vitrectomy probe, and endo-diathermy. The latter is useful when bleefing is judged to get worse and still more dissection is needed, to control the bleeding early before a clot forms.

- Be aware that endo-diathermy can create collateral damage to nearby vessels and full-thickness retinal holes.
- Large clots can then be removed to clear the fovea, but some clot could be trimmed down and left closing the bleeding point to mitigate postoperative re-bleeding. Usually most blood clots would resolve provided silicone oil tamponade was not used.

5.11   Laser

- Endolaser probes are available with a fixed curve, retractable curve, or articulating probe and as illuminated or non-illuminated.
- We like fixed curved illuminated laser probes; they are simple to use, and no manipulation is needed.
- Surgeons can cross to the opposite side without touching the crystalline lens.
- An efficient method for doing full PRP is to do the posterior laser with the light pipe in one hand and then turn the illuminated laser probe to do indented peripheral laser before switching hands. When starting the opposite side, the laser light is kept on, and indented laser is done first before switching back to doing posterior laser (Video 6).
- It is advisable to laser out to the pars plana under the trocar ports to decrease the incidence of entry site NVs. Caution is needed in phakic eyes so as not to touch the lens (Video 7).

5.12   Tamponade Choice

- Air: Filling the vitreous cavity with air may help with better port sealing and avoid hypotony and early hemostasis. Air re-absorbs within just a few days. We use this routinely.
- No tamponade: A saline fill can be used if surgery was limited with minimal bleeding or if it is the patient's only seeing eye and minimal downtime is required. Also, when combined cataract surgery is performed, a saline fill will not disturb the IOL implant as much as gas or air, which can push the IOL anteriorly.
- Gas: If small posterior or superior breaks are encountered, or there is a CTRD, non-expansile concentrations of SF6 (for superior retinal breaks) or C3F8 (for inferior breaks) can be used, depending on the extent and location of the breaks.
- Silicone oil: When there are multiple breaks, with unrelieved retinal traction, or retinectomies were done, we use silicone oil. Oil should be the last resort in diabetic vitrectomy, due to exaggerated retro-oil fibrous proliferation in diabetic eyes (Image 10) and increased rates of macular edema. This is likely because organic molecules, such as fibrogenic growth factors, are concentrated in the retro-oil fluid [20]. Visual outcomes are also worse in diabetics with silicone oil as compared to gas [21]. Silicone oil does not decrease the rate of

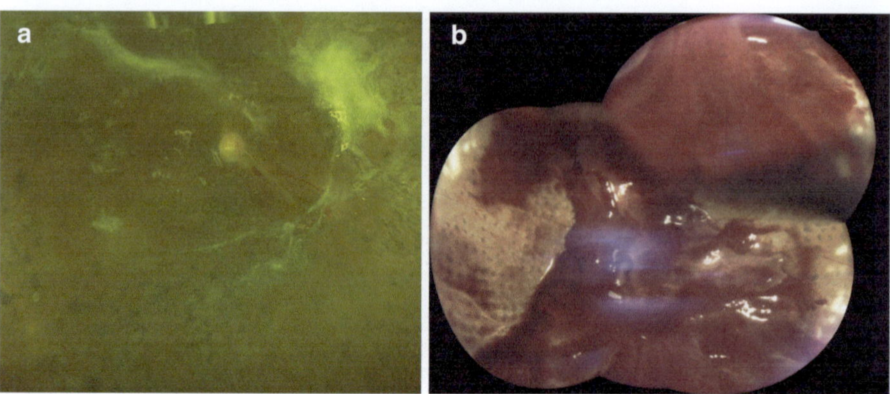

Image 10 A. Retro-oil epiretinal membrane in a diabetic eye operated with silicone oil. Note the membrane at the superior vascular arcade and nasal to the disc. B. Trapped preretinal blood under silicone oil after diabetic vitrectomy in another patient.

POVCH. However, it may compartmentalize postoperative bleeding (Image 10). While this limits the dispersion of retinal hemorrhage as compared to air/gas fill, it significantly delays the hemorrhage absorption, makes removal of this blood with surgery difficult with high rates of retinal tears and can also result in reproliferation and retinal detachment [22].

- Data from a UK national database registry that comprised 510 diabetic vitrectomies with delamination/segmentation showed that approximately 30% of eyes had one or more retina tears and 60% required internal tamponade use that included gas (mainly SF6) in 60% of eyes, air in 15%, and silicone oil in 15% [23].

6 Postoperative Considerations

1. **IOP** should be checked at the end of surgery or shortly after and should be <25 mmHg or less. Throughout the post-op course, the IOP may rise from NVG, hemolytic glaucoma, pupil synechiae with iris bombe, or gas expansion (if used). Using intravitreal steroids can also raise the eye pressure after surgery but usually not in the first week.
2. **Corneal healing**. If corneal debridement was done (which is best to avoid in diabetics), the cornea should also be monitored in the first week for delayed epithelial healing and the development of stromal infiltrates. We routinely spare the peripheral corneal epithelium and place a bandage contact lens at the end of surgery if we remove the epithelium during surgery.
3. **Inflammation and postoperative fibrin syndrome.** Intense inflammation is sometimes seen after prolonged surgery or intensive endolaser. Fibrinoid syndrome may develop, which if severe enough, may lead to traction/rhegmatogenous detachment with anterior PVR, neovascular glaucoma, and ultimately loss of the eye. This is uncommon/rare. Early treatment is important, and intensive

topical steroids usually reverse this condition in few days [8], but in severe cases, systemic steroids or intravitreal tissue plasminogen activator (tPA) is neeeded [12].

4. **Postoperative vitreous cavity hemorrhage (POVCH).** The most common complication after diabetic PPV is postoperative vitreous cavity hemorrhage or POVCH. This occurs in 50% or more of patients in the early postoperative period though most of these (90%) will resolve on their own in the first month [24]. Therefore, many can be observed.

Early POVCH (less than 1 month) is commonly from leeching from residual hemorrhage in the vitreous skirt or oozing from trimmed fibrovascular membranes or sheared veins. Later, POVCH can occur from vitreous contraction around pegs or new retinal or entry site NV.

If retinal detail is visible, the etiology of late POVCH can be determined. If veins are dilated and there is active NV, additional PRP may help to quiet the proliferative process. If veins are thin and no active NV can be seen, but there are areas of pre-retinal hemorrhage, the POVCH may be from residual traction on NV pegs. PRP is unlikely to be helpful in this setting. Persistent POVCH is treated with PPV. In the absence of residual traction, office-based air-fluid exchange may be a reasonable, cost-effective option for clearing the hemorrhage, particularly in pseudophakic eyes with recurrent bleeding [25] (Video 8).

6.1 Visual Outcome After Diabetic Delamination Surgery

- The outcome depends on several factors other than removing media opacity and retinal traction.
- Diabetic eyes are sick eyes, and worse outcome is seen in eyes with extensive proliferative disease and ischemia. When disrupted outer retinal layers (external limiting membrane and ellipsoid zone) can be seen on OCT, eyes tend to have poor visual outcome.
- A large national database study from the UK showed that in PPV with delamination, visual success ($\geq$ 3 Snellen lines gain) was achieved by 60% of eyes and visual loss occurred in 15%. Approximately, 15% of eyes required further PPV [26].

Key Points

- Be wary of the phenomenon of vitreoschisis in diabetic TRD. The posterior leaflet of the vitreous and the fibrovascular membranes are one fused layer.
- It is easier to get into the correct plane between the vitreous/fibrovascular membranes and the retina with "in-out" dissection.
- Common sense should prevail when dissecting diabetic membranes (Table 1).
- A "bad" scenario, in our view that we try to avoid at all costs, is when the surgeon "insists" on the removal of all fibrovascular membranes and ends up with multiple tears with surrounding traction.

References

1. Vander JF, Duker JS, Benson WE, Brown GC, McNamara JA, Rosenstein RB. Long-term stability and visual outcome after favorable initial response of proliferative diabetic retinopathy to panretinal photocoagulation. Ophthalmology. 1991;98(10):1575–9. PMID: 1961647.
2. Salman AG. Pascal laser versus conventional laser for treatment of diabetic retinopathy. Saudi J Ophthalmol. 2011;25(2):175–9.
3. Sun JK, Glassman AR, Beaulieu WT, et al. Rationale and application of the protocol S anti-vascular endothelial growth factor algorithm for proliferative diabetic retinopathy. Ophthalmology. 2019;126(1):87–95.
4. Tan Y, Fukutomi A, Sun MT, Durkin S, Gilhotra J, Chan WO. Anti-VEGF crunch syndrome in proliferative diabetic retinopathy: a review. Surv Ophthalmol. 2021;66(6):926–32. Epub 2021 Mar 8, 926.
5. Bressler NM, Beaulieu WT, Bressler SB, Glassman AR, Melia BM, Jampol LM, Jhaveri CD, Salehi-Had H, Velez G, Sun JK, DRCR Retina Network. ANTI-VASCULAR ENDOTHELIAL GROWTH FACTOR THERAPY AND RISK OF TRACTION RETINAL DETACHMENT IN EYES WITH PROLIFERATIVE DIABETIC RETINOPATHY: pooled analysis of five DRCR retina network randomized clinical trials. Retina. 2020;40(6):1021–8. PMID: 31567817; PMCID: PMC7075724.
6. Suresh R, Yu HJ, Thoveson A, Swisher J, Apolinario M, Zhou B, Shah AR, Fish RH, Wykoff CC. Loss to follow-up among patients with proliferative diabetic retinopathy in clinical practice. Am J Ophthalmol. 2020;215:66–71. Epub 2020 Mar 21.
7. Early vitrectomy for severe vitreous hemorrhage in diabetic retinopathy. Two-year results of a randomized trial. Diabetic retinopathy vitrectomy study report 2. The diabetic retinopathy vitrectomy study research group. Arch Ophthalmol. 1985;103(11):1644–52; PMID: 2865943.
8. Sebestyen JG. Fibrinoid syndrome: a severe complication of vitrectomy surgery in diabetics. Ann Ophthalmol. 1982;14(9):853–6; PMID: 7181348.
9. Haimann MH, Abrams GW. Prevention of lens opacification during diabetic vitrectomy. Ophthalmology. 1984;91:116–21.
10. Dong F, Yu C, Ding H, Shen L, Dingh L. Evaluation of intravitreal ranibizumab on the surgical outcome for diabetic retinopathy with tractional retinal detachment. Medicine (Baltimore). 2016;95(8):e2731; PMID: 26937902.
11. El-Sabagh HA, Abdelghaffar W, Labib AM, Mateo C, Hashem TM, Al-Tamimi DM, Selim AA. Preoperative intravitreal bevacizumab use as an adjuvant to diabetic vitrectomy: histopathologic findings and clinical implications. Ophthalmology. 2011;118(4):636–41.
12. McClellan AJ, Flynn HW, Smiddy WE, Gayer SI. The use of perioperative antithrombotics in posterior segment ocular surgery. Am J Ophthalmol. 2014;158(5):858–9.
13. Van Hecke MV, Dekker JM, Stehouwer CD, Polak BC, Fuller JH, Sjolie AK, Chaturvedi N. Diabetic retinopathy is associated with mortality and cardiovascular disease incidence: the EURODIAB prospective complications study. Diabetes Care. 2005;28(6):1383–9.
14. Shukla SY, Hariprasad AS, Hariprasad SM. Long-term mortality in diabetic patients with tractional retinal detachments. Ophthalmol Retina. 2017;1(1):8–11. Epub 2016 Nov 10.
15. Kumar CM, Seet E, Eke T, Dhatariya K, Joshi GP. Glycaemic control during cataract surgery under loco-regional anaesthesia: a growing problem and we are none the wiser. Br J Anaesth. 2016;117(6):687–91.
16. Schwatz SD, Alexander R, Hiscott P, Gregor ZJ. Recognition of vitreoschisis in proliferative diabetic retinopathy. A useful landmark in vitrectomy for diabetic traction retinal detachment. Ophthalmology. 1996;103:323–8.
17. El-Baha SM. Ahmed ISH trimanual vitrectomy for severe proliferative diabetic retinopathy. Int Ophthalmol. 2021;41(5):1717–27.
18. Wu RH, Xu MN, Lin K, Ren MX, Wen H, Feng KM, Zhou HJ, Moonasar N, Lin Z. Inner limiting membrane peeling prevents secondary epiretinal membrane after vitrectomy for proliferative diabetic retinopathy International Journal of Ophthalmology. 2022;15(9):1496–501.

19. Sung JY, Lee MW, Lim HB, Ryu CK, Yu HY, Kim JY. The Ganglion Cell-Inner Plexiform Layer Thickness/Vessel Density of Superficial Vascular Plexus Ratio According to the Progression of Diabetic Retinopathy. Invest Ophthalmol Vis Sci. 2022;63(6):4.
20. Asaria RHY, Kon CH, Bunce C, Sethi CS, Limb GA, Khaw PT, Aylward GW, Charteris DG. Silicone oil concentrates fibrogenic growth factors in the retro-oil fluid. Br J Ophthalmol. 2004;88:1439–42; PMID: 15489490.
21. Ryan B, Rush Agustin, Del Valle Penella Robert M, Reinauer Sloan W, Rush Pedro G, Bastar. SILICONE OIL VERSUS PERFLUOROPROPANE GAS TAMPONADE DURING VITRECTOMY FOR TRACTIONAL RETINAL DETACHMENT OR FIBROUS PROLIFERATION Retina 2021;41(7):1407–15.
22. Yeh PT, Yang CM, Yang CH. Distribution, reabsorption, and complications of preretinal blood under silicone oil after vitrectomy for severe proliferative diabetic retinopathy. Eye (Lond). 2012;26(4):601–8.
23. Jackson TL, Donachie PH, Sparrow JM, Johnston RL. United Kingdom National Ophthalmology Database Study of vitreoretinal surgery: report 1; case mix, complications, and cataract. Eye. 2013;27:644–51.
24. Smith JM, Steel JHW. Rebleeding after diabetic vitrectomy. Retin Physician. 2012;9:56–60.
25. Behrens AW, Uwaydat SH, Hardin JS, Sallam AB. Office-based air-fluid exchange for diabetic post-operative vitreous cavity hemorrhage. Med Hypothesis Discov Innov Ophthalmol. 2019;8(2):104–9; PMID: 31264998.
26. Jackson TL, Johnston RL, Donachie PH, Williamson TH, Sparrow JM, Steel DH. The Royal College of Ophthalmologists' National Ophthalmology Database Study of vitreoretinal surgery: report 6, diabetic vitrectomy. JAMA Ophthalmol. 2016;134:79–85.

Surgery for Sickle Cell Retinopathy

Riley Sanders and Kwesi Nyan Amissah-Arthur

1   Introduction

- Sickle cell disease (SCD) is a group of hemoglobinopathies caused by defective hemoglobin beta (β) chains, which results in abnormal "sickle"-shaped red blood cells (RBCs), intravascular hemolysis, and impaired oxygen transport [1].
- It is the most common inherited blood disorder, occurring commonly in people of African descent, as well as people of Caribbean, Mediterranean, South and Central American, Arabic, and East Indian descent. As many as 1 in 365 African Americans have sickle cell disease, and 1 in 13 has sickle cell trait [2].
- Normal adult hemoglobin (Hb A) comprises two α-globin subunits and two β-globin subunits. HbS and HbC are two abnormal variants of β-globin. Other abnormal hemoglobin variants, such as Hb E, O, and D, can cause similar presentations when inherited along with HbS [3]. Classic sickle cell disease is inherited in an autosomal recessive fashion, with two copies of Hb-S causing sickle cell disease (SS). A single copy of HbS and a normal β-globin chain results in sickle trait, which is usually asymptomatic [1].
- The most common and severe subtype of SCD worldwide is homozygous SS disease which is also referred to as sickle cell anemia.
- Heterozygous disorders of SCD arise due to coupling of the sickle gene with another hemoglobinopathy such as hemoglobin C, where there is a structural abnormality of the hemoglobin (HbSC) [1].

R. Sanders
Retina and Uveitis Services, Jones Eye Institute, University of Arkansas for Medical Sciences, Little Rock, AR, USA

K. N. Amissah-Arthur (✉)
Ophthalmology Unit, Department of Surgery, College of Health Sciences, University of Ghana Medical School, Korle Bu Teaching Hospital, Accra, Ghana
e-mail: kwesi@amissaharthur.com

   241

A. B. Sallam et al. (eds.), *Practical Manual of Vitreoretinal Surgery*,
https://doi.org/10.1007/978-3-031-47827-7_19

- It is of note that HbSC disease causes less severe systemic sickle cell disease affecting the body, but is associated with a higher rate and severity of retinopathy than HbSS.
- Sickling of blood cells causes painful vaso-occlusive crises, cerebrovascular accidents, splenic sequestration, and infarction with subsequent immune deficiency, priapism, and chronic anemia. SS disease portends a significant reduction in life expectancy [1]. Patients are also at risk of sickle cell retinopathy (SCR) and spontaneous hyphema and at greater risk of intraocular hypertension following hyphema.
- Retinal disease occurs more frequently and is considered to have more significant morbidity. The hallmark of SCR is peripheral ischemic retinopathy, although the macula is also involved with enlargement of the foveal avascular zone, thinning, and foveal depression/splaying notable on OCT [2].
- Sickle cell retinopathy can be divided into non-proliferative and proliferative changes. **Non-proliferative SCR** changes include *salmon patch hemorrhages* between the retina and internal limiting membrane *iridescent spots* or schisis cavities within areas of resolved hemorrhage containing hemosiderin-laden macrophages, and *black sunbursts*, thought to be ischemic damage to the RPE. **Proliferative SCR** typically progresses through five stages: (I) peripheral arteriolar occlusion, (II) arteriovenular anastomoses, (III) neovascular sea fans, (IV) vitreous hemorrhage, and (V) tractional retinal detachment [4]. Also, PSR can result in epiretinal membrane (ERM) and tractional macular holes (MH).
- The natural history of sickle cell retinopathy is variable in disease progression and severity, which makes its management challenging.
- In this chapter, we will discuss the main considerations and techniques for surgical intervention in sickle cell proliferative retinopathy.

2   Indications for Surgery in Sickle Cell Disease

2.1   Indications for Surgical Intervention

1. Anterior chamber washout for hyphema with intraocular hypertension (>24 for 24 h, or any intraocular pressure (IOP) >30). Sickling of RBCs in the anterior chamber makes these patients more prone to high IOP, corneal staining, and glaucomatous nerve damage.
2. Pars plana vitrectomy (PPV) for visually significant vitreous hemorrhage (stage IV SCR) (Fig. 1).
3. PPV for traction retinal detachment (TRD) (Fig. 2) or combined tractional rhegmatogenous retinal detachment (CTRD) (stage V SCR) (Fig. 3).
4. PPV surgery for ERM and MH.

Fig. 1 Chronic vitreous hemorrhage (de-hemoglobinized) and peripheral sea fan neovascularization

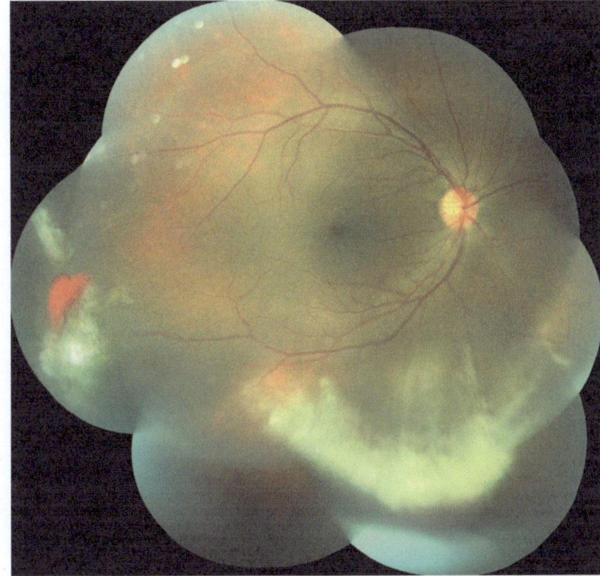

Fig. 2 Traction retinal detachment. Note the broad nature and the anterior location of the traction membranes in sickle cell retinopathy and the macular epiretinal membrane

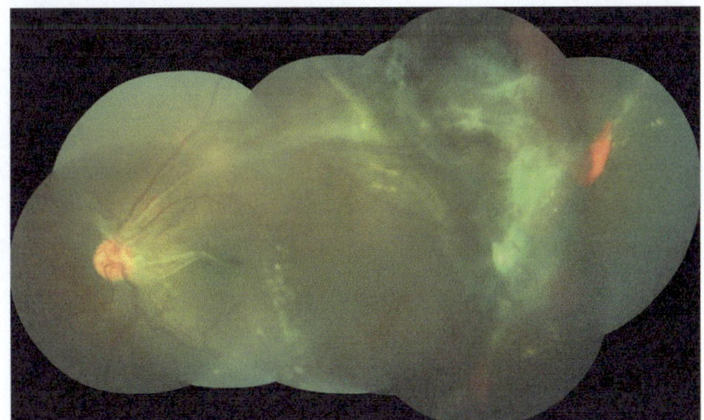

2.2   Possible Indications for Laser Intervention

- Progressive neovascularization (stage III SCR). Small neovascular (NV) sea fans will often auto-infarct.
- Laser photocoagulation [5] and anti-VEGF injections have been used with some success in hastening the involution of NV but have not been definitively shown to reduce the recurrence of new areas of NV or prevent progression to VH or TRD.
- In general, we only perform laser in eyes with large, progressive, florid NV (Fig. 4) or fellow eyes with active NV where there has been loss of vision in the contralateral eye.

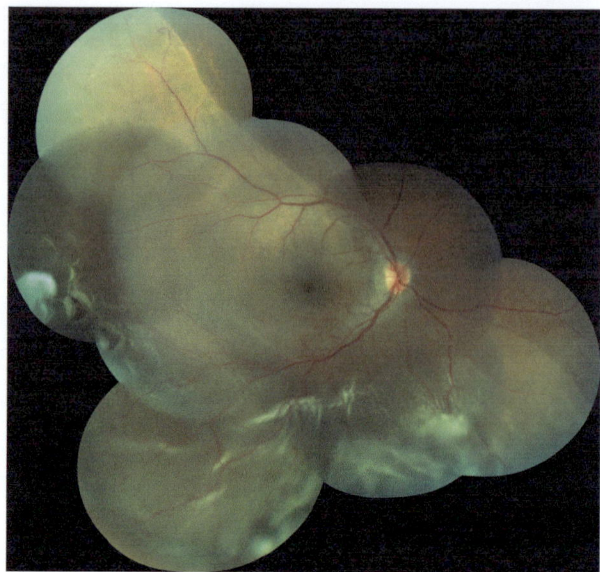

Fig. 3 Combined traction rhegmatogenous retinal detachment in sickle cell retinopathy

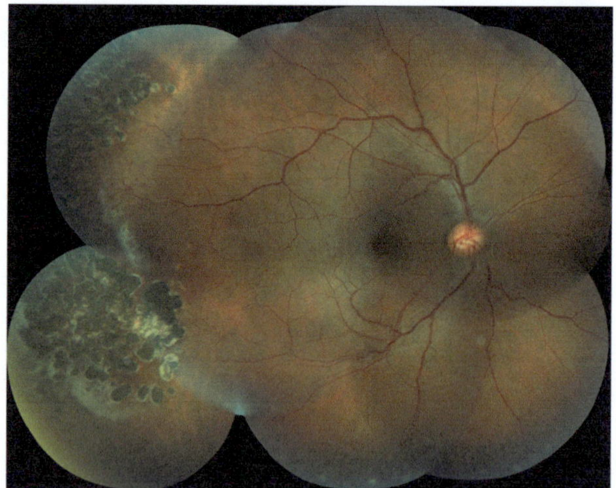

Fig. 4 Regression of peripheral neovascularization with laser treatment

3 Preoperative Considerations

- Efforts should be made to optimize hemoglobin level, oxygenation, and hydration to avoid intraoperative and/or early postoperative sickling.
- The ophthalmic surgeon should consult with the patient's primary care physician, anesthesiologist, and/or hematologist to do so.
- There is no consensus on whether preoperative exchange transfusions are necessary for reducing intra- or postoperative sickling complications, and transfusion itself carries significant risk [6].

- Similar to diabetic vitrectomy, preoperative anti-vascular endothelial growth factor (VEGF) medications may be injected within a week of surgery to help control intraoperative bleeding [7].

4   Surgical Procedure

- Because patients with SCD are usually young, general anesthesia is often used. Sub-tenon or peribulbar blocks may be used if GA is felt to be unsafe, without the use of a retrobulbar block, as SCD patients are at least at a theoretically higher risk of orbital compartmentalization and infarct.
- Induction of PVD is expected to be difficult in sickle cell retinopathy as patients are usually young. However, as opposed to diabetic delamination, vitreoschisis is usually not present, and tractional fibrovascular membranes are usually peripheral in location.
- We start by clearing the central vitreous then move on to induce PVD over the disc using suction to start with and a retinal pic or serrated forceps if the vitreous cannot be separated. The use of trypan blue or triamcinolone to stain the posterior hyaloid will help to visualize the hyaloid better in more challenging cases.
- Where there is a vitreous hemorrhage, be careful as the posterior hyaloid may still be attached to the detached retina, particularly near the peripheral neovascular complexes which tend to be in the temporal retina. As in diabetic cases, the surgeon needs to be careful of not putting too much traction on the peripheral retina.
- Following PVD induction, we continue with extending the separated posterior hyaloid to the mid-peripheral retinal stopping posterior to the areas of peripheral vascularization and fibrovascular traction.
- For the peripheral membranes, segmentation of anterior-to-posterior traction and segmentation of tangential membranes between vascular stalks (if possible) is preferable to attempted delamination. Unlike diabetic vascular pegs and membranes, epiretinal membranes in SCR are more challenging to delaminate. This is because the neovessels in SCR are of a greater caliber arising directly from arteriovenous anastomosis with hallmarks of a vein. Also, SCR membranes are more broadly adherent to the underlying retina (Fig. 2). They are located in the anterior retina, where the tissue is more ischemic and thinner and, thus, prone to iatrogenic breaks with even minimal manipulation.
- At all costs, avoid retinectomies in these eyes as they are associated with an increased risk of proliferative vitreoretinopathy and retinal detachment even worse than in diabetic eyes. Conservative dissection is the key to successful surgery!
- Epiretinal membranes can usually be peeled off the macula. However, one needs to be cautious as the macula can be thin in SCD. While peeling epiretinal membranes, be careful once the membrane gets to the border of the peripheral membranes, as excessive manipulative force may lead to breaks at the border of the membranes and the thin schitic retina.

- After segmentation of membranes, laser is applied to encircle any retinal breaks, under air or perfluorocarbon liquid if needed.
- We also tend to do peripheral scatter laser photocoagulation of the ischemic retinal periphery, although this is not proven to reduce recurrent NV. Some surgeons advocate sparing the ciliary vessels at the 3′ and 9 o'clock location to reduce the risk of ocular ischemic crisis postoperatively.
- Like diabetic TRD, in the absence of retinal tears, subretinal fluid does not need to be drained.
- Tamponade choice depends on the extent of retinal breaks and residual traction on the retina, particularly near the breaks. If no retinal tear is present, the eye can be left filled with saline or air. Non-expansile gas may be used to tamponade retinal tears after clearing any traction at or around the tears. Breaks with unrelieved traction around them can be supported by a segmental buckle; however, be cautious about excessive extra ocular muscle manipulation during buckle surgery to reduce the risk of postoperative ocular ischemic crises. Silicone oil can be used as a last resort in cases of extensive unrelieved traction with multiple breaks or after retinectomy. These situations are best avoided by following a conservative approach during membrane dissection.

4.1 Other Intraoperative and Postoperative Considerations

- Scleral buckles can be performed without a significant risk of anterior segment ischemia [10] but care should be taken to avoid broad and tight encircling buckles [8].
- It is important to be judicious with the use of high IOP as a measure to decrease intraoperative bleeding, as prolonged intraocular hypertension can lead to sickling and retinal arterial occlusion.
- Serious thought should be given before combining cataract surgery with retinal surgery due to the enhanced inflammation following the breach of the blood-aqueous barrier.
- Also, if a patient develops systemic hypotension during surgery, hydration is preferable to vasopressors to elevate the blood pressure.
- Postoperatively, watch out for IOP elevation, hyphema, and postoperative vitreous cavity hemorrhage.

5 Surgery Outcome

- This depends on several factors, most notably the severity of vitreoretinal pathology [9].
- Macular hole closure rate is nearly comparable to idiopathic macular hole closure rate.
- The best outcomes are seen in uncomplicated vitreous hemorrhages.

- The worst outcome appears in cases with TRD and CTRD with a final reattachment rate of approximately 80%. Vision improvement is minimal, but stabilization of vision can be achieved in nearly 80%.
- Retinectomy and silicone oil are associated with worse outcomes. It is important to note that most data come from retrospective studies so there may be a selection bias and these were done in more complex cases.
- The rate of iatrogenic retinal breaks ranges from 12% to 30% in cases with retinal detachment.
- Small-gauge vitrectomy systems may be associated with fewer intraoperative complications than 20-g PPV.

Key Points
- PSR can present with a broad-spectrum vitreoretinal interface disease, the worst being TRD and CTRD.
- There is no consensus on the benefit of laser treatment for retinal NV, and many eyes can be observed.
- When operating on tractional retinal detachment due to SCD, it is best to follow a conservative approach for membrane dissection.
- Iatrogenic retinal breaks with unrelieved traction and retinectomies result in poor anatomical and visual outcomes.

References

1. Stuart MJ, Nagel RL. Sickle-cell disease. Lancet. 2004;364(9442):1343–60.
2. Hoang QV, Chau FY, Shahidi M, Lim JI. Central macular splaying and outer retinal thinning in asymptomatic sickle cell patients by spectral-domain optical coherence tomography. Am J Ophthalmol. 2011;151(6):990–4.
3. Daniel YA, Turner C, Haynes RM, Hunt BJ, Dalton RN. Rapid and specific detection of clinically significant haemoglobinopathies using electrospray mass spectrometry. Br J Haematol. 2005;130(4):635–43.
4. Goldberg MF. Natural history of untreated proliferative sickle retinopathy. Arch Ophthalmol. 1971;85(4):428–37.
5. Myint KKT, Sahoo S, Thein AW, Moe S, Ni H. Laser therapy for retinopathy in sickle cell disease. Cochrane Database Syst Rev. 2015;9:10.
6. Estcourt LJ, Kimber C, Trivella M, Doree C, Hopewell S. Preoperative blood transfusions for sickle cell disease. Cochrane Database Syst Rev. 2020;(7)
7. Moshiri A, Ha NK, Ko FS, Scott AW. Bevacizumab presurgical treatment for proliferative sickle-cell retinopathy-related retinal detachment. Retin Cases Brief Rep. 2013;7(3):204–5.
8. Rohowetz LJ, Panneerselvam S, Williams BK Jr, Smiddy WE, Berrocal AM, Townsend JH, Gayer S, Palte HD, Flynn HW Jr; Proliferative Sickle Cell Retinopathy Study Group. Proliferative Sickle Cell Retinopathy: Outcomes of Vitreoretinal Surgery. Ophthalmol Retina. 2024:S2468–6530(24)00049-6.
9. Chen RW, Flynn HW Jr, Lee WH, et al. Vitreoretinal management and surgical outcomes in proliferative sickle retinopathy: a case series. Am J Ophthalmol. 2014;157(4):870–5.
10. Ho J, Grabowska A, Ugarte M, Muqit MM. A comparison of 23-gauge and 20-gauge vitrectomy for proliferative sickle cell retinopathy—clinical outcomes and surgical management. Eye (Lond). 2018;32(9):1449–54.

Suprachoroidal Hemorrhage

Ehab El Rayes and Mahmoud Leila

This chapter discusses surgery-related suprachoroidal hemorrhage (SCH), its definition, epidemiology, risk factors, and management.

1 Definition and Epidemiology

- SCH is an uncommon but potentially devastating complication of intraocular surgery.
- Suprachoroidal hemorrhage (SCH) is caused by rupturing one or more of the posterior ciliary arteries that traverse the suprachoroidal space.
- SCH is associated mainly with ophthalmic surgery. Less commonly, it can develop secondary to trauma or spontaneously.
- The incidence of SCH in ophthalmic surgery is small ranging from 0.06% to 1.9%. SCH occurs less commonly in association with modern techniques of cataract surgery and PPV than in surgeries where IOP is less maintained such as old-style large incision extracapsular cataract extraction (ECCE), trabeculectomy and glaucoma tube surgery and penetrating keratoplasty [1, 2].

Supplementary Information The online version contains supplementary material available at https://doi.org/10.1007/978-3-031-47827-7_20.

E. El Rayes (✉) · M. Leila
Retina Department, Research Institute of Ophthalmology, Giza, Egypt

A. B. Sallam et al. (eds.), *Practical Manual of Vitreoretinal Surgery*, https://doi.org/10.1007/978-3-031-47827-7_20

- The extent of SCH ranges from localized, self-limiting hemorrhage to expulsion of intraocular contents.
- Early recognition of this complication can save the patient's eye and preserve vision.

2 Risk Factors for SCH

Two main sets of risk factors can induce SCH, either through producing direct weakening of the arterial wall or setting the stage for arterial rupture by toppling the equilibrium between intravascular pressure and intraocular pressure (IOP).

2.1 High-Risk Patient Profile

- Patients with deranged coagulation profiles associated with blood diseases or anticoagulant therapy are prone to uncontrolled bleeding intraoperatively.
- Chronic systemic hypertension, arteriosclerosis, advanced age, and vasculitis are associated with underlying weakening of the arterial wall and put the patient at risk of developing SCH.
- Anatomical features that alter the normal scleral rigidity can either induce or perpetuate SCH. High myopia is associated with abnormally low scleral rigidity, thus offering less support to the posterior ciliary arteries in the event of overstretching of these vessels by blood or fluid accumulating in the suprachoroidal space. Nanophthalmic eyes have abnormally increased scleral thickness. Consequently, these eyes have relatively lower uveoscleral outflow and hence less albumin clearance accumulating in the suprachoroidal space from extravasation from the intravascular compartment [3].
- Aphakic eyes have a loss of normal ocular compartmentalization into anterior and posterior chambers. This predisposes to an easier separation of the uvea from the sclera in the event of blood or fluid accumulating in the suprachoroidal space.

2.2 Intraoperative Risk Factors

- Valsalva maneuver associated with coughing, nausea, vomiting, or bucking effect during general anesthesia increases the episcleral venous pressure and subsequently the choroidal venous pressure that increases shear stress on the vascular wall that might cause its rupture.
- A high volume of retrobulbar anesthetic or uncontrolled glaucoma increases the IOP and predisposes to rupture of the posterior ciliary arteries due to sudden decompression of the globe upon placement of the surgical incision.

- Direct mechanical injury of the choroid by surgical instruments as in pars plana vitrectomy (PPV) or scleral buckle.
- Large surgical incision, inadequate sealing of the postoperative wound with subsequent aqueous leakage, or application of aqueous shunt devices that cause over-filtration of the aqueous and prolonged hypotony in the postoperative period.

3 Pathophysiology: How Does SCH Develop and How Does it Cause Loss of Vision?

- Animal and human histopathologic studies suggest that prolonged ocular hypotony combined with one or more of the aforementioned risk factors induces the development of a suprachoroidal serous effusion. SCH ensues either due to direct rupture of the posterior ciliary arteries due to excessive shear stress inflicted on the vessel wall by the choroidal effusion/detachment or the unabated intravascular systemic blood pressure [3–5].
- There are different mechanisms for vision loss in SCH. The most drastic would be an expulsive hemorrhage with loss of all intraocular contents and blindness. Long-standing massive SCH may cause cyclodialysis, hypotony and may end up in phthisis bulbi. Conversely high intraocular pressure from SCH can result in accelerated optic nerve damage. Blood in the suprachoroidal space can break through the choroid and the retina resulting in vitreous hemorrhage and hyphema. This can also result in a retinal tear and rhegmatogenous retinal detachment. In a study of surgery related to SCH, retinal detachment was present in 35% and there was a high rate of proliferative vitreoretinopathy [6]. Of note, some degree of exudative retinal detachment may happen over the SCH. This does not require any intervention and it self-corrects as the hemorrhage resolves. Direct toxicity or hypoxia to the foveal photoreceptors may occur with macular involving SCH [1].

4 Prophylactic Measures to Prevent SCH

- Liaison with the patient's physician in the preoperative period for adequate control of the systemic conditions that increase the risk of SCH as blood pressure and blood dyscrasias is essential. Ideally, anticoagulants should be stopped before the surgery, and the international normalized ratio (INR) of the patient should be less than 2. In real-world practice, this is not possible to achieve in many cases due to the high likelihood of major cardiovascular adverse events if anticoagulation is lessened.
- Patients with conditions that might cause Valsalva maneuver as bronchial asthma or other causes of chronic cough should be referred to the internist for control of

these parameters before admission for surgery. There should be liaison with the anesthesiologist to induce local anesthesia combined with sedation whenever possible instead of general anesthesia to avoid the bucking effect. Adequate lid akinesia is essential to avoid the rise of IOP due to lid squeezing. Adequate ocular massage using the Honan balloon is mandatory after delivering local anesthesia, particularly the retrobulbar approach.

- Patients with uncontrolled glaucoma should have adequate IOP control prior to surgery. Perioperative intravenous hyperosmotic agents or systemic carbonic anhydrase inhibitors might be necessary.
- Intraoperatively, the surgical time should be kept to the minimum possible for a safe and effective procedure. All surgical wounds should be adequately sealed to avoid postoperative hypotony.
- Finally, in some high-risk patients, additional steps may need to be taken. For example, several authors have proposed performing sclerotomy at the time of cataract surgery to reduce the risk of uveal effusion in nanophthalmic eyes [7].

5   Clinical Picture of SCH

- Acute SCH is characterized by its sudden onset and very rapid progression. It is the sum of all ocular emergencies, and unless an adequate and swift response is initiated, expulsion of ocular contents may ensue. A typical scenario is during a large incision ECCE, after delivery of the nucleus. The surgeon notices a dark mound rapidly replacing the red reflex with the rapid rise of IOP, progressive shallowing of the anterior chamber, and extrusion of the lens capsule followed by extrusion of the vitreous and even the entire intraocular contents, hence the term "expulsive hemorrhage." Because of the closed nature of phacoemulsification, the progression tempo is less severe than in ECCE, and the surgeon can usually control the situation and close the eye. In severe cases, choroidal bullae overstretched by blood could come into apposition, hence the term kissing choroidals.
- SCH during PPV surgery is usually localized in nature and tends to occur more during surgery in already vitrectomized eyes such as silicone oil removal and secondary IOL procedures. In these cases, there is a lack of vitreous support and fluctuation of intraocular pressure is more likely to happen than during primary PPV [8].
- Delayed SCH is more common than the acute variant. It typically develops 1–4 days after surgery and is most seen following glaucoma surgery, particularly with the use of aqueous drainage devices [9].

6   Management of SCH

- Intraoperatively, once the surgeon detects incipient SCH, the lid speculum is released, and the incision is tightly closed. In large incision surgery, often closure of the wound is difficult due to back pressure, and the assistant is asked to apply pressure on the wound with their thumb while the surgeon rapidly closes the wound. The surgeon should aim for water-tight closure of the wound and reformation of the anterior chamber using balanced salt saline (BSS) or air.
- The anesthesiologist should administer sedating agents and control the systemic blood pressure.
- Draining the SCH at the time of surgery through drainage sclerotomies should be reserved only for cases with extremely high back pressure and the inability of repositioning prolapsed intraocular content despite the aforementioned measures. SCH drainage might induce hypotony and trigger more bleeding. In addition, bleeding from the posterior ciliary arteries is known to be self-limiting due to early clotting.
- If SCH happens during PPV, the surgeon should raise the infusion pressure for a few minutes till the bleeding stops and then concludes the surgery without delay. It is crucial to avoid postoperative hypotony by ensuring that all scleral ports are sealed at the end of the surgery.
- Postoperatively, topical steroids, cycloplegics, and analgesics are prescribed to control inflammation and pain. A serial ultrasound examination is performed to monitor the evolution of the SCH and to detect signs that warrant secondary intervention to drain the SCH.
- Indications for drainage of SCH are ultrasound evidence of massive non-resolving SCH causing kissing choroidals with retinal apposition, macular involvement with the hemorrhage, or intractable IOP rise that is unresponsive to medical therapy.
- If drainage of SCH is indicated, it is usually best to wait for 10–14 days to allow time for liquefaction of the blood clot [10, 11]. Earlier intervention might be considered in cases with severe ocular hypertension and when rhegmatogenous retinal detachment coexists.
- Concurrent PPV with drainage may be needed if there is coexisting pathology, such as vitreous hemorrhage or rhegmatogenous retinal detachment [1, 10]. Some surgeons have also advocated performing PPV with drainage for SCH regardless of the presence of retinal complications [5], but the benefit remains unclear. While PPV may allow more complete drainage of the SCH and insertion of a tamponading agent, visualization and access to the vitreous cavity are usually difficult in this context and PPV may be associated with an increased risk of complication most importantly retinal tears and rhegmatogenous detachment (Fig. 1).

Fig. 1 Color photograph of marked three-quadrant suprachoroidal hemorrhage during phacoemulsification. The surgeon promptly stopped the surgery and sutured the wound. This patient was managed conservatively as there was no retinal apposition, intraocular pressure was well-controlled with medical treatment, and the macula was spared

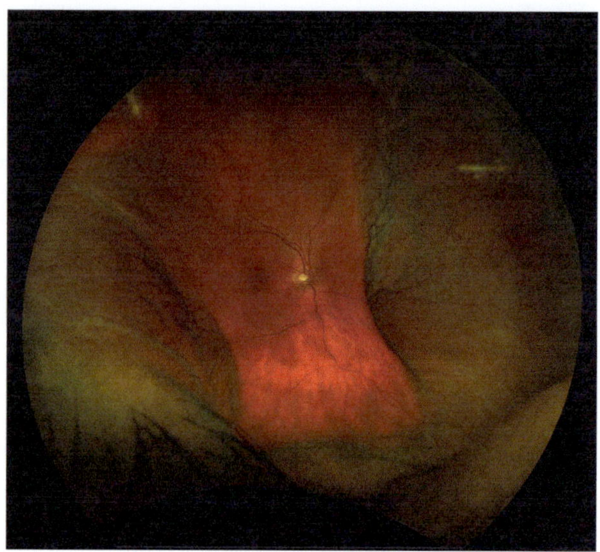

6.1   Steps of Surgical Drainage of SCH (Video 1)

- Preoperatively, identify the quadrant(s) with the maximum collection of blood using ultrasound.
- At the start of surgery, close any identifiable wound leaks.
- Apply an anterior chamber maintainer or 25-gauge infusion cannula. If using the latter, always make sure you can see the tip of the cannula inside the eye before turning the infusion on.
- Set the IOP at 30 mmHg. This will help the egress of suprachoroidal blood when the surgeon performs the drainage sclerotomy. Care should be taken to avoid excessive IOP rise, which may cause incarceration of the choroid into the drainage sclerotomies and impede blood drainage. In addition, excess IOP could cause cloudiness of the cornea and impede visualization during the ensuing PPV.
- Perform a limited peritomy in the quadrant(s) selected for drainage, followed by bridling of the respective recti muscles.
- Perform one or more radial sclerotomies at 6–8 mm posterior to the limbus. The sclerotomy should be 2–3 mm long and extends posteriorly from the equator but anterior to the vortex veins [1].
- Initially, the surgeon should partially drain the blood to avoid excessive hypotony. A Colibri forceps is used to separate the edges of the sclerotomy while applying slight pressure to help the egress of blood. A blunt spatula could be carefully introduced into the suprachoroidal space through the sclerotomies to aid in extruding the blood. Typically, the extruded blood is dark in color and is mixed with blood clots.

- After the choroidal bullae have receded, the infusion cannula could be removed from the anterior chamber and inserted into the pars plana to start PPV if needed. Before starting the infusion, check that the tip of the infusion cannula is clearly seen inside the vitreous cavity and that it is not clogged by blood clots or exudates.
- During PPV, you might need to inject perfluorocarbon liquid (PFCL) to help displace the blood in the suprachoroidal space away from the posterior pole and through the open sclerotomies.
- Manage any retinal breaks and/or retinal detachment and use gas or silicone oil tamponade as needed.
- At the end of the procedure, the radial sclerotomies are left without suturing and the conjunctiva is closed.
- 23-g cannulas can be used for SCH drainage instead of creating sclerotomies (Video 2). This avoids the need for conjunctival and scleral dissection. However, drainage can be slower and less complete than in cut-down sclerotomies. Care is also taken to insert the trocar at a 15° angle from the sclera to avoid penetration of the RPE of the retina [12].
- Suprachoroidal injection of alteplase (tPA) has also been suggested when attempting early drainage of the SCH to help liquefy the blood clot and facilitate drainage [11, 13] without PPV. Suprachoroidal dose of tPA equals the intravitreal dose, 50 mcg in 0.05 ml (Video 3).

7 Outcome of SCH

Overall, SCH is associated with poor vision [5]. In non-expulsive hemorrhage cases, some vision can be saved by timely management. In a UK-based study, only 60% of patients with post-cataract surgery SCH attained a vision of >20/200 with poor prognostic criteria being SCH in 3–4 quadrants, ECCE surgery, retinal apposition, and retinal detachment [2]. For PPV, SCH is usually localized in nature and has a relatively good prognosis [8].

8 Case Scenario

A 58-year-old man with a history of systemic hypertension and primary open-angle glaucoma was operated on for ECCE in the right eye. The patient was on aspirin for the past 5 years. Preoperative best-corrected acuity was 20/400. The axial length was 29 mm. Intraoperatively, the cataract surgeon noticed excessive back pressure immediately after delivery of the nucleus with forward bowing of the posterior capsule, progressive shallowing of the anterior chamber, dimming of the red reflex, and a black mound appearing behind the pupil. The surgeon immediately closed the limbal incision using 8/0 nylon sutures. The patient was left aphakic. Postoperatively, an ultrasound examination revealed vitreous hemorrhage and 360° choroidal detachment. The maximum elevation of choroidal detachment was detected in the inferotemporal and nasal quadrants (Fig. 2). Two weeks later, the ultrasound showed minimal resolution of SCH choroidal detachment necessitating surgery. The surgeon performed two radial sclerotomies in the inferotemporal quadrant and nasal quadrants. The surgeon proceeded with PPV to remove the vitreous hemorrhage. PFCL was injected to help displace the remaining SCH peripherally and its release through the open sclerotomies. The retinal periphery was inspected for retinal breaks. Finally, the surgeon performed fluid/air exchange and air/SF6 gas exchange (Fig. 3).

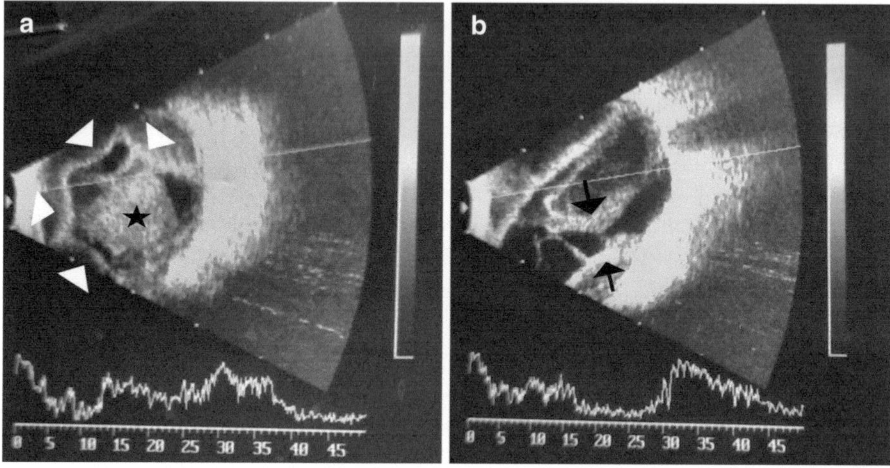

Fig. 2 (**a**) Preoperative ultrasound image, transverse scan of the right eye of a 58-year-old male with suprachoroidal hemorrhage. Note the characteristic scalloped appearance of 360° choroidal detachment (white arrowheads) and the densely dispersed hemorrhage in the suprachoroidal space with a corresponding low chain of spikes on the A-scan. The vitreous cavity is occupied with dense hemorrhage (black asterisk). (**b**) Oblique scan mode shows high choroidal bullae almost in contact with each other; kissing choroidals (black arrows)

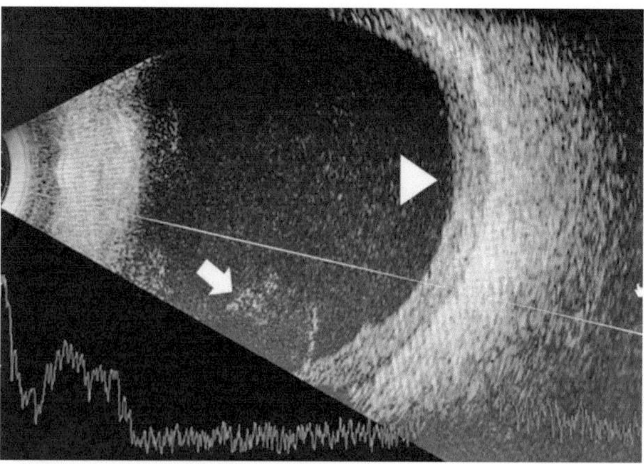

Fig. 3 Postoperative ultrasound image in a transverse scan mode of the same eye in Fig. 2 after drainage of suprachoroidal hemorrhage (SCH) through drainage sclerotomies and pars plana vitrectomy. Previously noted choroidal bullae and SCH resolved. Note the choroidal thickening (white arrowhead) and residual cuff of vitreous (white arrow)

Key Points

- Preoperative patient assessment for identifying patients at high risk of developing SCH is important.
- Prolonged intraoperative hypotony associated with large incision surgery is a significant risk factor for developing SCH.
- SCH during PPV is usually localized and is more commonly encountered during procedures in already vitrectomized eyes.
- In the event of SCH, prompt correction of hypotony and increasing the IOP will help stop further bleeding from the posterior ciliary arteries.
- Intraoperative drainage of SCH should be the last resort because it could trigger a vicious circle due to hypotony and cause further bleeding.
- Postoperative drainage of SCH should be performed only whenever a permanent visual loss is imminent.

References

1. Chu TG, Green RL. Suprachoroidal hemorrhage. Surv Ophthalmol. 1999;43(6):471–86.
2. Ling R, Cole M, James C, Kamalarajah S, Foot B, Shaw S. Suprachoroidal haemorrhage complicating cataract surgery in the UK: epidemiology, clinical features, management, and outcomes. Br J Ophthalmol. 2004;88(4):478–80.
3. Jackson TL, Hussain A, Salisbury J, Sherwood R, Sullivan PM, Marshall J. Transscleral albumin diffusion and suprachoroidal albumin concentration in uveal effusion syndrome. Retina. 2012;32(1):177–82.
4. Wolter JR, Garfinkel RA. Ciliochoroidal effusion as precursor of suprachoroidal hemorrhage: a pathologic study. Ophthalmic Surg. 1988;19(5):344–9.
5. Liu T, Elnahry AG, Tauqeer Z, Yu Y, Ying GS, Kim BJ. Visual and anatomic outcomes of suprachoroidal Hemorrhage: a systematic review and meta-analysis. Ophthalmol Retina. Published online February 27. 2023.
6. Spaeth GL, Baez KA. Long-term prognosis of eyes having had operative suprachoroidal expulsive hemorrhage. Ger J Ophthalmol. 1994;3(3):159–63.
7. Rajendrababu S, Babu N, Sinha S, et al. A randomized controlled trial comparing outcomes of cataract surgery in nanophthalmos with and without prophylactic sclerostomy. Am J Ophthalmol. 2017;183:125–33.
8. Mo B, Li SF, Liu Y, et al. Suprachoroidal hemorrhage associated with pars plana vitrectomy. BMC Ophthalmol. 2021;21:295.
9. Tuli SS, WuDunn D, Ciulla TA, Cantor LB. Delayed suprachoroidal hemorrhage after glaucoma filtration procedures. Ophthalmology. 2001;108(10):1808–11.
10. Garcia-Arumi J. Massive suprachoroidal hemorrhage. In: Ryan SJ, editor. Retina. 6th ed. Philadelphia: Saunders; 2018. p. 2371.
11. Kwon OW, Kang SJ, Lee JB, Lee SC, Yoon YD, Oh JH. Treatment of suprachoroidal hemorrhage with tissue plasminogen activator. Ophthalmologica. 1998;212(2):120–5.
12. Rezende FA, Kickinger MC, Li G, Prado RF. Regis LG transconjunctival drainage of serous and hemorrhagic choroidal detachment. Retina. 2012;32(242):9.
13. Murata T, Kikushima W, Imai A, Toriyama Y, Tokimitsu M, Kurokawa T. Tissue-type plasminogen activator-assisted drainage of suprachoroidal hemorrhage showing a kissing configuration. Jpn J Ophthalmol. 2011;55(4):431–2.

Submacular Hemorrhage

Rachid Tahiri Joutei Hassani, Otman Sandali, and Mohamed Tawfik

Submacular hemorrhage (SMH) refers to bleeding under the macula. In this chapter, we discuss the management of SMH with significant visual symptoms.

1 Causes, Pathogenesis, and Natural Cause

- Several causes can lead to SMH. The most common is neovascular age related macular degneration (nAMD) (Fig. 1). In the IVAN study around 50% had some degree of SMH at presentation. However, only 10% were greater than 2.5 mm [1]. Other causes include idiopathic polypoidal choroidal vasculopathy (IPCV), peripheral exudative hemorrhagic chorioretinopathy (PEHCR), macroaneurysm, trauma, and traumatic CNV, as well as anticoagulants use [2].
- The presence of hemorrhage under the retina can result in permanent damage with atrophy of the photoreceptors and retinal pigment epithelium (RPE).
- The natural course of untreated eyes is loss of approximately ≥ 3 lines of vision and poor vision of <20/200 in most cases [3].

Supplementary Information The online version contains supplementary material available at https://doi.org/10.1007/978-3-031-47827-7_21.

R. T. J. Hassani (✉)
Ambulatory Surgery Department, Avranches Granville Hospital, Granville, France

O. Sandali
Ophthalmology, National Quinze-vingts Institute, Paris, France

M. Tawfik
Vitreoretinal Department, Memorial Institute of Ophthalmic Research, Giza, Egypt

- Retinal degeneration over areas of dense fibrin occurs at approximately 3–14 days in an experimental model [4], highlighting the importance of early management of SMH.

2   Clinical Features

- SMH due to nAMD is usually seen in older patients and traumatic SH in younger ages. It is important to ask for bleeding disorders and anticoagulants use.
- Patients usually complain of significant metamorphopsia, decreased vision, and central scotoma.
- The duration of symptoms is critical to record as early cases (within 1–2 weeks) gain more vision with treatment.
- Some cases may be associated with vitreous, intraretinal or suprachoroidal hemorrhage.
- Optical coherence tomography (OCT) particularly vertical scans can help localization of the level of the hemorrhage and other associated signs. However, its utility can be limited in the presence of dense retinal hemorrhage.
- Flourescein and indocyanin green angiograoghy can be helpful when the diagnosis is not clear, particularly in the context of PEHCR.
- Examination of the other eye is essential and may help diagnose the cause of SH such as nAMD and PEHCR.

3   Treatment and Outcomes

- Previous attempts of direct removal of SMH in the past did not result in satisfactory outcomes due to damage of the retinal/RPE with the removal of the blood clot [5].
- The main lines of treatment of significant SMH currently range from the intravitreal injection of anti-vascular endothelial growth factor (anti-VEGF), non-surgical pneumatic displacement with intravitreal expansile gas bubble +/intravitreal tissue plasminogen activator (tPA) and anti-VEGF, and pars plana vitrectomy (PPV) with subretinal displacement with balanced salt solution (BSS) +/− subretinal or intravitreal tPA +/− subretinal air +/− subretinal/ or intravitreal anti-VEFG. Subretinal air has been suggested to aid the subretinal displacement of blood [6].
- Anti-VEGF use to decrease re-bleeding is recommended in patients with nAMD, IPCV, and possibly PECHR.

- Intravitreal anti-VEGF alone without displacement for thin (<450 μm) SMH due to nAMD appears to be associated with good visual results that are not inferior to pneumatic displacement [7].
- PPV provides at least some theoretical advantages over non-surgical pneumatic displacement with gas including greater success for blood displacement, and less need for postoperative positioning owing to a large air/gas fill. However, the cost and the risks of surgery are more than in-office pneumatic displacement. PPV also alters the pharmacokinetics of anti-VEGF resulting in rapid elimination from the vitreous cavity. Subretinal injection of fluid can also increase the risk of macular holes. This risk appears to be higher with rapid injection rates and large volumes of subretinal fluid and with the use of subretinal air [8].
- Intravitreal and subretinal tPA helps liquefy the subretinal blood, minimizing the shearing stress on the photoreceptors caused by the displacement with gas only with improved anatomical and functional outcomes [9]. Subretinal use of tPA is thought to be more efficient than through the intravitreal route but carries a higher risk of retinal/RPE toxicity and macular hole formation (Video 1). tPA can also increase the risk of bleeding. Although differing the route and dosages would influence its efficacy, tPA achieves its action of liquefaction in around 1 h [5, 9]. Table 1 shows the dosages for intravitreal and subretinal tPA.

Table 1 Tissue plasminogen activator (Alteplase) for ophthalmology use

Intracameral alteplase (TPA)
- Dose recommended = 25 mcg in 0.05 ml.
- Commercially available product = 20 mg powder for infusion.
- Reconstitute a 20 mg vial with 20 ml water for injection.
- Withdraw 1 ml and make up to 2 ml with sodium chloride to give a concentration of 500 mcg/ml.
- Administer 0.05 ml.

Intravitreal and suprachoroidal alteplase (TPA)
- Dose recommended = 50 mcg in 0.05 ml.
- Commercially available product = 20 mg powder for infusion.
- Reconstitute a 20 mg vial with 20 ml water for injection to give a concentration of 1 mg/ml.
- Administer 0.05 ml.

Subretinal alteplase (TPA)
- Dose recommended = 0.1–0.2 ml of 125 mcg/ml concentration.
- Toxic dose is 40–50 mcg.
- Commercially available product = 20 mg powder for infusion.
- Reconstitute a 20 mg vial with 20 ml water for injection.
- Withdraw 1 ml and make up to 8 ml with sodium chloride to give a concentration of 125 mcg/ml.
- Administer 0.1–0.2 ml.

- Regarding postoperative positioning, while prone positioning was suggested with pneumatic displacement, 40° gaze down or sitting up (45°) in the first few days appears to be more optimal for the pneumatic displacement of a subretinal hemorrhage in the macula [10].
- There is controversy regarding the efficacy of non-surgical pneumatic displacement vs. displacement with PPV. Anatomically, both techniques are effective in displacing blood off the fovea, but surgery may be more effective [11]. Functionally, improvement of vision after displacement of blood is usually modest with one study showing an improvement of 3 Snellen lines in only 40% of patients [12]. There appears to be no difference in visual outcomes between the non-surgical pneumatic displacement and PPV even after accounting for subretinal hemorrhage size and presenting VA [13, 14, 15].
- A study by Chew et al. [11] showed that using a stepwise approach, performing pneumatic displacement for SMH with gas first, and moving on to PPV if the former procedure fails achieved displacement of foveal blood in 75% of cases without the need for PPV. In this study, the factors that were predictive of non-surgical pneumatic displacement success were better initial visual acuity (1.34 LogMAR vs. 1.81, $p = 0.02$), hemorrhages of size <10 disc diameter area (DDA) (71.4% vs. 52.2%, $p = 0.43$) and were more likely to be predominantly subretinal (62.5 vs. 14.3%, $p = 0.02$), and a smaller central retinal thickness (630 vs. 1369 mm, $p = 0.01$).
- While displacement can sometimes result in a shift of sub-RPE hemorrhage component together with the subretinal hemorrhage, most retina specialists would not treat predominantly sub-RPE hemorrhages as they are difficult to displace [11, 16].
- Based on our understanding of the current evidence and until we have results of well-powered randomized trials, we have adopt a more conservative approach that consists of the following: (1) intravitreal anti-VEGF alone for patients with small (≤ 2 DDA) and/or thin submacular hemorrhage (<450 μm) from nAMD; (2) for SMH up to 10 DDA we treat with pneumatic displacement using 0.3 ml of 100% C3F8 or C2F6 gas +50 μg/0.05 ml tPA + intravitreal bevacizumab 1.25 mg/0.05 ml. We perform a paracentesis before and after the procedure to limit the IOP rise. We position the patient at 45° upright for 3 days; and (3) for cases with vitreous hemorrhage, failed pneumatic displacement, or large SMH >10 DD area or SMH with a considerable sub-RPE component, we perform PPV. Following PVD induction and vitrectomy without vitreous base shaving, we perform subretinal injection of 0.1–0.15 ml of tPA at a concentration of 12.5 μg /0.1 ml in 1–4 blebs over the blood clot around the fovea followed by air-fluid exchange. Some of us only use BSS for the subretinal injection and place the tPA intravitreally after the eye is filled with air to limit possible toxicity. Postoperatively, we ask the patient to maintain 45° posturing for 3 days (Fig. 1).

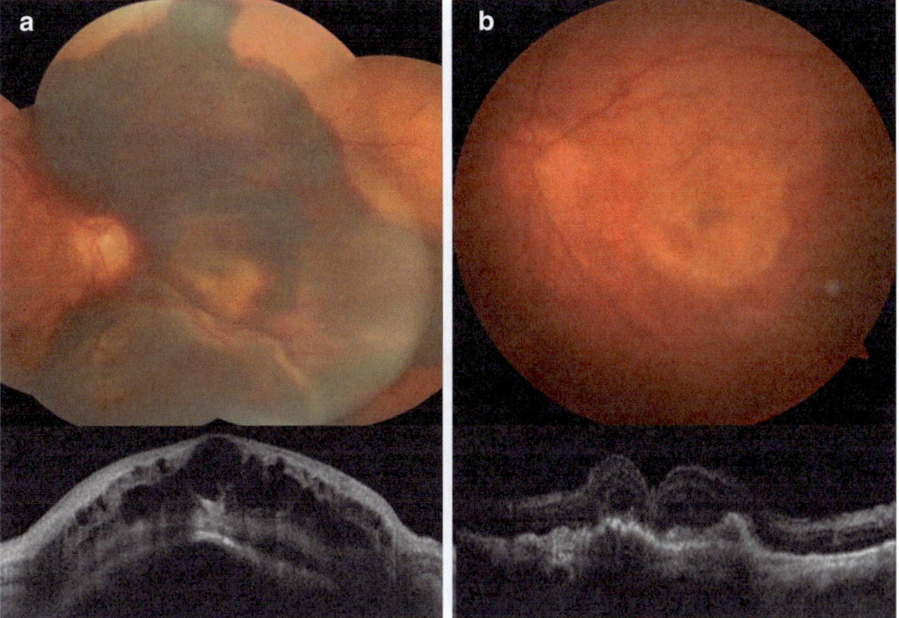

Fig. 1 Pre-displacement (**a**) and 2-day post-displacement (**b**) color images and optical coherence tomography scans of submacular hemorrhage due to neovascular age related macular degeneration treated with vitrectomy and subretinal tissue plasminogen activator (tPA). The blood was successfully displaced with modest improvement of vision from CF to 20/200 at 1 month

Key Points

- Treatment of SMH is timely to avoid retinal toxicity from blood.
- For thin SMH due to nAMD, anti-VEGF treatment alone appears to be sufficient.
- Non-surgical pneumatic displacement is effective for SMH in most cases and PPV may not be superior.
- Subretinal injection should be done slowly to avoid the formation of a macular hole (Video 2).
- Be aware of the dose and the potential toxicity of tPA on the retina, particularly when used subretinally.

References

1. Mehta A, Steel DH, Muldrew A, Peto T, Reeves BC, Evans R, Chakravarthy U, IVAN Study Investigators. Associations and outcomes of patients with submacular Hemorrhage secondary to age-related macular degeneration in the IVAN trial. Am J Ophthalmol. 2022;236:89–98.
2. Sun MT, Wood MK, Chan W, et al. Risk of Intraocular Bleeding With Novel Oral Anticoagulants Compared With Warfarin: A Systematic Review and Meta-analysis. JAMA Ophthalmol. 2017;135(8):864–70.

3. Scupola A, Coscas G, Soubrane G, Balestrazzi E. Natural history of macular subretinal hemorrhage in age-related macular degeneration. Ophthalmologica. 1999;213:97–102.
4. Toth CA, Morse LS, Hjelmeland LM, Landers MB. Fibrin directs early retinal damage after experimental subretinal hemorrhage. Arch Ophthalmol. 1991;109(5):723–9.
5. Bressler NM, Bressler SB, Childs AL, et al. Submacular surgery trials (SST) research group: surgery for hemorrhagic choroidal neovascular lesions of age-related macular degeneration: ophthalmic findings: SST report no. 13. Ophthalmology. 2004;111:1993–2006.
6. Martel JN, Mahmoud TH. Subretinal pneumatic displacement of subretinal hemorrhage. JAMA Ophthalmol. 2013;131(12):1632–5.
7. Shin JY, Lee JM, Byeon SH. Anti-vascular endothelial growth factor with or without pneumatic displacement for submacular hemorrhage. Am J Ophthalmol. 2015;159:904–914e1.
8. Obeid A, Talcott KE, Ali FS, Gao X, Sioufi K, Wibbelsman TD, Ho AC. Macular hole following subretinal tissue plasminogen activator for submacular Hemorrhage secondary to neovascular AMD. Ophthalmic Surg Lasers Imaging Retina. 2019;50(9):e257–9.
9. Fassbender JM, Sherman MP, Barr CC, Schaal S. Tissue plasminogen activator for subfoveal hemorrhage due to age-related macular degeneration: comparison of 3 treatment modalities. Retina. 2016;36(10):1860–5.
10. Lincoff H, Kreissig I, Stopa M, Uram D. A 40 degrees gaze down position for pneumatic displacement of submacular hemorrhage: clinical application and results. Retina. 2008;28(1):56–9.
11. Chew GWM, Ivanova T, Patton N, Dhawahir-Scala F, Jasani KM, Turner G, Charles S, Jalil A. Step-wise approach to the management of submacular hemorrhage using pneumatic displacement and vitrectomy: the Manchester protocol. Retina. 2022;42(1):11–8.
12. Wilkins CS, Mehta N, Wu CY, Barash A, Deobhakta AA, Rosen RB. Outcomes of pars plana vitrectomy with subretinal tissue plasminogen activator injection and pneumatic displacement of fovea-involving submacular haemorrhage. BMJ Open Ophthalmol. 2020;5(1):e000394.
13. de Jong JH, et al. Intravitreal versus subretinal administration of recombinant tissue plasminogen activator combined with gas for acute submacular hemorrhages due to age-related macular degeneration: an exploratory prospective study. Retina. 2016;36:914–25.
14. Mun Y, Park KH, Park SJ, et al. Comparison of treatment methods for submacular hemorrhage in neovascular age-related macular degeneration: conservative versus active surgical strategy. Sci Rep. 2022;12:14875.
15. Gabrielle PH, Delyfer MN, Glacet-Bernard A, et al. Surgery, Tissue Plasminogen Activator, Antiangiogenic Agents, and Age-Related Macular Degeneration Study: A Randomized Controlled Trial for Submacular Hemorrhage Secondary to Age-Related Macular Degeneration, Ophthalmology. 2023;130(9):947–57.
16. Sandhu SS, Manvikar S, Steel DH. Displacement of submacular hemorrhage associated with age-related macular degeneration using vitrectomy and submacular tPA injection followed by intravitreal ranibizumab. Clin Ophthalmol. 2010;4:637–42.

Idiopathic Uveal Effusion Syndrome

Loubna M. Radwan and Nicola G. Ghazi

1 Introduction

Idiopathic effusion syndrome (UES) is a rare (approximately, 1 in 10 million), idiopathic, relapsing, and remitting cause of choroidal and serous retinal detachment [1]. The exact pathogenesis is unclear, most likely involving a primary scleral abnormality that impedes the drainage of the vortex vein and the uveoscleral outflow. This chapter discusses the surgical management of idiopathic uveal effusion syndrome.

2 Types of UES [2]

	Type 1	Type 2	Type 3
Axial length	Nanophthalmic (less than 19 mm)	Normal (average 21 mm)	Normal
Scleral histology	- Thickened - Disorganized collagen bundles - Deposits of glycosaminoglycans (GAG)	- Thickened - Disorganized collagen bundles - Deposits of glycosaminoglycans (GAG)	Normal

Supplementary Information The online version contains supplementary material available at https://doi.org/10.1007/978-3-031-47827-7_22.

L. M. Radwan
Ophthalmology Department, Lebanese American University, Medical Center, Beirut, Lebanon
e-mail: Loubna.radwan@lau.edu

N. G. Ghazi (✉)
Eye Institute, Cleveland Clinic Abu Dhabi, Abu Dhabi, UAE

3   Signs and Symptoms

- Blurry vision and metamorphopsia.
- Vision/visual field loss.
- Retinal and choroidal effusions.
- Narrow angle.
- Vitreous cells.
- Dilated episcleral vessels.
- Blood in Schlemm's canal.
- Normal IOP.

4   Diagnostic Criteria

- Serous retinal detachment (no retinal break).
- Subretinal shifting fluid (high in protein content).
- Peripheral flat or annular choroidal and ciliary body detachment.
- Choroidal elevation.
- Elevation of the ora serrata.
- No significant leakage into subretinal space on fluorescein angiography (FA).
- Retinal pigment epithelium pigmentation (leopard spots) in chronic cases.
- Exclusion of other causes of ciliochoroidal detachment.

5   Differential Diagnosis

- Inflammatory conditions such as scleritis, Vogt-Koyanagi-Harada disease, as well as various causes of vasculitis and choroiditis.
- Intraocular tumors such as intraocular lymphoma, choroidal hemangioma, and choroidal melanoma.
- Idiopathic conditions such as Coats disease and central serous chorioretinopathy (CSCR).
- Vascular diseases such as hypertensive choroidopathy, pregnancy hypertensive disorders, chronic renal disease, and carotid cavernous fistula (CCF).
- Post-surgical complications such as hypotony, hemorrhagic choroidal detachment, post-pan-retinal photocoagulation, and post-retinal detachment repair.
- Medications, especially sulfa derivatives [3].
- Rhegmatogenous retinal detachment.

6 Multimodal Imaging

- Fluorescein angiography (FA): hypofluorescent spots corresponding to leopard spots, slow choroidal perfusion, prolonged choroidal fluorescence, focal areas of leakage.
- Fundus autofluorescence (FAF): persistent mixed hyper- and hypoautofluorescent spots corresponding to leopard spots.
- Indocyanin green (ICG): dilated choroidal vessels.
- Ultrasound (US):

   B-scan to document retinal/choroidal detachment, thickened choroid/sclera. A-scan to measure the axial length.

- US biomicroscopy: annular thickening of the anterior choroid. Rule out other causes of detachment.
- Optical coherence tomography (OCT): RPE thickening through the leopard spots, subretinal fluid, choroidal thickening.
- Enhanced-depth OCT: increased choroidal thickness with large areas of hyporeflectivity corresponding to engorged choroidal veins or suprachoroidal space expansion.

7 Work-up Tips

- Ask for intake of *medications* to exclude sulfa derivatives.
- Look carefully for a tumor:

   - History.
   - Transillumination, B-scan, and MRI patterns may be critical.

- Orbital auscultation to look for signs of a CCF.
- Rule out an inflammatory condition:

   - Treatment is non-surgical.
   - Responds to corticosteroids (therapeutic test, when in doubt).
   - Scleritis is the most relevant masquerade:

      B-scan and MRI may be helpful.

- If you decide to obtain an MRI:

   - T1 with contrast and T2 sequences can help differentiate between scleritis and tumors (Fig. 1). T1 sequence with contrast may be the most helpful as it isolates the normally dark sclera between the bright choroid and bright orbital fat.
   - May include MRI angiography if CCF is suspected.

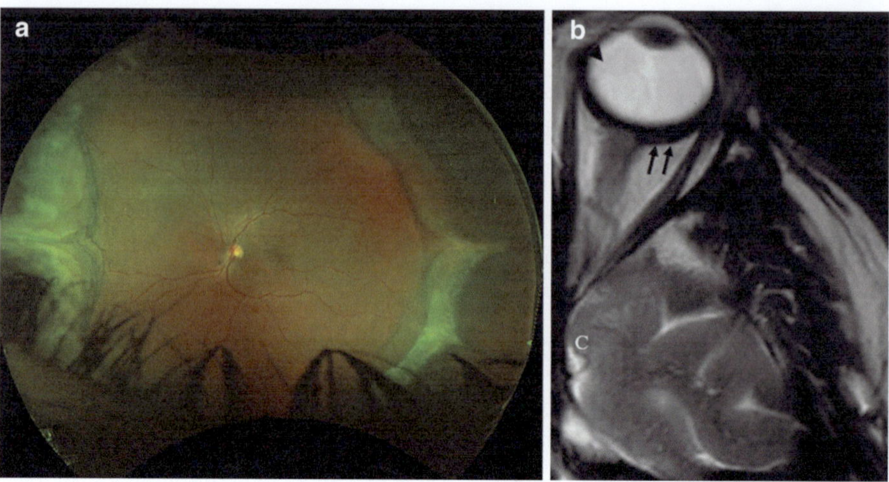

Fig. 1 A 57-year-old patient with type 2 uveal effusion syndrome. (**a**) Ultra-wide field fundus image of the left eye discloses peripheral 360° of annular choroidal thickening without retinal detachment. (**b**) Axial T2-weighted magnetic resonance imaging scan-Turbo spin Echo (T2-TSE) of the left orbit showing abnormally thickened sclera (double arrows) despite an axial length of 22.60 mm

8   Indications for Surgery

The UES is a surgical disease that generally does not respond to medical therapy. The two main indications for surgery are:

- Persistent retinal detachment with macular involvement and decreased vision: spontaneous reattachment may occur over weeks to months. Careful judgment is needed as the final visual outcome depends on the degree and duration of detachment.
- Anterior chamber angle closure or appositional angles.

9   Types of Surgical Procedures

The surgical approach to treating UES has evolved over time. Four main categories of approaches have been described:

9.1   Vortex Vein Decompression by Brockhurst RJ (1980) (Fig. 2) [4]

- Sclerectomy at the insertion of the rectus muscles extending to the exit of the vortex veins was made in each quadrant.
- In each scleral dissection bed, sclerotomies were done close to the horizontal meridians to avoid injury to the long posterior ciliary arteries, nerves, and vortex ampulla branches.
- A separate full-thickness sclerotomy was used to drain subretinal fluid in cases of total RD.

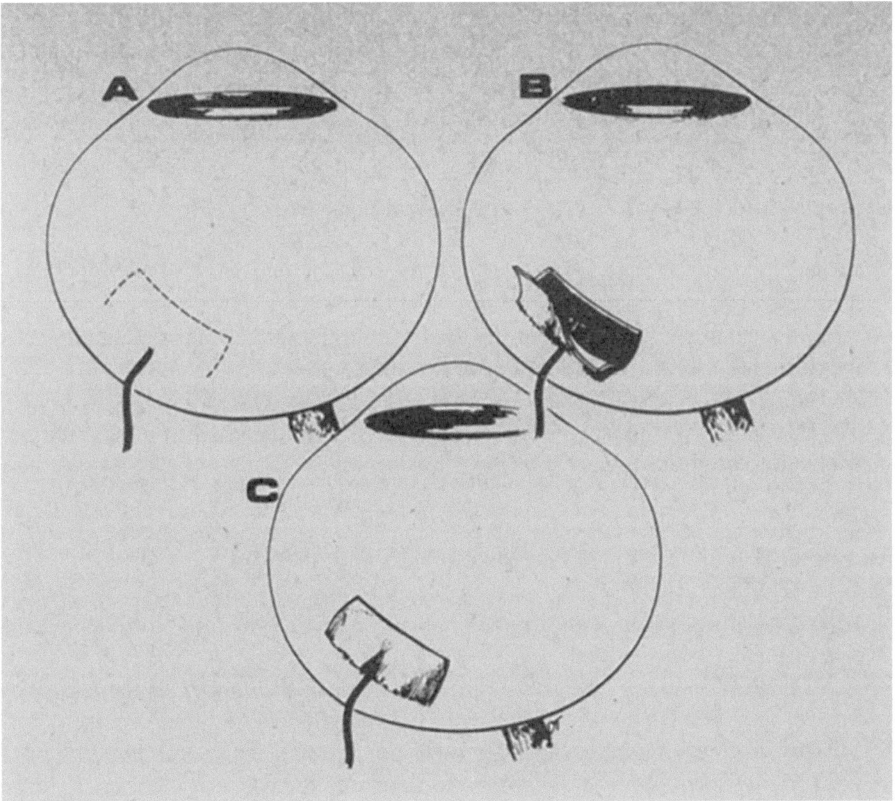

Fig. 2 Sketch showing steps in vortex vein decompression. (**a**) Initial flap incisions; (**b**) dissection of scleral flap exposing intra-scleral course of vortex vein; and (**c**) excess scleral flap tissue excised. Published with Permission from American Medical Association. Brockhurst RJ. Vortex vein decompression for nanophthalmic uveal effusion. Arch Ophthalmol 1980;98 (11): 1987–1990. https://jamanetwork.com/journals/jamaophthalmology/article-abstract/633581

9.2 Localized Scleral Surgery with Sclerectomy/Sclerotomy/Sclerostomy

Gass JD and Co-Workers (1983) [5, 6]

They noted that vortex vein decompression is not only risky (high risk of ocular hemorrhage) but also not necessary.

- Four rectangular 5 × 7 mm, half to two-thirds thickness sclerotomies were made, one in each quadrant taking care to avoid the areas anterior to the exit sites of the vortex veins.
- The sclerotomies were centered 1–2 mm anterior to the equator with the long axis oriented circumferentially.
- A linear 2-mm sclerostomy was made in the center of each sclerectomy, and a punch was used to enlarge the scleral opening.
- No attempt was made to perforate the choroid.

Uyama M and Co-Workers 2000 (Subscleral Sclerectomy) (Fig. 3) [2]

- At the equator of the inferotemporal and inferonasal quadrants, two-thirds thickness scleral flaps measuring 4 × 5 mm were made.
- Under the scleral flap, the remaining thickness of the sclera was excised in pieces measuring 3 × 4 mm, and the choroid was exposed.
- The edges of the scleral wound were cauterized to avoid scarring.
- The scleral flap was loosely sutured, but Tenon's capsule and the bulbar conjunctiva were closed tightly.

Akduman L et al. (1997) [7] and Suzuki Y Et al. (2007) [8]

- Scleral window surgery and topical application of mitomycin C to reduce scarring of the sclerectomy bed.
- A 2/3 thickness scleral flap (4 × 4 mm) was made at the equator in the temporoinferior quadrant (Suzuki et al.) or in all four quadrants (Akduman et al.).
- Mitomycin C was applied using a surgical sponge under the scleral flap for 5 min.
- A 2 × 3 mm sclerectomy was then performed, and the flap was closed.

Faulborn J and Kölli H (1999) (Fig. 4) [9]

- 4 mm posterior to the limbus, a 2 × 8-mm full-thickness sclerotomy without sclerectomy was made in each quadrant.
- The sclerotomies were not sutured.

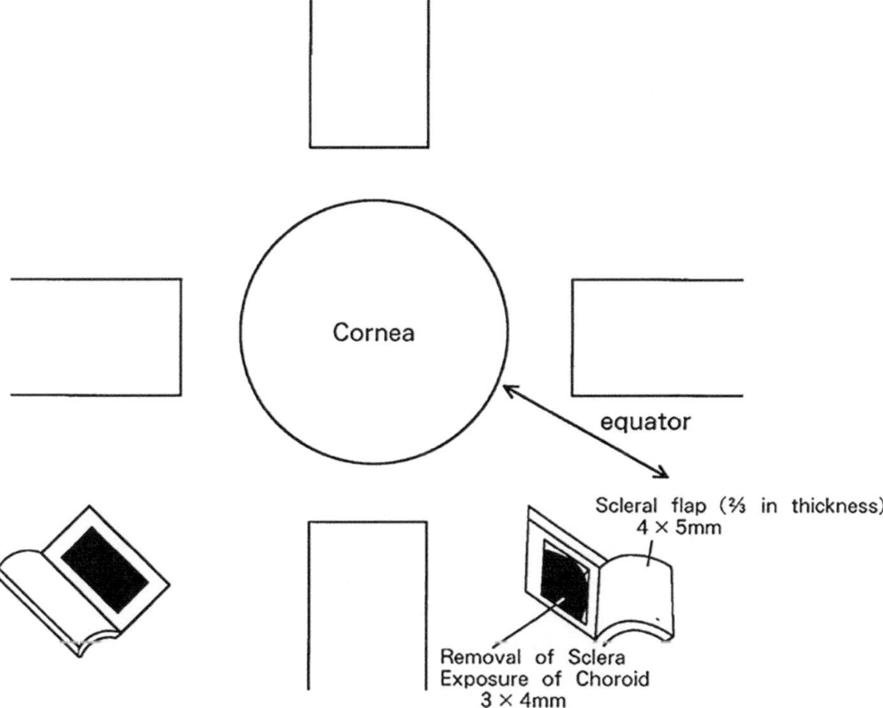

Fig. 3 Schematic drawing of the surgical procedure, subscleral sclerectomy. Primary surgery was performed at two sites at the equator in the lower quadrants, and a scleral window was opened under the scleral flap. Published with Permission from Elsevier. Uyama M, Takahashi K, Kozaki J, Tagami N, Takada Y, Ohkuma H, et al. Uveal effusion syndrome: clinical features, surgical treatment, histologic examination of the sclera, and pathophysiology. Ophthalmology. 2000; 107(3):441–449. https://www.aaojournal.org/article/S0161–6420(99)00141–4/fulltext

Fig. 4 Localization of sclerotomies. Published with Permission from Wolters Kluwer. Faulborn J, Kölli H. SCLEROTOMY IN UVEAL EFFUSION SYNDROME: Retina.1999; 19 (6). P504–507. https://journals.lww.com/retinajournal/Abstract/1999/19060/SCLEROTOMY_IN_UVEAL_EFFUSION_SYNDROME.4.aspx

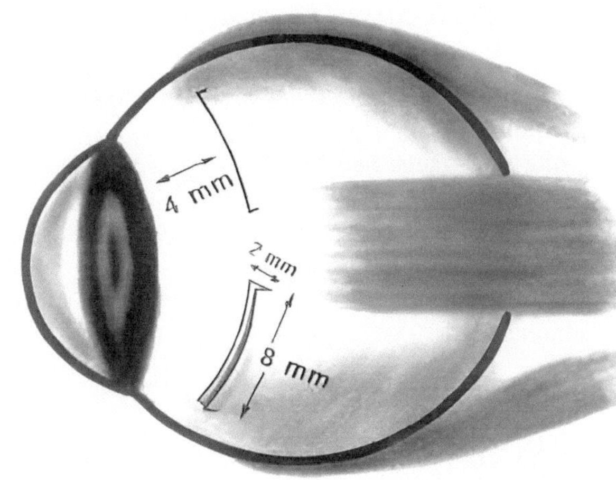

- The conjunctiva was then secured to the limbus.

Bausili MM et al. (2017) [10]

- 6 mm posterior to the limbus, two partial-thickness fornix-based flaps were performed in the nasal quadrants.
- Sclerotomy was done using a fiberoptic-guided CO_2 laser. This exposed the choroid while avoiding bleeding. The flap was then removed.
- Then another full-thickness sclerotomy was done in the inferotemporal quadrant using the same laser.

Ghazi NG et al. Procedure (2013) (Fig. 5) (Video 1) [11]

- An ultrasound-guided hybrid technique.
- B-scan ultrasonography was used preoperatively and intraoperatively to localize the areas of maximal choroidal swelling.
- Single sclerostomy placement in each involved quadrant subjacent to the area of maximal choroidal swelling as guided by ultrasound.
- No scleral flaps or vortex vein decompression.
- Anterior pathology: a 4-mm full-thickness circumferential scleral incision was fashioned subjacent to the area of maximal choroidal swelling. A sclerostomy was then done in the center of the incision using a Kelly punch.
- Posterior pathology: equatorial partial-thickness sclerectomy (4 × 4 mm, 2/3 scleral thickness) was made. Then a full-thickness radial incision was made through the remaining sclera, and a Kelly punch was used to place a sclerostomy in the center.

9.3 Ex-Press Shunt by Yepez JB and Arevalo JF (2015) [12]

- Preop B-scan ultrasonography was used to determine the quadrant with the most effusion.
- Using a 25-gauge needle, an oblique sclerotomy was done 13 mm posterior to the limbus.
- The Ex-Press shunt was placed obliquely in the sclerotomy to help drain excessive suprachoroidal fluid.
- The conjunctiva was then sutured, and subconjunctival antibiotics were administered.

9.4 Extensive Circumferential Partial-Thickness Sclerectomy by Mansour a Et al. (2018) (Fig. 6) [13]

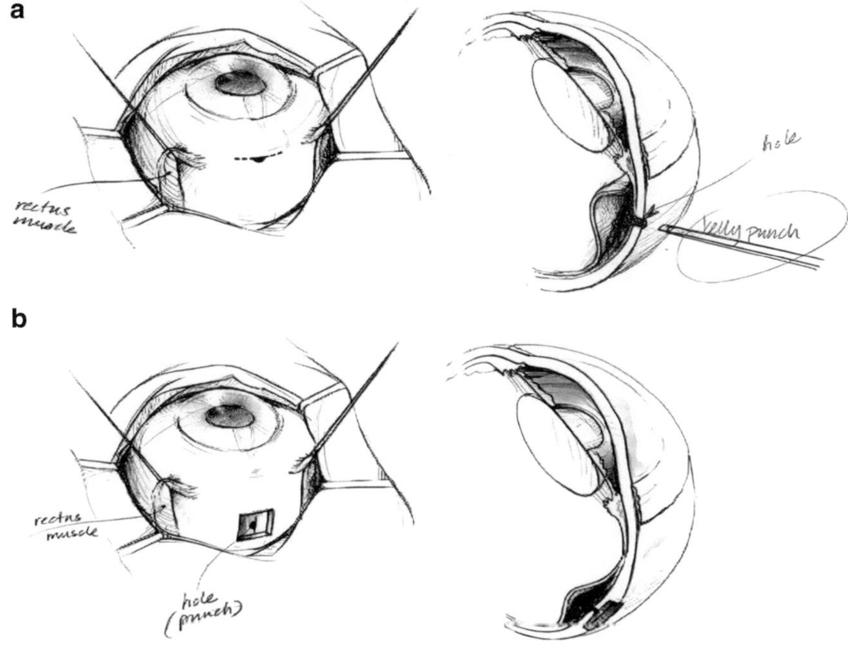

Fig. 5 Schematic representation of the surgical procedure. (**a**) Topographical and cross-sectional illustration of the circumferential scleral incision with anterior sclerostomy. (**b**) Topographical and cross-sectional illustration of the equatorial partial-thickness sclerectomy and sclerostomy. The sclerostomy is localized subjacent to the area of maximal choroidal swelling and is created using a Kelly punch in either approach. Published with permission from Wolters Kluwer; Ghazi NG, Richards CP, Abazari A. A modified ultrasound-guided surgical technique for the management of the uveal effusion syndrome in patients with normal axial length and scleral thickness. Retina. 2013; 33 (6) - P 1211-1219. https://journals.lww.com/retinajournal/Abstract/2013/06000/A_ MODIFIED_ULTRASOUND_GUIDED_SURGICAL_TECHNIQUE.18.aspx

- Scleral dissection began immediately behind the muscle insertions and extended posteriorly past the vortex veins.
- A 90% depth scleral window was excised over 3 and 1/4 quadrants.
- 3/4 of the superior-temporal quadrant was excluded to avoid damaging the superior oblique muscle.
- A hockey stick-shaped scleral knife was used to incise the boundaries of the window deep enough to see the bluish hue of the choroid.
- An angled 2-mm crescent blade and serrated forceps were used to bimanually dissect and remove the outer wall of the sclera.
- A small rim of the sclera was left intact for areas of the globe with limited exposure, such as under the rectus muscles.

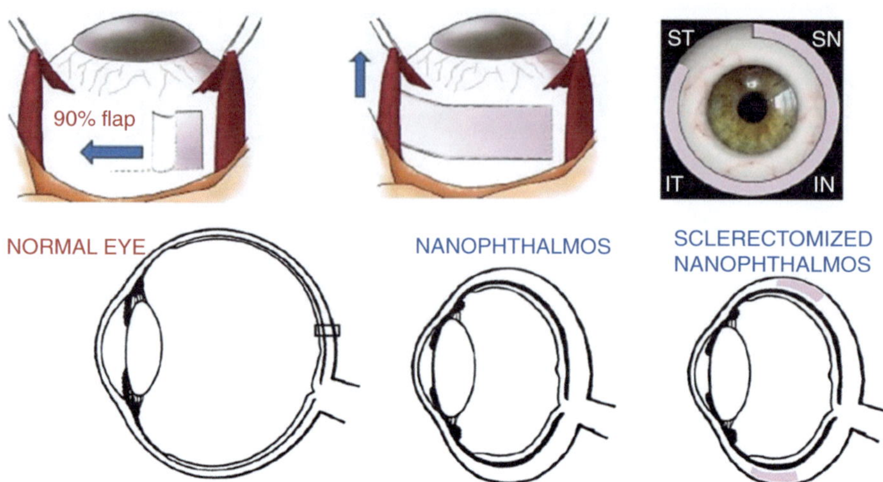

Fig. 6 Top row: A three-quadrant-plus, subtotal (90%), scleral excision is performed with sparing of most of the superior-temporal quadrant to avoid damage to the superior oblique muscle. Bottom row: The cartoons compare a normal eye, a nanophthalmic eye, and a nanophthalmic eye that has undergone extensive scleral excision. ST, superotemporal; SN, superonasal; IT, inferotemporal; IN, inferonasal. Published with Permission from BMJ; Mansour A, Stewart MW, Shields CL, Hamam R, Abdul Fattah M, Sheheitli H, et al. Extensive circumferential partial-thickness sclerectomy in eyes with extreme nanophthalmos and spontaneous uveal effusion. Br J Ophthalmol. 2019; 103 (2) P 1862–1867, https://bjo.bmj.com/content/103/12/1862

10 Prognosis

The techniques described by Faulborn and Kölli [9] and that described by Ghazi et al. [11] are simple, easy to perform, and reproducible. In approximately 85% of cases, the effusuion resolves with one surgery. They are the techniques of choice for the authors. The technique of Faulborn and Kölli was described in nanophthalmic eyes only, whereas that of Ghazi et al. was successful even in type 3 cases with normal sclera and axial length. It also adapts the location of scleral surgery to the location of maximal choroidal swelling as guided by ultrasound.

11 Intraoperative and Postoperative Complications

– Choroidal detachment or trauma.
– Vortex vein rupture.
– Cauterization of the vortex vein.
– Hypotony.
– Choroidal bleeding.
– Choroid/retinal penetration.

- Hyphema.
- Intraoperative retinal hemorrhage.
- Scleral ectasia.
- Scleral fibrosis.
- Scleral rupture with minor trauma.
- Vitreous leakage and incarceration leading to fibrous ingrowth, macular edema and retinal tears.

Key Points

- UES occurs in small or normal-sized eyes. There are three types of UES.
- UES is generally due to primary scleral abnormality.
- The list of differential diagnoses is extensive: keep in mind scleritis, CSCR, tumors, medications, and CCF.
- Thorough history and examination details, ultrasound, MRI, and retinal/brain angiography findings are critical in the workup.
- The treatment is surgical.

References

1. Sharma R, Foot B, Jackson TL. A prospective, population-based, surveillance (BOSU) study of uveal effusion syndrome in the UK. Eur J Ophthalmol. 2021;31(5):2451–56.
2. Uyama M, Takahashi K, Kozaki J, Tagami N, Takada Y, Ohkuma H, et al. Uveal effusion syndrome: clinical features, surgical treatment, histologic examination of the sclera, and pathophysiology. Ophthalmology. 2000;107(3):441–9.
3. Ikeda N, Ikeda T, Nagata M, Mimura O. Ciliochoroidal effusion syndrome induced by sulfa derivatives. Arch Ophthalmol Chic Ill 1960. 2002;120(12):1775.
4. Brockhurst RJ. Vortex vein decompression for Nanophthalmic uveal effusion. Arch Ophthalmol. 1980;98(11):1987–90.
5. Gass JD. Uveal effusion syndrome: a new hypothesis concerning pathogenesis and technique of surgical treatment. Trans Am Ophthalmol Soc. 1983;81:246–60.
6. Johnson MW, Gass JDM. Surgical Management of the Idiopathic Uveal Effusion Syndrome. Ophthalmology. 1990;97(6):778–85.
7. Akduman L, Adelberg DA, Del Priore LV. Nanophthalmic uveal effusion managed with scleral windows and topical mitomycin-C. Ophthalmic Surg Lasers. 1997;28(4):325–7.
8. Suzuki Y, Nishina S, Azuma N. Scleral window surgery and topical mitomycin C for nanophthalmic uveal effusion complicated by renal failure: case report. Graefes Arch Clin Exp Ophthalmol. 2007;245(5):755–7.
9. Faulborn J, Kölli H. Sclerotomy in uveal effusion syndrome. Retina. 1999;19(6):504.
10. Bausili MM, Raja H, Kotowski J, Nadal J, Salomao DR, Keenum D, et al. Use of FIBEROPTIC-guided CO2 laser in the treatment of uveal effusion. Retin Cases Brief Rep. 2017;11(3):191–4.
11. Ghazi NG, Richards CP, Abazari A. A modified ultrasound-guided surgical technique for the management of the uveal effusion syndrome in patients with normal axial length and scleral thickness. Retina. 2013;33(6):1211–9.
12. Yepez JB, Arevalo JF. Ex-PRESS shunt for choroidal fluid drainage in uveal effusion syndrome type 2: a potentially novel technique. JAMA Ophthalmol. 2015;133(4):470.
13. Mansour A, Stewart MW, Shields CL, Hamam R, Abdul Fattah M, Sheheitli H, et al. Extensive circumferential partial-thickness sclerectomy in eyes with extreme nanophthalmos and spontaneous uveal effusion. Br J Ophthalmol. 2019; bjophthalmol-2018-313702

Retinal Pigment Epithelium and Choroid Transplantation

Barbara Parolini and Michele Palmieri

1 Introduction

This chapter discusses the use of retinal pigment epithelium (RPE) and choroidal patch transplantation to treat advanced age related macular degeneration (AMD). The aim is to provide a practical guide to understanding the indications of surgery and to describe the surgical technique we use.

1.1 *The Rationale for Surgery*

The underlying concept of RPE-choroid patch transplantation resides in the idea that a healthy choriocapillaris-RPE complex is crucial for oxygen and metabolic demand of retinal photoreceptors. In maculopathies that primarily affect the choroid and RPE before affecting the retina, we could preserve the photoreceptor function by moving the fovea on top and in contact with healthy RPE [1, 2]. Thus, surgery should be performed before the retina is irreversibly damaged by the disease. This complex surgical technique was commonly proposed to end-stage diseases and to patients with very low visual acuity (VA). However, it has been demonstrated that it should be offered in a phase of the disease when the preoperative visual function is still present and when the outer retina is still recognizable on OCT scans.

Supplementary Information The online version contains supplementary material available at https://doi.org/10.1007/978-3-031-47827-7_23.

B. Parolini (✉) · M. Palmieri
Eyecare Clinic, Brescia, Italy

A. B. Sallam et al. (eds.), *Practical Manual of Vitreoretinal Surgery*, https://doi.org/10.1007/978-3-031-47827-7_23

2 Potential Indications

Anti-vascular endothelial growth factor (anti-VEGF) intravitreal injections represent the standard of treatment for neovascular age related macular degeneration (nAMD). However, the different retrospective analyses revealed that long-term visual outcomes of patients who poorly responded to anti-VEGF were due to disruption of retinal anatomy [3, 4]. Moreover, anti-VEGF therapy is less effective in patients suffering of submacular hemorrhage or RPE tear because the anatomy of the outer retina is compromised [5–7].

Good case selection is important for good functional results, specifically with relatively intact external limiting membrane (ELM) and of the ellipsoid zone (EZ) on OCT.

Thus, patients affected by:

- Exudative maculopathies of various origins (i.e., nAMD, myopia, angioid streaks, idiopathic choroidal neovascular membrane (CNV)).
- Recent submacular hemorrhage.
- CNV not responding to repeated anti-VEGF.

Considering the possible postoperative complications with this surgery, we recommend surgery only to patients with vision ≤20/100.

Atrophic maculopathy may also be treated with RPE-choroid patch transplantation but only as a last resource for patients with poor vision in the fellow eye. A very guarded outcome should be given in this context [8].

2.1 Contraindication of RPE-Choroid Patch

1. Atrophic macula on OCT.
2. In case of significant hemorrhagic retinal detachment secondary to AMD, it is not always possible to determine the status of the macula. In those cases, multiple choices can be selected:

   (a) Perform surgery just to remove the hemorrhage, reevaluate the macula, and perform RPE-choroid patch only if it is considered beneficial.
   (b) Perform surgery to remove the hemorrhage and RPE-choroid patch simultaneously (preferably with intraoperative OCT to evaluate the macula at the time of surgery).

3 Surgical Technique [8]

3.1 Anesthesia

Our preferred protocol for anesthesia is sedation and subtenon injection of 2 cc of lidocaine and 5 cc of bupivacaine.

3.2 Surgery Step (Video 1)

23-gauge (g) Trocar System

The superior trocars are placed at 9.30 and 2.30, to allow easier maneuvers at 12 o'clock.

Risk Related to this Maneuver

If the trocars are too anterior, you can touch the lens (if the lens is still in place). If the trocars are too posterior, you can enter in the retina and prematurely detach it with the infusion. If the superior trocars are too close to each other, you will not be able to perform maneuvers at 12 o'clock.

Insert a Chandelier

Insert a chandelier, which is necessary to allow bimanual maneuvers. We recommend inserting it at 12 o'clock at 3.5 mm from the limbus.

Phacoemulsification and Intraocular Lens (IOL) Implantation

We recommend using a three-piece intraocular lens (IOL) implanted in the capsular bag. The reason is linked to the need to perform a very peripheral vitrectomy and this could lead to breaking the capsular bag during vitrectomy. If this happens, the plate of the three-piece IOL can be moved to the ciliary sulcus.

Risk Related to this Maneuver

Induced miosis.

Complete Vitrectomy and Posterior Vitreous Detachment

Start with a core pars plana vitrectomy (PPV) and identify the posterior hyaloid to verify if posterior vitreous detachment (PVD) is already present. Staining the vitreous with triamcinolone improves the posterior hyaloid visualization. Extend the PVD to the midperiphery and complete the vitrectomy assisted by scleral indentation. In this surgery shaving of the vitreous base is necessary to reduce the risk of postoperative proliperative vitreoretinopathy (PVR), in our view. We recommend to repeat the use of diluted triamcinolone, to verify the completeness of vitrectomy and the removal of the posterior hyaloid.

Risk Related to this Maneuver

Retinal break that will prevent an easy detachment of the retina (see phase 6).
   Posterior capsular break.
   Inability to remove completely the hyaloid or the vitreous.
   Vitreous strands in the sclerotomies.

Induction of Retinal Detachment

Induce a retinal detachment (RD) by injecting balanced salt solution (BSS) into the subretinal space, using a 41-g needle connected to the active pump (we set the injection pressure at 30 mmHg). IOP should be kept at 10–15 mmHg. We recommend choosing the spot for the first subretinal injection in the peripheral area for two main reasons. First, because when the bubble of the detached retina increases in size, you will still be able to see the tip of the 41-g needle. Second the injection will be less violent in the macular area, lowering the risk of inducing a macular hole as compared to injection near the macula. The retina should be detached in the whole temporal quadrant superior and inferior or from the inferotemporal to the superonasal area. The aim is to be able to uncover the whole temporal macular area of the choroid to perform submacular maneuvers. If an iatrogenic retinal break happens during the induction of retinal detachment or during vitrectomy, it will be more difficult to detach the retina in the desired area, since the subretinal fluid will exit through the break into the vitreous chamber.

Risk Related to this Maneuver

Iatrogenic macular hole.

Fluid-Air Exchange

This maneuver extends the RD. The IOP should be kept at 30 mmHg.

Risk Related to this Maneuver

Iatrogenic retinal breaks by touching the retina with the backflush needle or with the tip of the chandelier.

Peripheral Retinotomy and Exposure of the Subretinal Space

Once the retina is detached, perform an approximately 200° peripheral retinotomy with scissors or with the vitrector near to the ora serrata in the inferotemporal, superotemporal, and superonasal quadrants. In case of bleeding use diathermy to coagulate blood vessels. However, bleeding in the extremely peripheral retina rarely occurs. The injection of perfluorocarbon liquid (PFCL) till the equator helps to stabilize the retina. PFCL has to be removed before step 9.

Risk Related to this Maneuver

Retinal incarceration into the sclerotomies and into the instruments (even the scissors create a vacuum effect) after completing the retinotomy. This happens more with large sclerotomies.

Unfold the Retina

Use the end-gripping forceps or the backflush needle to fold the temporal retina nasally and expose the subretinal space. Remember that the retina could be firmly attached to the CNV or to the choroid if areas of RPE atrophy are present. Use a spatula, a scraper, or a loop to gently separate the retina from the CNV or from the RPE.

Risk Related to this Maneuver

Tearing the retina.
Bleeding (note that blood has a glue-like effect on the retina and might create retinal folds which are difficult to open without creating a iatrogenic break).

Drainage of Subretinal Hemorrhage

After exposing the subretinal space, proceed to drain any subretinal debris or hemorrhage, when present. If the amount of blood is significant, and the visibility is compromised, pay attention so as not to inadvertently aspirate the retina. You need to find the right balance between an IOP high enough to stop active bleeding and low enough to avoid retina incarceration into the backflush and/or into the sclerotomies.

Risk Related to this Maneuver

Retinal damage and incarceration.

CNV Removal and Endodiathermy

The CNV, when present, can be removed from the choroid using retinal forceps, a diamond dust scraper, or the backflush. It is advisable to leave the CNV lying over the retina or RPE and take care of the bleeding from the CNV feeder vessels. To do so, you can use a bimanual technique, having in one hand an endodiathermy and in the other the backflush, or you can use a special tool that combine endodiathermy and aspiration in one tip. Endodiathermy should be applied, after CNV removal, not only to stop the feeder vessel but also in multiple spots to the macular choroidal bed, to create micro-trauma to the choriocapillaris and stimulate the revascularization of the RPE-choroid patch. After completion of endodiathermy, the CNV has to be removed. Small CNV are easily cut and aspirated with the vitrectomy probe. Large CNV with a significant fibrotic component cannot be removed by the vitrector and need to be segmented with scissors to create small portions. Very often a dedicated sclerotomy is needed to remove the CNV.

Risk Related to this Maneuver

Inability to remove the CNV without opening an extra sclerotomy, with risk of retina incarceration.

Prepare the RPE-Choroid Patch

The location of the harvesting site of the patch is chosen by selecting an area of healthy-appearing RPE in the exposed quadrants, avoiding the vortex veins. Mark the margins of the intended patch location with diathermy. This step helps for both delineating the area of the patch and limiting choroidal bleeding. The ideal size of the patch should be large enough to cover the whole atrophic macular area (approximately 3–4 optic disc diameters). Once positioned, the edge of the patch should get in touch with healthy choriocapillaris. Using vertical scissors, isolate a full-thickness patch of RPE and choroid, until the bear white sclera is visible within the margins of the diathermy burns. We suggest started cutting the patch on the posterior side, toward the posterior pole. After isolating the posterior half of the patch, inject PFCL into the subretinal space to cover and stabilize the patch. The edge of the patch tends to roll up and elevate. Subsequently, complete the dissection of the anterior half of the patch.

Risk Related to this Maneuver

Losing the rolled-up patch into the vitreous chamber.
Excessive bleeding while cutting the choroid is uncommon and more frequent in patients on anticoagulant therapy.

RPE-Choroid Patch Transplant

The patch should be transplanted onto the submacular area, under PFCL, using a vitreoretinal forceps with blunt tips. The edge of the patch should be mildly elevated over the choroidal plane, to avoid scratching the choroid. An excessive elevation will result in rolling of the patch. Pull one edge of the patch toward the optic nerve for a distance of 2–3 mm. Then leave that edge and pull a different edge toward the final position in order to avoid folding the patch. To unfold the edges of the patch, grasp it in different spots and stretch\unfold the edges.

The areas of the patch touched by the instruments will be inevitably damaged and that is why it is important to isolate a large patch, to save a healthy RPE area under the fovea. Center the patch on the fovea and let it under PFCL for about 1 min to favor adhesion.

Remove the remaining residues of choroid, from the area of bare sclera, with aspiration and/or forceps, and treat the borders of incised RPE-choroid with intense endodiathermy.

Risk Related to this Maneuver

To scratch the choroid while translocating the patch.
  Losing the patch into the vitreous chamber.

Reattach the Retina with PFCL

Slowly and progressively aspirate the subretinal PFCL with the same syringe and cannula used to inject it and reinject it on the epiretinal space, to flatten the retina. Do not aspirate the entire quantity of subretinal PFCL all at once, but gradually. Start repositioning PFCL on the optic nerve head and keep the cannula in the growing bubble of PFCL. While reinjecting PFCL, keep in the other hand the backflush at the edge of the subretinal space, to aspirate fluid, stabilize the IOP, and reattach the retina. When PFCL covers the fovea, check the centration of the patch (Fig. 1). If it is not centered, move the PFCL again subretinally, re-center the patch, and repeat the sequence of steps.

Risk Related to this Maneuver

Decentration of the patch with respect to the fovea.
  Subretinal PFCL.

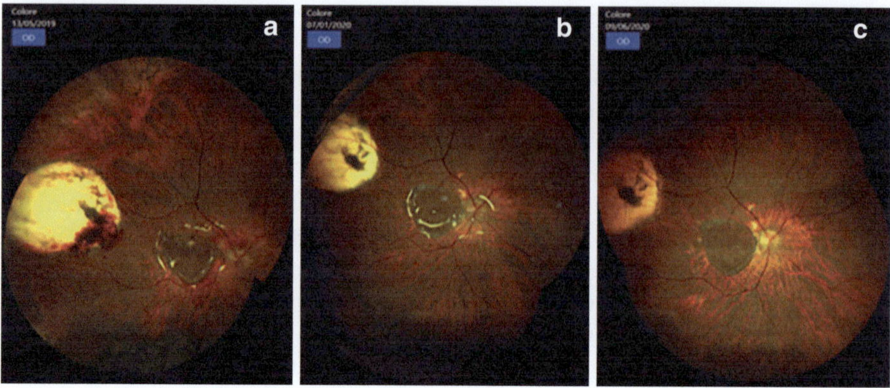

Fig. 1 Color fundus widefield image of an eye operated with autologous choroidal transplant 1 week (**a**) and 6 months (**b**) after surgery and after silicone oil removal (**c**). In the temporal area, a whitish area shows the harvesting site of the bare sclera covered by the retina. The choroidal patch is well placed under the macula and looks more pigmented than the surrounding choroid

Remove the Anterior Edge of the Retina

Once the retina is completely reattached under PFCL, the anterior edge of the retinotomy should be removed by the cutter. If the retinotomy was initially performed with the cutter, there is usually no edge left at this point. Keep IOP around 20 mmHg to avoid turbulence. When releasing the scleral indentation, do it very slowly, to avoid detaching the retina and getting some of the PFCL bubbles to go subretinally.

Risk Related to this Maneuver

Decentration of the patch with respect to the fovea.
Subretinal PFCL.

Endolaser

Seal the retinotomy, which should be covered completely with PFCL at this point, with 3–5 rows of confluent laser spots. We suggest a 360° laser retinopexy.

Risk Related to this Maneuver

To touch the retina with laser tip.
To leave untreated areas.

PFCL/Tamponade Exchange

We usually complete the procedure with a direct PFCL/1000 cSt silicone oil exchange as described in Vitreous Substitutes Chap. 5.

Risk Related to this Maneuver

BSS slipping under the retina and re-detachment.
  Aspirate the retina with aspirating tools.
  Silicone migration to the anterior chamber with a displacement of IOL.
  In some selected cases we used PFCL-air exchange and then injection of 1 cc of pure SF6 gas to get a concentration of about 25% SF6.

Risk Related to this Maneuver

Retina slippage.

Removal of Trocars

We apply external diathermy at the edges of the sclerotomies, to stretch and seal them. 7-0 Vicryl is used for leaking sclerotomies.

3.3 *Prognosis for Vision after Surgery [8]*

In our long-term study of 88 eyes operated for various exudative and atrophic chorioretinal pathology, we found the mean preoperative and postoperative VA to be 20/320 (1.2 logMAR) and 20/200 (0.94), respectively (p = 0.009). Reading ability recovered in 43% of cases and a gain of at least 15 letters was obtained in 40% of the eyes. The eyes with atrophic (dry) AMD did not gain vision. Integrity of external limiting membrane and higher preoperative VA ($\geq$ 20/200) predicted better long-term VA. Note that the surgery outcome is poor in atrophic maculopathies.

3.4 *Potential Complications of Surgery [8]*

– Retinal detachment (11.4%).
– Progressive atrophy of the RPE-choroid patch (7%).

- Epiretinal membrane (4.5%), extrafoveal CNV recurrence (4.5%), and subretinal hemorrhage (4.5%) (observed only in patients with preoperative hemorrhagic CNV).
- Cystoid macular edema (3%).
- Off-centered patch (2.3%).
- Absence of graft revascularization (1.1%).
- Partial graft revascularization with atrophy of the non-perfused area (1.1%).
- Loss of vision: 11% of eyes had postoperative BCVA lower than preoperative.
- Atrophy of the RPE-choroid patch.

3.5 Case Scenario

A 77-year-old woman with a sudden vision drop in her right eye with a submacular hemorrhage due to neovascular age related macular degeneration. She was on anticoagulants for atrial fibrillation. Preoperative VA was counting fingers. Pars plana vitrectomy with subretinal hemorrhage drainage, a retinal pigment epithelium-choroidal patch, and silicone oil tamponade was performed. At 1-month she gained her vision up to 20/50. Few weeks later, she had postoperative macular edema managed with topical steroids and non steroidal drops. Silicone oil removal was performed 6 months after the first surgery. At 1 year follow-up, she had a stable VA of 20/50 with good perfusion of the patch, demonstrated by the OCT angiography (Fig. 2).

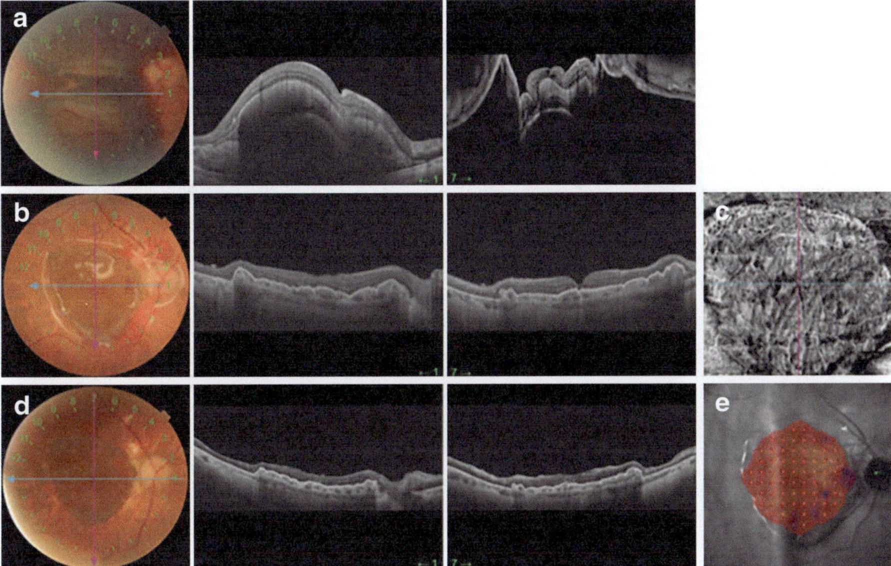

Fig. 2 Evolution of one eye affected by massive subretinal hemorrhage secondary to neovascular age related macular degeneration. (**a**) preoperative color fundus image and optical coherence tomography (OCT) horizontal and vertical scans. (**b**) 1 month postoperatively, the fundus image shows the total resolution of the subretinal hemorrhage with the autologous choroidal patch well positioned under the macula. OCT scans show the choroidal patch under a well-preserved retina. (**c**) OCT angiography depicts the revascularization of the patch. (**d**) 6 months after original surgery and 1 month after silicone oil removal, the choroidal patch remaining well positioned. (**e**) Microperimetry shows good retinal sensitivity over the patch

References

1. Peyman GA, Blinder KJ, Paris CL, Alturki W, Nelson NCDU. A technique for retinal pigment epithelium transplantation for age-related macular degeneration secondary to extensive subfoveal scarring. Ophthalmic Surg. 1991;22(2):102–8.
2. Stanga PE, Kychenthal A, Fitzke FW, et al. Retinal pigment epithelium translocation and central visual function in age related macular degeneration: preliminary results. Int Ophthalmol. 2001;23(4-6):297–307.
3. Rosenfeld PJ, Shapiro H, Tuomi L, Webster M, Elledge J, Blodi B. Characteristics of patients losing vision after 2 years of monthly dosing in the phase III ranibizumab clinical trials. Ophthalmology. 2011.
4. Rofagha S, Bhisitkul RB, Boyer DS, Sadda SR, Zhang K. Seven-year outcomes in ranibizumab-treated patients in ANCHOR, MARINA, and HORIZON: A multicenter cohort study (SEVEN-UP). Ophthalmology. 2013.
5. Van Meurs JC, Van Den Biesen PR. Autologous retinal pigment epithelium and choroid translocation in patients with exudative age-related macular degeneration: short-term follow-up. Am J Ophthalmol. 2003;136(4):688–95.

6. Cereda MG, Parolini B, Bellesini E, Pertile G. Surgery for CNV and autologous choroidal RPE patch transplantation: exposing the submacular space. Graefes Arch Clin Exp Ophthalmol. 2010;248(1):37–47.
7. van Romunde SHM, Polito A, Peroglio Deiro A, Guerriero M, Pertile G. Retinal pigment epithelium–choroid graft with a peripheral retinotomy for exudative age-related macular degeneration. Retina. 2017:1.
8. Parolini B, Di Salvatore A, Pinackatt SJ, et al. Long-term results of autologous retinal pigment epithelium and choroid transplantation for the treatment of exudative and atrophic maculopathies. Retina. 2018.

Pressure-Dependent Optic Neuropathy (Ocular Hypertension/Glaucoma) and Vitreoretinal Surgery

Giampaolo Gini

- The goal of intraocular ophthalmic surgery is to preserve/improve visual function.
- As retina surgeons, we are more focused on retinal pathology, and we may overlook other components of the eye's pathophysiology which may significantly impact the vision.
- One of the most important aspects is represented by the damage suffered by the optic nerve because of increased intraocular pressure (IOP) in association with vitreoretinal surgery.
- While long-term glaucoma management for these patients must be entrusted to a glaucoma specialist, the retina surgeon needs to be aware of situations where vitreoretinal procedures can cause raised IOP and address them in a timely fashion. The present chapter aims to identify such situations.

1 Assessing the Patient before the Surgery

The following information is essential:

- Preexisting glaucoma. Is the patient on any eye drops? Optic nerve status/previous visual fields if available.
- Family history of glaucoma (first-degree relative with primary open angle glaucoma).
- History of previous steroid-induced ocular hypertension.
- Myopia; previous corneal refractive surgery.

Supplementary Information The online version contains supplementary material available at https://doi.org/10.1007/978-3-031-47827-7_24.

G. Gini (✉)
Department of Ophthalmology, University Hospitals Sussex NHS Foundation Trust, Worthing, West Sussex, UK

- Lens status: phakic, pseudophakic, aphakic.
- If phakic, is a narrow angle present?
- If pseudophakic, are there indications of zonular weakness?

2 Optic Nerve Damage Results from the Summation of Raised IOP Events

- Optic nerve damage may become clinically relevant even years after the initial insult.
- Glaucoma damage related to vitreoretinal surgery results from a combination of repeated spikes in ocular pressure or prolonged periods of raised IOP.
- We can therefore consider raised IOP as occurring either during or after surgery.

3 During Surgery

The use of an appropriate surgical technique can prevent damage to the optic nerve:

- Valved trocars provide greater stability to the fluidics inside the vitreous cavity, but they have also created a truly "closed" system with relatively few opportunities for venting.
- Using a relatively high infusion pressure (> 30 mmHg) during pars plana vitrectomy (PPV) can result in an insult to the optic nerve. Although fragile eyes such as ones with high myopia and eyes with preexisting glaucoma or diabetic retinopathy may show manifest damage afterward, this generally goes unnoticed in most eyes. Some telltale signs that could alert the surgeon that IOP is above physiological levels include fine corneal haze from epithelial edema.
- Scleral indentation during surgery should be gentle and continuous rather than abrupt and discontinuous. This will allow for backflow in the infusion tubing until the preset infusion gradient is reached and will prevent spikes in IOP created by repeated compression/decompression maneuvers.
- Dual-bore cannulas should always be used when injecting heavy liquids. Repeated injecting with a traditional cannula until the optic artery pulsates and then venting is suboptimal as it puts the optic nerve at risk of damage.
- Raising intraocular pressure to control bleeding may also be disputable in diabetic patients and those with significant cardiovascular risk. IOP elevation should be kept to a minimum during surgery whether under fluid or air. Localized compression on the bleeding vessel, diathermy, or a combination of air/fluid exchange and diathermy should be considered as an alternative.
- Attention to other surgical steps that may increase the risk of ganglion cell damage such internal limiting membrane peel [1].

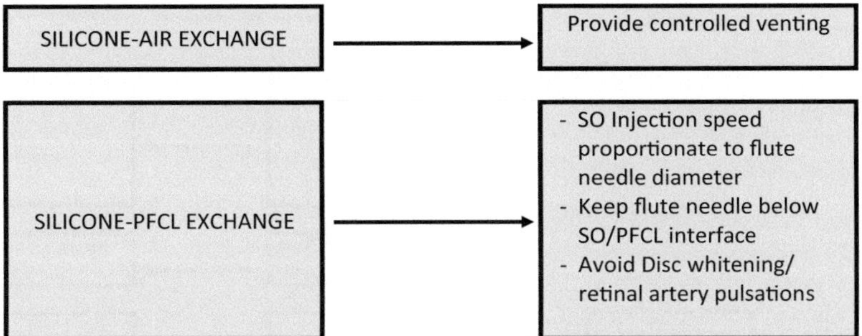

Fig. 1 Pearls aimed at preventing raised intraocular pressure during silicone oil (SO) injection

- Silicone oil (SO) injection can increase the risk of damage to the optic nerve. One must remember that silicone pumps operate with very high-pressure gradients to overcome SO viscosity. Settings are expressed in "psi" rather than in "mmHg" where 1 psi is equal to 52 mmHg. Since pumps operate within a range of 0–30 psi, it is easy to see how we can have a pressure in the pump of up to 1560 mmHg! What this tells us is that, while we have nothing to worry about as long as there is space within the eye for the silicone to fill, the pressure in the eye will increase abruptly and dramatically once this space is filled. It is therefore essential to maintain air venting during air-silicone and silicone-PFCL exchanges (Fig. 1).

4 After Surgery

Raised intraocular pressure following vitreoretinal surgery can be seen as transitory, intermittent, or permanent.

5 Transitory Raised IOP

- A raised IOP may present itself within a time spanning from a few hours to a few weeks.
- There is evidence that up to 50% of eyes affected with RRD (rhegmatogenous retinal detachment) treated with PPV and either gas (C3F8 more than SF6) or silicone oil tamponade may develop clinically significant raised IOP within the first week post-op [2, 3].
- This highlights the need for close post-op monitoring of IOP.
- In line with this principle, IOP readings should be obtained (preferably with applanation tonometry) on day 1 and day 7/8 post-op.
- Gonioscopy can guide the diagnosis and therapeutic approach in eyes with high IOP (Fig. 2).

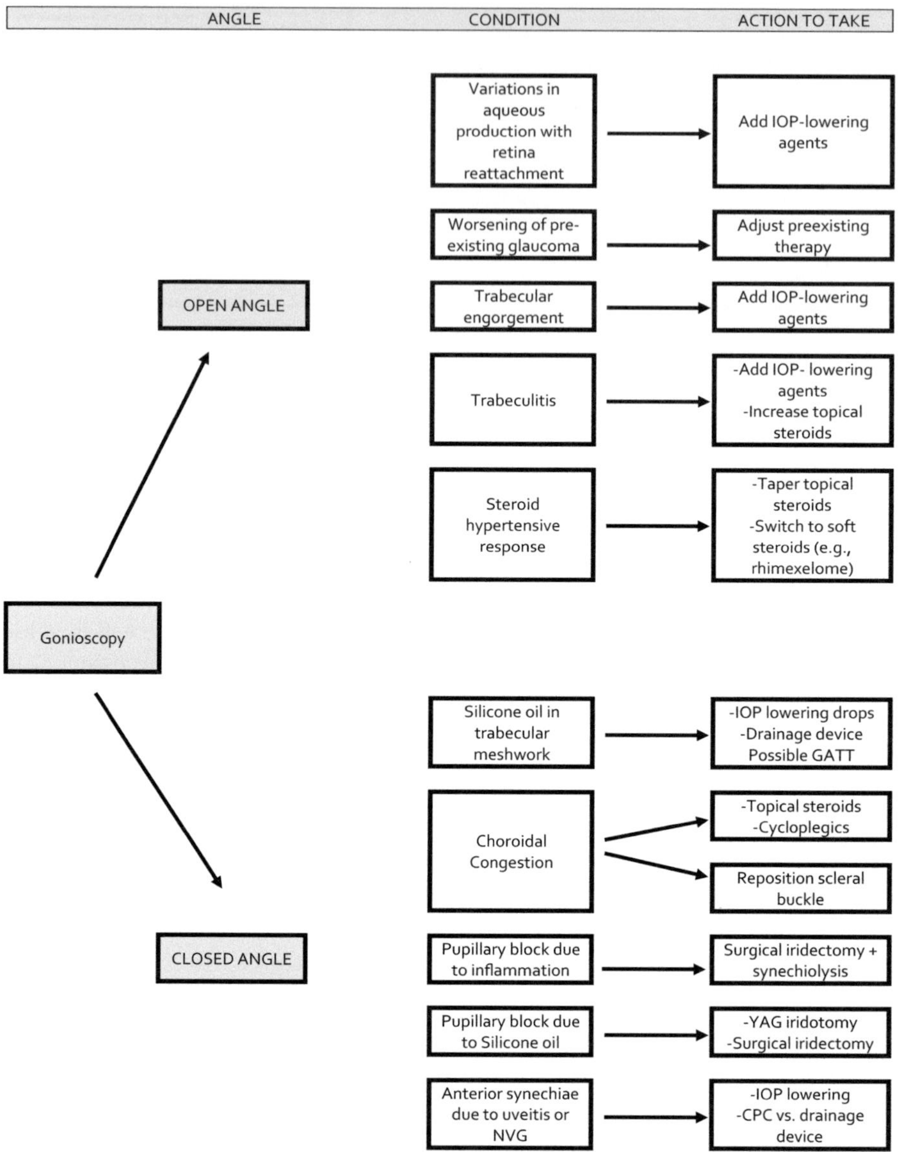

Fig. 2 Gonioscopy findings and corresponding actions to take in eyes with raised intraocular pressure (IOP). *GATT* gonioscopy-assisted transluminal trabeculotomy, *CPC* cyclophotocoagulation, *NVG* neovascular glaucoma

5.1   Open Angle

- Eyes in which considerable bleeding has occurred or where intense inflammatory reaction took place are prone to develop raised IOP early due to a combination of trabecular engorgement and trabecular swelling. Treatment with steroids and anti-glaucoma agents is generally sufficient to control this condition.
- A brisk spike in IOP may be seen in steroid responders earlier than generally thought in the past. Those eyes can develop surprisingly high IOPs even after 1 week of treatment. Patients with eyes with preexisting glaucoma, myopia, and diabetes are more susceptible to develop steroid-induced IOP rise than the average population. Steroid responders represent up to 30% of the normal population but considering that many of the patients who require retina surgery are diabetics or myopes, the proportion of eyes with steroid-induced ocular hypertension that the retina surgeon encounters could be significant.

5.2   Closed Angle

- Positional angle closure:

  - It is advised to avoid supine positioning in patients with intravitreal gas or SO tamponade.
  - This is to decrease crystalline lens opacification, maximize tamponade contact with the retina, and avoid 2ry angle closure from the tamponade pushing forward on the ciliary body.
  - The latter problem is more significant in pseudophakic and aphakic eyes, as compared to phakics.

- Choroidal congestion:

  - Extensive laser retinal photocoagulation especially when combined with SO tamponade can result in choroidal congestion.
  - This could lead to anterior rotation of the ciliary body and displacement of the iridolenticular diaphragm. As a result, the AC shallows with an impaired aqueous outflow or even angle closure in predisposed eyes.
  - Choroidal congestion may also be the result of scleral buckling especially when an encircling band is used.
  - A conservative approach based on the use of topical IOP-lowering agents, steroids, and cycloplegics is generally sufficient.
  - If pharmacological treatment of the increased IOP fails, repositioning the buckle and possibly draining the choroidal effusion may become necessary.
  - Conventional and ultrasound biomicroscopy (UBM) can help guide the therapeutic approach.
  - A peripheral iridotomy (PI) is useless in these cases as the angle closure is not associated with a pupillary block.

- An intense inflammatory reaction can result in posterior synechiae, a pupillary block, and a closed angle:

  - A YAG-iridotomy may be attempted in such cases.
  - Laser iridotomy is not always successful or advisable for several reasons:

    The laser impulse often "bounces off" the iris of eyes containing a silicone or gas tamponade.
    An edematous iris becomes more difficult to perforate.
    P.I. cannot be placed peripherally enough.
    A YAG-iridotomy in a severely inflamed eye may cause bleeding or exacerbate the inflammatory condition.

  - When the YAG fails or as a first-instance alternative to it, a surgical peripheral iridotomy +/− synechiolysis is a safe and effective procedure.

- Pupil block:

  - When an eye is aphakic, SO tamponade will result in pupillary block [3].
  - To prevent this, a peripheral iridectomy is performed during surgery.
  - The same is true when an eye is pseudophakic with weak zonules or for a phakic eye with weak zonules and/or a shallow anterior chamber (AC).
  - It is worth remembering that a 6 o'clock iridectomy must be used for SO (1000 Cs and 5000 Cs) and a 12 o'clock iridectomy for heavy SO.
  - Gas in the aphakic eye can also cause pupillary block but much less so than SO.
  - When failure to perform the initial intra-operatory iridectomy results in post-op pupil block, either a YAG-iridotomy or a surgical iridectomy must be carried out.
  - In the face of severe inflammation or proliferative vitreoretinopathy, iridectomies can be closed by fibrous tissue.
  - Depending on the severity of the fibrosis and the possible iris displacement, a YAG iridotomy can be attempted. If this fails surgical revision must be performed.

- Overfilling the eye with SO is another possible cause of ocular hypertension.

  - This can be avoided by leaving a small bubble of air 0.2 cc in the SO.
  - Regardless of how the oil is injected (through one of the ports or through the infusion line) or what sort of exchange is being performed, the air bubble will float to the top.

- Incorrect gas dilution:

  - This is a *"never"* event that should not occur and is totally avoidable.
  - *At least two* persons should witness the process of gas dilution.
  - If it does occur and the pressure is high, a complete washout of the eye with air and subsequent reintroduction of the gas at the proper dilution must be carried out urgently in the operating room.

6   Intermittent Raised IOP

- This is a clinical entity which can often go unnoticed.
- The spikes in IOP occur at night with the patient in supine position due to intermittent angle closure in eyes having either gas tamponade or oil tamponade with no iridectomy (Video 1).
- Eventually telltale signs of this phenomenon will develop and include the dispersion of iris pigment on the trabecular meshwork and the formation of anterior synechiae.
- While it is necessary for an anatomic predisposition to be present for this to happen, it is often difficult to know which patients will be affected.
- It would therefore seem wise to recommend that patients with a tamponade present sleep with a few pillows behind their head (unless another positioning is necessary to support retinal breaks) rather than supine.

7   Permanently Raised IOP

- Permanently raised IOP occurs when the trabecular meshwork is irreversibly damaged and unable to function.
- Treatment options are essentially surgical, with the possible adjunct of long-term glaucoma medication.
- Comparing tamponades, SO is associated with a higher likelihood of chronic IOP rise (that may be up to 10%) and glaucoma compared to gas [4] (Fig. 3).
- What sort of procedure will be carried out depends mainly on the visual potential of the eye and the type of glaucoma (Fig. 4).
- For example, a blind eye with neovascular glaucoma (NVG) will be treated with cyclo-destruction (laser cyclophotocoagulation (CPC) or cryotherapy). In contrast, an eye with visual potential may benefit from PPV, panretinal photocoagu-

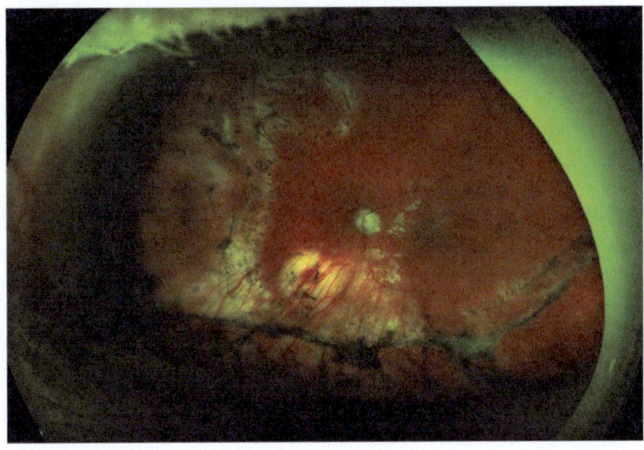

Fig. 3 Advanced glaucomatous disc cupping in a patient with permanent silicone oil tamponade for recurrent retinal detachment

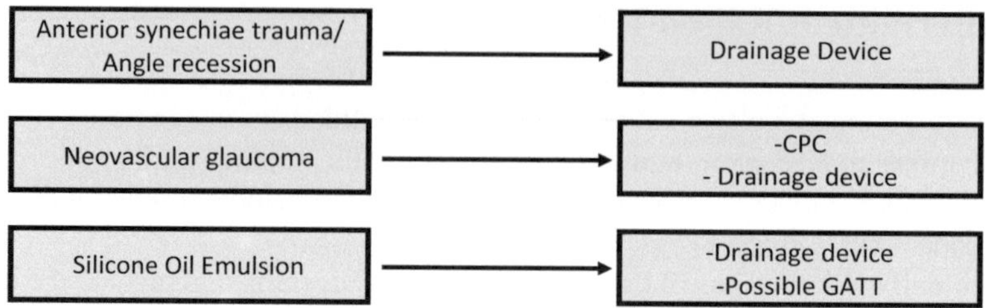

Fig. 4 Glaucoma surgery techniques for different clinical presentations related to vitreoretinal conditions

lation laser, and the implant of a glaucoma drainage device. As detailed in the diabetic vitrectomy chapter, intravitreal anti-VEGF is important in the initial management of NVG.

- It is of note that PPV even without the use of tamponade may increase the risk of subsequent primary open angle glaucoma compared to the general population (9% vs 1%) [5].

8 IOP Drops in Glaucoma: General Rule

- The use of IOP drop after retina surgery follows the same line for raised IOP in uveitis.
- There is usually no role for miotic eye drops as pupillary block glaucoma in this case is secondary and requires cycloplegic drops.
- In an eye with elevated IOP and no preexisting damage, the following algorithm can help guide use of drops in the short term:

  - Up to 25 mmHg: watch.
  - 25–30 mmHg: add 1 drop (usually a β blocker or prostaglandin analogue).
  - 30–35 mmHg: add 2 drops.
  - 35 mmHg: add 2 drops + systemic acetazolamide.

- ≥40 mmHg should be treated in the clinic with the IOP lowered to <40 before they leave.

9 Drainage Devices

- Drainage devices are designed to bypass trabecular block.
- The drainage tube can still be placed in the AC even when a complete angle closure is present.

- Positioning the tube in the vitreous cavity in vitrectomized eyes is possible but results may be less predictable. Pars plana placement could benefit eyes with completely obliterated AC or significant uveitis and NVG and is contraindicated in SO-filled eyes.
- Silicone-induced trabecular block can also be treated with these devices. One should remember to position the tube 4–5 mm into the AC far away from the angle where silicone droplets tend to collect. Alternatively in such eyes, the implant can be placed in the inferior part of the globe (generally inferotemporally).
- A detailed discussion of glaucoma drainage choice is beyond the scope of this chapter. In general, tubes with valves such as Ahmed shunt are easier to place, provide more immediate IOP control, and have a lower rate of hypotony. Non-valved implants such as Baerveldt implant may take 4–6 weeks to achieve full effect but have better long-term surgical success with less need for additional IOP-lowering drops [6].

10   Paracentesis and Vitreous Tap

- Paracentesis can achieve an instantaneous short-term reduction of IOP in eyes with intractable high IOP that is resistant to treatment.
- A good example of cases in which paracentesis could be helpful is in eyes with NVG or vitreous hemorrhage and very high IOP. It is of note that paracentesis is not of help in eyes filled with SO or gas and may lead to further IOP rise due to AC shallowing and 2ry angle closure.
- In gas-filled eyes and eyes with very high IOP, a vitreous tap of gas can be done (see Chap. 5). However, one needs to be careful to do gradual decompression of the eye to avoid the risk of suprachoroidal hemorrhage.
- Vitreous tap in eyes with silicone overfill usually does not work even with using large, bored needles. These cases are best taken to the operating room for controlled oil removal as previously mentioned.

References

1. Gelman R, Stevenson W, Prospero Ponce C, Agarwal D, Christoforidis JB. Retinal Damage Induced by Internal Limiting Membrane Removal Journal of Ophthalmology. 2015;1–10.
2. Muether PS, Hoerster R, Kirchhof B, Fauser S. Course of intraocular pressure after vitreoretinal surgery: is early postoperative intraocular pressure elevation predictable? Retina (Philadelphia, Pa). 2011;31(8):1545–52.
3. Zhang X, Hao X, Xie L. Intraocular pressure elevation within six days after vitreoretinal surgery with silicone oil injection for rhegmatogenous retinal detachment.
4. Al-Jazzaf AM, Netland PA, Charles S. Incidence and management of elevated intraocular pressure after silicone oil injection journal of glaucoma. 2005;14(1):40–6.

5. Mansukhani SA, Barkmeier AJ, Bakri SJ, Iezzi R, Pulido JS, Khanna CL, Bennett JR, Hodge DO, Sit AJ. The Risk of Primary Open-Angle Glaucoma Following Vitreoretinal Surgery—A Population-based Study American Journal of Ophthalmology. 2018;19(3):143–155.
6. Wang S, Gao X, Qian N. The Ahmed shunt versus the Baerveldt shunt for refractory glaucoma: a meta-analysis. BMC Ophthalmol. 2016;16:83.

Posterior Segment Complications of Cataract Surgery: When the Anterior Segment Meets the Posterior

Giampaolo Gini, Ahmed M. Alkaliby, Abdulrahman Rageh, and Ahmed B. Sallam

1 Introduction

- In cataract surgery when the vitreous prolapses in the anterior chamber (AC), it may become incarcerated in the corneal wounds.
- Contraction of the vitreous collagen fibers may result in complications including cystoid macular edema (CME), retinal tears, and retinal detachment.

2 Vitreous Loss/Prolapse (Video 1)

- Vitreous prolapse may occur through zonular dialysis or a posterior capsular tear (PCR). Posterior capsule rupture can occur at any stage of the surgery, but is more common to happen during removing the last portion of the nucleus and cortex removal.

Supplementary Information The online version contains supplementary material available at https://doi.org/10.1007/978-3-031-47827-7_25.

G. Gini (✉)
Department of Ophthalmology, University Hospitals Sussex NHS Foundation Trust, Worthing, West Sussex, UK

A. M. Alkaliby
Ophthalmology, Cincinnati Eye Institute (CEI) Vision Partners, Maumee, OH, USA

A. Rageh
Ophthalmology, Prairie Eye Center, HSHS Medical Group, Springfield, IL, USA

A. B. Sallam
Jones Eye Institute, University of Arkansas for Medical Sciences, Little Rock, AR, USA

A. B. Sallam et al. (eds.), *Practical Manual of Vitreoretinal Surgery*, https://doi.org/10.1007/978-3-031-47827-7_25

- The initial reaction of the surgeon when zonular dialysis or PCR is encountered should be to stop aspiration, maintain irrigation, and place an ophthalmic visco-elastic device through the side port before withdrawing the instrument from the eye. Maintaining the AC pressure helps prevent/limit vitreous prolapse.
- We use diluted triamcinolone (1 part +3 parts balanced salt solution (BSS)) to help visualize the vitreous [1].
- The first step consists in removing the connection between the vitreous prolapsed in the AC and the main vitreous body.
- We advise using a one port pars plana approach for a limited vitrectomy (Fig. 1a). By placing the infusion in the AC, the vitreous is pushed back toward the vitreous cavity while the pars plana approach guarantees a cutting plane that is parallel and immediately posterior to the iris attracting the vitreous back from the anterior segment. This procedure should be within reach of any cataract surgeon with a solid background. It is best to place a trocar rather than to perform a sclerotomy to decrease the risk of entry site retinal breaks associated with non-trocar sclerotomy and simplifies access to the vitreous cavity.
- The vitreous cutter should be moved in a plane parallel to the iris, with the port turned away from the iris to avoid damaging it.
- Once the connections between the main vitreous body and the prolapsed vitreous have been severed, the residual vitreous present in the AC is removed. This can be done by introducing the vitrectomy probe through one of the side ports while maintaining the AC infusion in the contralateral port.
- If the surgeon is uncomfortable with the pars plana approach, they can carry out the anterior vitrectomy procedure through the two limbal paracenteses (Fig. 1b). After clearing the prolapsed vitreous from the AC, the cutter should be passed through the pupil and the breach in the posterior capsule to remove the vitreous immediately behind the iris. Care must be taken not to damage the anterior capsule if the plan is to use it for a support for intraocular lens (IOL) implant. Limbal approach is also needed when vitreous prolapse occurs from a zonular dialysis.
- For the vitrectomy setting, one must remember to use low to moderate vacuum (300 mmHg) and a high cutting rate (the highest on the machine, approx. 4000 cut/min as we write) to minimize traction on the retina. Irrigation is set to physiological IOP or slightly higher, to what is needed to maintain the depth of the AC during the procedure.
- Lastly, attention can be given to residual lens matter. We do this by using the vitrectomy probe with the cutting function switched off to preserve the anterior capsule. We proceed as we would with standard irrigation aspiration during routine phacoemulsification, aiming to engage the lens material from the capsular fornix using low vacuum then, with increased vacuum, we peel off the cortex with a centripetal motion.
- Table 1 summarizes the additional management strategies for eyes with different grades of zonular dialysis.

Zonulopathy grade	Extent of dialysis	Management
Mild	≤ 1 quadrant	+/- CTR
Moderate	1-2 quadrant	CTR
Severe	2-3 quadrants	Capsular segments + CTR
Extreme	>3 quadrants	Treat as aphakia

Tab. 1 Management plan for eyes with different grades of zonular dialysis (CTR = capsule tension ring)

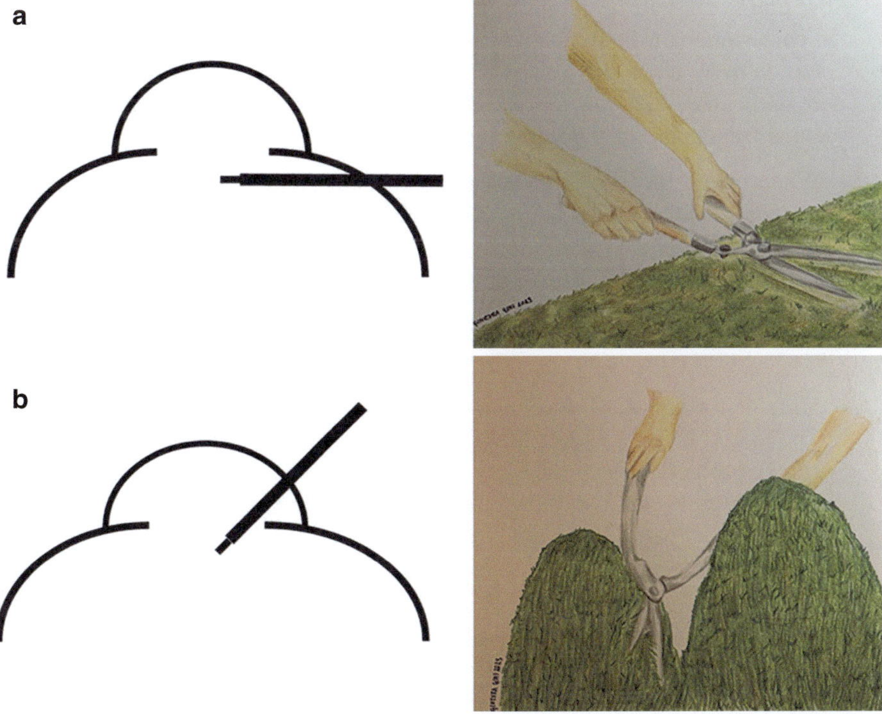

Fig. 1 Pars plana approach versus limbal approach for anterior vitrectomy. The horizontal cutting plane achieved with the pars plana approach (**a**) is more efficient in separating the vitreous from the anterior segment structures than the vertical cutting plane provided by the limbal approach (**b**). This concept is exemplified by the results obtained from cutting a hedge with the two different approaches. The efficiency of the pars plana approach is further enhanced by the presence of an anterior chamber infusion which compresses the vitreous behind the iris plane

3 Removing Lens Fragments from the Vitreous

- The management of the dropped lens fragment is twofold: first to defuse the potential vitreous tractional hazard, and second to remove the retained nuclear fragment in a timely fashion to prevent the occurrence of adverse events such as increased IOP, uveitis, rhegmatogenous retinal detchment (RRD), epiretinal membrane, and CME [2, 3].
- In general, we advise early removal of the dropped nucleus to avoid complications such as uveitis and raised IOP from retained fragments. If delays happen due to the unavailability of a retina surgeon, poor corneal view, or other logistic issues, appropriate treatment with anti-inflammatory and IOP-lowering agents needs to be initiated.
- How fragments will be removed from the vitreous largely depends on the size and consistency of the retained material.
- Common to all three techniques is the need to induce posterior vitreous detachment and carry out a complete pars plana vitrectomy (PPV) *before tackling* the retained fragments for the following reasons:

  - When using the fragmatome the vitreous cavity must be completely free of any vitreous strands so as not to place traction on the retina.
  - Lens matter tend to settle down into the peripheral vitreous and not only on the posterior pole. Failure to remove it will result in symptomatic floaters and ongoing inflammation.

- Vitreous cutter removal:

  - Suitable for non-hard/small pieces.
  - The larger the gauge, the higher the efficiency but even smaller 25-gauge (g) can be used effectively [4].
  - Use of high vacuum and low cutting rate (long duty cycle) makes removal of lens material more efficient (Video 2).

- Fragmatome:

  - Most efficient technique for hard and large fragments.
  - Available fragmatomes range from 19 to 23-g. Even 23-g fragmatomes will not fit into a 23-g trocar so trocar must be removed when using the fragmatome and replaced when reverting back to vitrectomy.
  - Remember to adjust infusion pressure accordingly, particularly with a large gauge fragmatome.
  - One of us favors protecting the macula with a small amount of PFCL (GG).
  - Aspirate fragment with *no* ultrasound, take it into central part of vitreous cavity, and activate ultrasound.
  - For the setting, best to use high vacuum (200–300 mmHg) and low pulse ultrasound (10–20%) to avoid chattering "spitting" of lens fragments (Video 3).
  - The fragmatome or a sleeveless phacoemulsification tip can also be placed through a limbal incision (Video 4).

- Floating the nucleus into the AC:

  - This technique is rarely needed as even most hard nuclei can be dealt with by the fragmatome with no fear of retinal injury.
  - However, in some instances, the technique may still be used due to unavailability of fragmatome or because of reluctance of the surgeon to use fragmatome for specific clinical reasons such as a coexisting retinal detachment.
  - Fill the eye with PFCL to the iris plane.
  - Protect the corneal endothelium with a dispersive viscoelastic device.
  - Because of the slope of the PFCL bubble (meniscus), the nucleus may tend to slide to the periphery under the iris base. This can be corrected by maneuvering the nucleus into the pupillary area and then into the AC with the help of the light probe inserted in one of the trocars (generally best to use your nondominant hand). If the anterior capsule is present, the nucleus will generally pass through even a relatively small capsulorhexis.
  - Keep the posterior segment infusion on.
  - Mark the intended width of the corneal incision and extract the lens through a large incision using a lens loop (vectis) as in extracapsular cataract surgery.
  - An alternative technique is to perform phacoemulsification in the posterior chamber over the PFCL bubble through a standard corneal phacoemulsification wound.

- Final remark: Following nucleus removal, it is important to search the retinal periphery to make sure there are no retinal tears and to remove any retained lens material from the vitreous base.

4   Dropped IOL in the Vitreous Cavity

- Similar to dropped nuclear fragments, PPV needs to be undertaken for dropped IOL with emphasis on first freeing the IOL from vitreous to avoid putting traction on the retinal periphery as the IOL is removed.
- As a part of the preoperative examination of patients with dropped IOL, it is best to examine the patient while lying flat. An IOL that appears to be slightly decentered in the anterior vitreous while the patient is sitting up at the slit lamp may move to the mid-vitreous cavity as they lie supine at the time of surgery.
- At the time of surgery, if the IOL is present in the anterior vitreous within reach, it could be grasped gently with an end-grasping forceps followed by freeing it from the vitreous using the vitrectomy probe before pulling it into the AC.
- Staining with diluted triamcinolone helps vitreous visualization.
- If the IOL is in the mid vitreous cavity, it is best not to attempt grasping it and focus on core vitrectomy and freeing the IOL. As vitrectomy continues the IOL becomes loose and moves over the posterior retina.
- Most dropped IOLs would settle over the posterior pole or onto the inferior retina, with the haptics attached to the vitreous base. Scleral indentation (either with

an assistant or with a chandelier) is usually needed in the latter scenario to release the trapped haptic(s) from the vitreous but care is taken not to hit the peripheral retina with the vitrectome.

- There are several techniques for retrieving the dropped IOL. We favor picking the IOL with the nasally situated hand using the active suction by backflush. This decreases the risk of retina injury if a forceps is used to grasp the IOL. The IOL is then brought anteriorly and handed to a forceps introduced by the temporal hand through a limbal side port. The IOL is then placed over the iris. Finally, a 3 mm corneal wound is fashioned, and the lens is either folded in the AC or cut by a lens cutter and pulled out of the eye. Alternatively, if an ACIOL placement is contemplated, a 6 mm wound is created without the need for cutting the IOL (Video 5).

- Detailed discussion of IOL options for correction of aphakia is beyond the scope of this chapter. In general, in the presence of capsular support, we opt for in-the-bag or sulcus IOL fixation with or without optic capture, depending on the amount of anterior and posterior capsule present. In the absence of capsular support, we prefer ACIOL or iris claw IOL fixation (not available in the USA) if normal iris/angle status exists and where a good endothelial cell count is present. A four-point Akreos IOL scleral fixation may be used in young patients or those with iris/angle abnormalities. A rather recent addition to our selection of IOLs is the Carlevale, a sutureless scleral-fixated IOL designed for use in the absence of capsular support [5]. We are generally not in favor of all techniques that involve two-point scleral fixation including Yamane scleral tunnel technique. It is of note that evidence from recent studies shows no superiority of any single IOL implantation technique in the absence of capsular support in terms of vision or safety outcomes [6].

5 Ocular Perforation

- Inadvertent globe perforation is a rare complication of local anesthesia with sharp needles.
- It is more common with retrobulbar anesthesia (1/10,000) but still can happen with peribulbar anesthesia (1/16,000) [7].
- It can be avoided using subtenon's or topical anesthesia for cataract surgery.
- Risk factors that increase the risk of ocular perforation include using longer needle, high myopia, previous scleral buckle surgery, and a non-ophthalmologist performing the anesthesia.
- Needle injury can result in choroidal hemorrhage, subretinal or retinal hemorrhage, and retinal detachment, with incarceration and vitreous hemorrhage. There is high risk of epiretinal membrane development and RRD with proliferative vitroretinopathy. Trauma to the optic nerve can also occur.
- There is also concern regarding chemical toxicity from the local anesthetic. Cases of retinal artery occlusion and vein occlusion have been reported.
- Signs that should raise suspicion for an ocular perforation after the administration of anesthesia include hyphema, soft eye, and loss of red reflex from vitreous

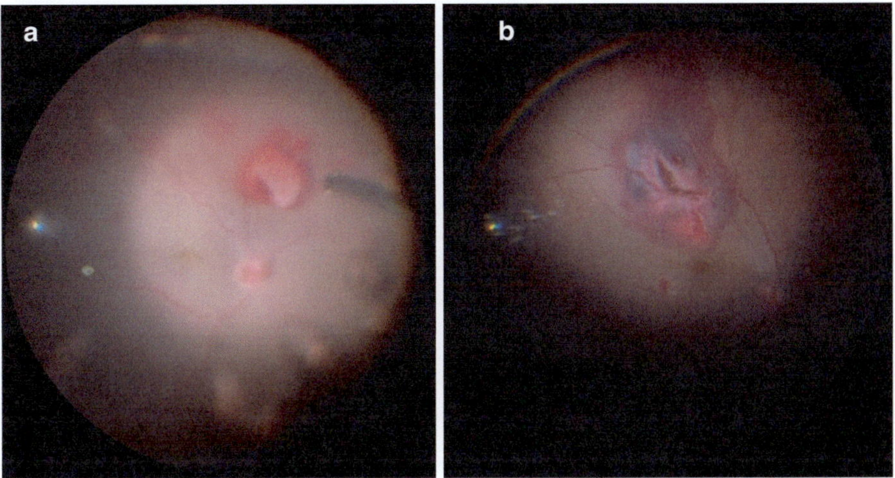

Fig. 2 Intraoperative photographs, surgeon's view of two cases with ocular perforation following sharp needle anesthesia for cataract surgery (Courtesy of Ahmed Habib, MD, Egypt)

hemorrhage. Other less common signs include a very firm eye with or without corneal edema and the presence of small air bubbles behind the lens.

- Given that the most common site for local anesthesia is inferotemporal, the most common site of perforation is usually inferonasal. The fovea can be also involved, and double perforations may happen (Fig. 2).
- Treatment depends on the nature of the injury and the clarity of the media. This can range from laser treatment to a retinal break to the perforation site to PPV for vitreous hemorrhage, retinal incarceration, or retinal detachment.
- Because of the high risk of RRD with proliferative vitroretinopathy in these types of injuries, early intervention is advisable.
- During PPV in early cases, it is best to trim the retinal blood clot to the perforation site and leave the stump sealing the perforation (Video 6) rather than pluck the clot out completely.
- The final vision outcome is variable and is mainly dependent on the location and the extent of the injury. In one series, >50% of eyes achieved acuity $\geq$20/80, while 25% were between 20/120 and 20/200 [8].

6   Suprachoroidal Hemorrhage

- SCH is an uncommon but potentially devastating complication of intraocular surgery including cataract and retina surgery (Fig. 3).
- This entity is covered in suprachoroidal hemorrhage mangement chapter, Chap. 20.
- In the context of cataract surgery, it is important to be aware of other causes of shallow AC with increased eye pressure and to have a management plan (Fig. 3). SCH can well mimic acute aqueous misdirection in presentation. Because

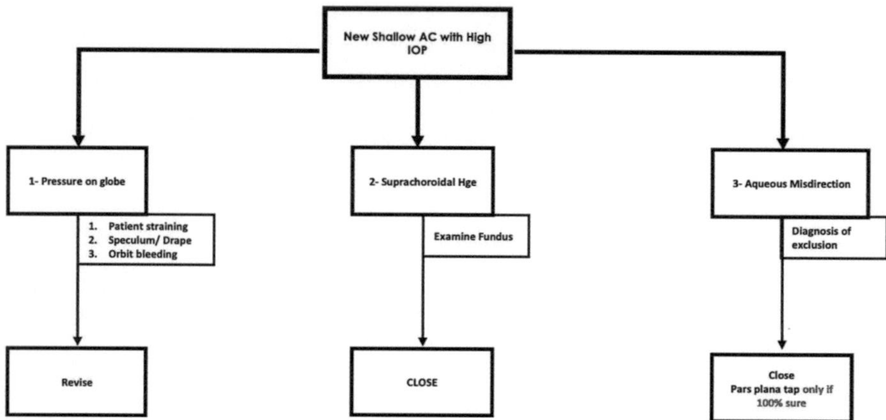

Fig. 3 Causes and management plan for increased eye pressure and shallow anterior chamber during cataract surgery

decreasing the IOP can result in SCH progression, one should not proceed with a vitreous tap or anterior vitrectomy (to treat a presumed aqueous misdirection) before SCH is excluded. If this is not possible, it is safer to close the eye and reassess later.

Key Points
- Vitreous prolapse during cataract surgery requires immediate action, such as stopping aspiration, maintaining irrigation, and performing vitrectomy to prevent tractional complications.
- Although more involving, anterior vitrectomy through a pars plana approach is more efficient in removing the prolapsed vitreous than the limbal approach.
- Dropped lens fragments require early PPV surgery.
- In ocular perforation prompt surgical intervention is crucial to lessen the severity of retinal complications.
- Suprachoroidal hemorrhage may mimic aqueous misdirection and requires careful assessment before considering intraoperative surgical interventions.

References

1. Burk SE, Da Mata AP, Snyder ME, Schneider S, Osher RH, Cionni RJ. Visualizing vitreous using Kenalog suspension. J Cataract Refract Surg. 2003;29(4):645–51.
2. Mirataollah, Salabati Raziyeh, Mahmoudzadeh Taku, Wakabayashi John W, Hinkle Allen C, Ho. Indications for surgical management of retained lens fragments Current Opinion in Ophthalmology. 2022;33(1):15–20.
3. Yousef A, Fouad Sayena, Jabbehdari Adam, Neuhouser Mohamed K, Soliman Aman, Chandra Yit C, Yang Ahmed B, Sallam. Visual outcomes and postoperative complications of eyes with

dropped lens fragments during cataract surgery: multicenter database study Journal of Cataract and Refractive Surgery. 2023;49(5):485–491.

4. Ho LY, Walsh MK, Hassan TE. 25-gauge pars plana vitrectomy for retained lens fragments. Retina. 2010;30(6):843–9.
5. Fiore T, Messina M, Muzi A, et al. Comparison of two different scleral fixation techniques of posterior chamber Carlevale lens. Medicine (Baltimore) 2021;100(32):e26728.
6. Shen JF, Deng S, Hammersmith KM, Kuo AN, Li JY, Weikert MP, Shtein RM. Intraocular lens implantation in the absence of zonular support: an outcomes and safety update: a report by the American Academy of Ophthalmology. Ophthalmology. 2020;127(9):1234–58.
7. Eke T, Thompson JR. Serious complications of local anaesthesia for cataract surgery: a 1 year national survey in the United Kingdom. Br J Ophthalmol. 2007;91(4):470–5. Epub 2006
8. Babu N, Kumar J, Kohli P, Ahuja A, Shah P, Ramasamy K. Clinical presentation and management of eyes with globe perforation during peribulbar and retrobulbar anesthesia: a retrospective case series. Korean J Ophthalmol. 2022;36(1):16–25.

Vitreoretinal Surgery in Uveitis

Shree K. Kurup and Vishali Gupta

This chapter focuses on the critical uveitis information that is relevant for the vitreo-retinal surgeon including the role of vitreoretinal surgery in making diagnosis as well as treatment of uveitis.

1 Differential Diagnosis of Uveitis or the Posterior Segment

- The first step is to identify the phenotype and characterize the lesion as retinitis, choroiditis, retinochoroiditis, chorioretinitis, etc. as this characterization helps narrow the differential diagnosis. Optical coherence tomography (OCT) cuts through the lesion may help in this characterization, if possible, along with wide-field autofluorescence, fluorescein angiography (FA), and indocyanine green angiography (ICG), particularly when choroidal disease is suspected (Fig. 1).

Supplementary Information The online version contains supplementary material available at https://doi.org/10.1007/978-3-031-47827-7_26.

S. K. Kurup (✉)
University Hospitals of Cleveland, Vitreoretinal Diseases and Surgery, Uveitis, Cleveland, OH, USA

V. Gupta
Advanced Eye Centre, Post Graduate Institute of Medical Education and Research, Chandigarh, India

A. B. Sallam et al. (eds.), *Practical Manual of Vitreoretinal Surgery*, https://doi.org/10.1007/978-3-031-47827-7_26

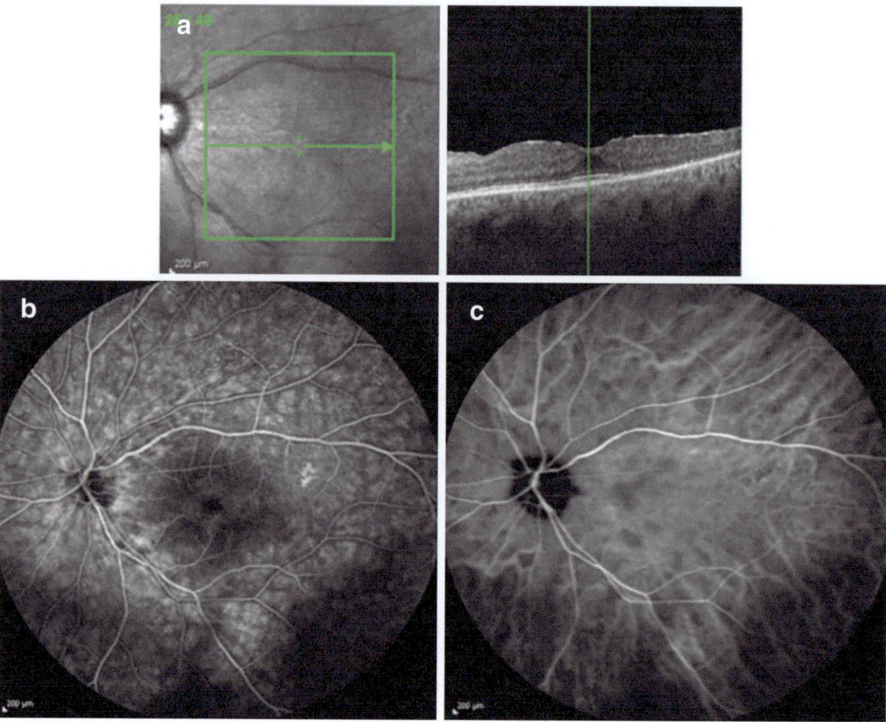

Fig. 1 Optical coherence tomography (OCT) image of a patient who was referred for decreased vision and epiretinal membrane peel (ERM) to consider pars plana vitrectomy (PPV) and ERM peel surgery. (**a**) the outer retinal bands were significantly thinned around the fovea, prompting a fluorescein angiogram (FA) (**b**) and an indocyanine green (ICG) tests (**c**) that were consistent with birdshot choroiditis and 2ry ERM. Note the subtle late staining on FA and the well-delineated hypocyanescent spots at mid phase of ICG

- After the phenotypic characterization, the goal would be specifying the disease, e.g., "a 20-year-old boy, unilateral, first episode of focal retinitis with overlying vitritis." This description will automatically trigger naming "meshing" toxoplasmosis as one of the leading differential diagnosis (Fig. 2a). Specifying a disease like this will narrow down the list of differential diagnoses and order targeted laboratory investigations.
- It is always best to categorize uveitis causes under three groups as far as etiologic diagnosis is concerned: infection, inflammation, and masquerade (including neoplastic and nonneoplastic causes).
- Table 1. Differential diagnosis of retinitis and choroiditis (Fig. 2) and vitritis (Fig. 3).

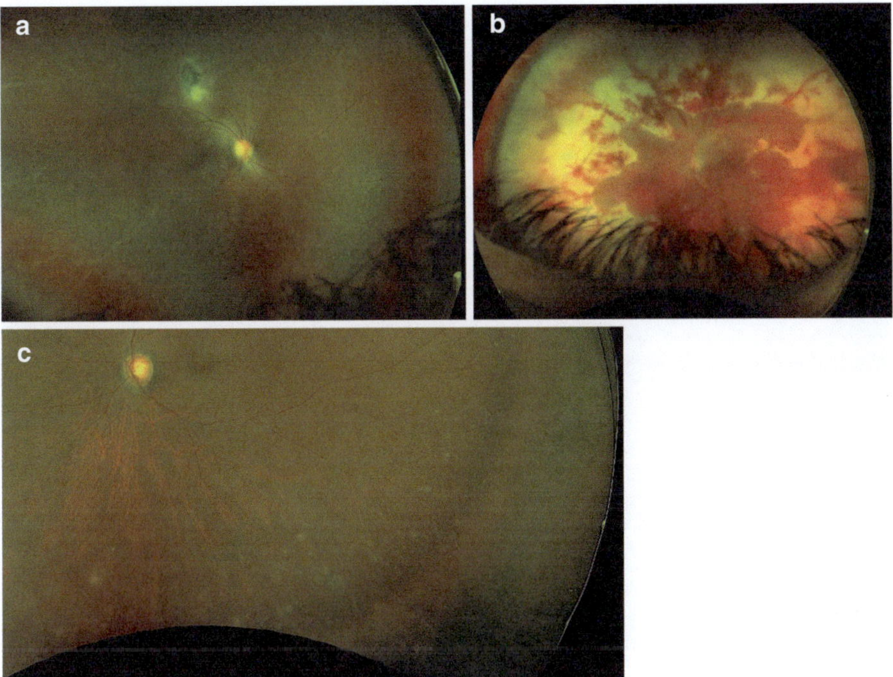

Fig. 2 Different phenotypical patterns of posterior uveitis. Unifocal retinitis next to a chorioretinal scar with retinal vasculitis typical of reactivated toxoplasma retinitis (**a**). Multifocal retinitis spreading from the periphery to the central with occlusive vasculitis suggestive of acute retinal necrosis (**b**). Multifocal choroiditis involving the inferior part of the choroid (**c**). Note the deep location of the choroiditis as compared to retinitis

Table 1 Important causes of posterior uveitis

	Vitritis	Retinitis	Choroiditis
(1) Infective			
• Bacterial	Bacteremia, syphilis, tuberculosis (TB), cat scratch	Bacteremia, syphilis, TB, cat scratch	Bacteremia, syphilis, TB, cat scratch
• Fungal	Molds, filamentous	Molds, filamentous	Molds, filamentous
• Viral	Herpes simplex virus (HSV), varicella zoster virus (VZV), cytomegalovirus (CMV)	HSV, VZV, CMV	
• Protozoal	Toxoplasma	Toxoplasma	Toxoplasma, Toxocara
(2) Inflammatory	Behçet's disease Sarcoidosis Others	Behçet's disease Sarcoidosis Others	Vogt-Koyanagi-Harada disease (VKH) Sympathetic ophthalmitis Sarcoidosis White dot syndromes—birdshot, acute posterior multifocal placoid pigment epitheliopathy (APMPPE), etc.
(3) Masquerade	Lymphoma Posterior vitreous detachment (PVD) Vitreous hemorrhage	Lymphoma	Lymphoma

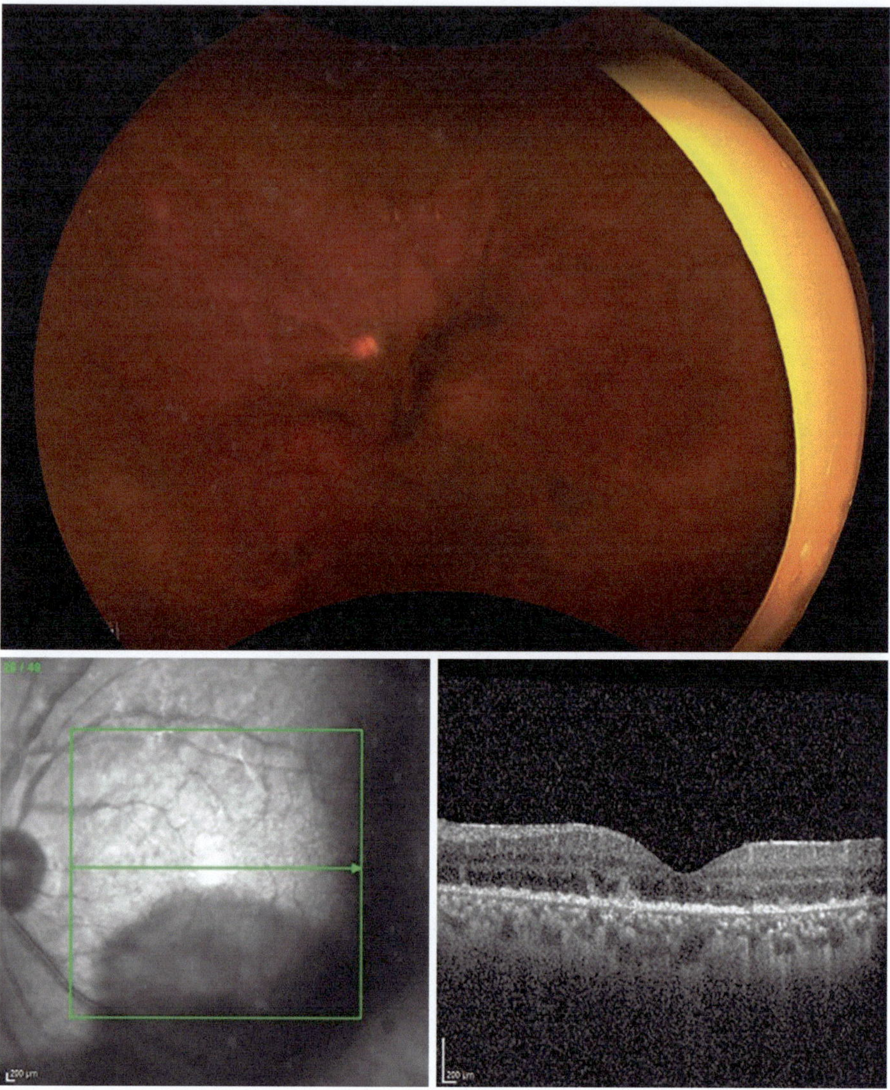

Fig. 3 Color fundus photograph (above) of a patient presenting with acute floaters. The examination was suggestive of hemorrhagic posterior vitreous detachment (PVD). However, optical coherence tomography scan (inferior) showed significant interruption of the outer retinal bands, more consistent with vitritis and choroiditis, particularly syphilis. The other crucial differential diagnosis in this context is intraocular lymphoma

2 Vitritis

– Of note, chronic vitreous hemorrhage and acute posterior vitreous detachment (PVD) with vitreous collapse (Fig. 4) are important differential diagnoses of vitritis.

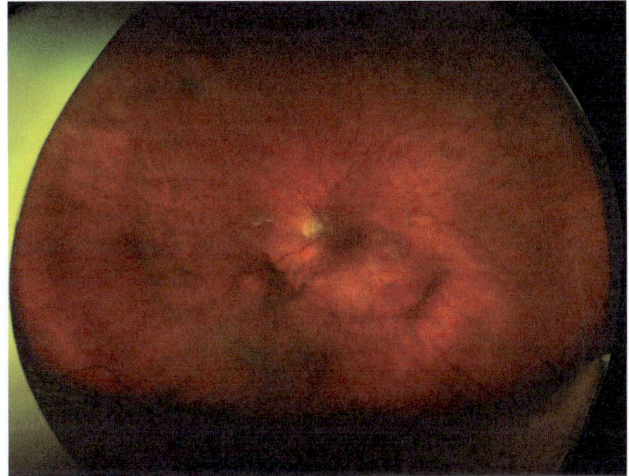

Fig. 4 Color fundus photograph of a patient with an acute posterior vitreous detachment and mild vitreous hemorrhage mimicking vitritis

- There are many causes of vitritis, but the most important is to exclude infection first, particularly herpes viruses (Fig. 2b), toxoplasmosis (Fig. 2a), and syphilis.
- When faced with unexplained vitreous opacities/vitritis in an elderly patient, it is important to consider intraocular lymphoma.
- Many patients with Fuchs uveitis would have vitreous opacities that may be mis taken for other causes of vitritis, particularly since this type of uveitis is chronic and can be asymptomatic.

3 Red Flags that May Indicate that Uveitis Is Due to an Infection

1. History of systemic comorbidities resulting in immunosuppression.
2. Sexual history of men having sex with men or multiple sexual partners.
3. Social history of intravenous drug use.
4. Retinitis: of note, in the absence of Behcet's disease, retinitis is most likely due to an infection or lymphoma.
5. Acute posterior multifocal pigmented epitheliopathy/serpiginous choroiditis, always exclude syphilis and tuberculosis (TB).
6. Worsening or no improvement on systemic steroids: most inflammation, even severe cases, would improve on systemic steroids. Failure to improve should alert the clinician about possible infection (or masquerade), although a temporary improvement in some infections can be seen.
7. Many times, infections like acute retinal necrosis need a prompt clinical diagnosis, and treatment needs to be initiated at the earliest suspicion without waiting for any laboratory confirmations.

8. In many cases, it is a pattern recognition based on experience. That is why we advise that uveitis-trained specialists best manage complicated uveitis or uveitis involving the posterior segment.

4 Intraocular Lymphoma

- A detailed discussion of intraocular lymphoma is beyond the scope of this chapter. We want to highlight three main ocular presentations so that the retina surgeon will be aware of the following: (1) vitritis unexplained by other causes; (2) indolent retinitis, especially after toxoplasma and lymphoma have been excluded; and (3) subretinal infiltrates and sub-retinal pigment epithelium infiltrates (Fig. 5).
- A high index of suspicion is needed. Diagnosis is based mainly on vitreous biopsy. Pars plana vitrectomy (PPV) with vitreous biopsy has a yield of around 65%. If results are negative and suspicion is still present, then repeat vitreous biopsy could be taken followed by chorioretinal biopsy (CRB). If accessible, vitreous IL6-IL10 ratio can be assayed. IL10 is elevated in lymphomas and IL6 in inflammations and infections [1]. Looking for MYD88 and LP265 from the vitreous specimen too can help in diagnosing lymphoma. Expert cytologists

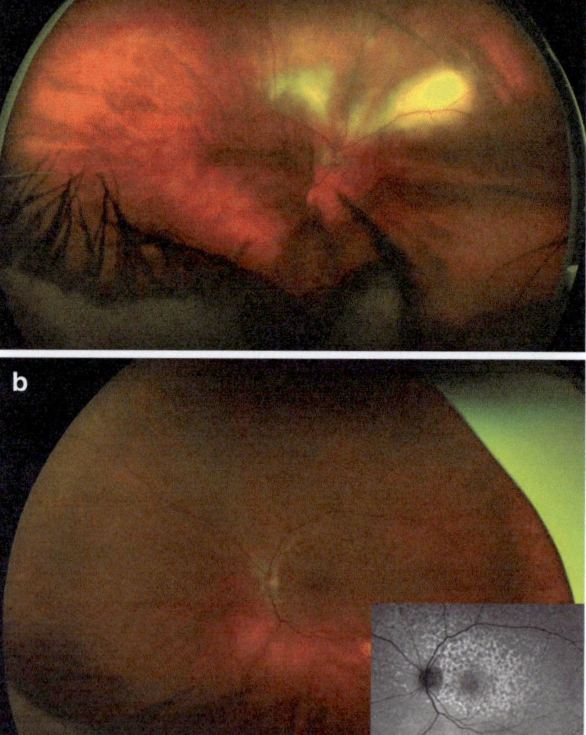

Fig. 5 Different presentations of intraocular lymphoma from two different patients showing vitritis and subretinal infiltration (**a**) and retinal pigment epithelium infiltration highlighted by fundus autofluorescence (**b**)

should be ready to receive the sample as the cells degenerate very fast and these cells are scant in the vitreous. Aspiration and analysis of subretinal aspirate could also be undertaken.

5 Chorioretinal Biopsy

5.1 Indications

- Intraocular lymphoma with non-revealing vitreous biopsy is the main indication. The yield is about 66% [2]. The yield of CRB is higher if vitritis is present [3].
- Severe retinitis with suspicion of infections and non-contributory vitreous biopsy.

5.2 Preoperative Considerations

- Perform vitreous biopsy first and consider the CRB at another session if vitreous biopsy is non-contributory.
- Ensure your laboratory has the expertise and is familiar with PCR and immuno-histochemistry techniques to process and interpret the sample.
- Communicate with the laboratory in advance regarding the specimen, handle the samples carefully, and deliver them to a laboratory familiar with testing for these samples with PCR.
- Stopping oral corticosteroids for two weeks before collecting the intraocular sample increases the yield.

5.3 Technique [2]

- Usually, we start with a vitreous biopsy under air. After PPV and PVD induction, we select the CRB site, ensuring it involves both abnormal and adjacent normal tissue.
- It is best to stay away from major vessels and, for easier access, avoid peripheral superior areas.
- CRB must be performed on a flat retina, so if the retina is detached, the biopsy must be performed after flattening the retina under a limited amount of perfluorocarbon liquid to harvest the retina and the choroid together.
- We start by surrounding the intended biopsy area with 2–3 rows of heavy lasers to decrease bleeding and perform retinopexy, Video 1. Diode lasers are preferred over argon lasers due to their deeper penetration. Retinopexy could also be performed later after harvesting the biopsy, but we prefer to do it early while the view is still good.

- We use a 23-g vertical scissor to cut the biopsy, ensuring we are in the plane between the choroid and the white sclera. You can perform a punch biopsy using a 23-g vitreous cutter, but we do not prefer this technique as the sample is usually small and may be difficult to retrieve from the suction line.
- Dissect the biopsy all around using a horizontal scissor, but leave a small part attached until you are ready to remove it from the eye.
- It is better to place a chandelier light from the beginning, as bimanual dissection with forceps may be needed for the above step.
- Next, we remove the 23-g trocar and enlarge the sclerotomy. We then switch off the infusion, and using intraocular forceps, we sever the remaining attachment of the CRB from its bed and remove it from the eye.
- Elevate IOP before cutting the specimen and place diathermy on the bleeding retina and choroidal vessels, as cutting takes place to control the intraocular bleeding. Some authors use diathermy to surround the biopsy site before cutting, but this is usually not needed if a heavy laser is applied before cutting the biopsy.
- Finally, we apply more laser retinopexy if needed, check for peripheral retinal breaks, and place silicone (SO).
- It is important to use SO as a tamponade, not gas, and to perform direct fluid/SO exchange without going through the air when a large CRB is performed. This avoids the rare but lethal risk of air embolism through the incised choroid [4]. Also, avoiding PFCL in these cases is best for the same reason [5].

5.4 Complications

- Overall complication rate is approximately 15%. Vitreous hemorrhage and retinal detachment are reported in 10% of cases [2]. There is a controversial risk of causing metastases in malignant lesions.

6 Which Is Better, Systemic Immunosuppression or Intravitreal Therapy for Noninfectious Uveitis of the Posterior Segment?

The Multicenter Uveitis Steroid Treatment (MUST) randomized patients with active noninfectious uveitis involving the posterior segment for systemic corticosteroid and immunosuppression therapy vs. fluocinolone acetonide intravitreal implant, 0.56 mg (Retisert™) [6].

- At the 2-year primary end point, while vision improvement was similar in both groups, +6.0 and + 3.2 ETDRS letters ($p = 0.16$), significantly fewer eyes had active uveitis in the implant group, 12% and 29%, respectively ($p = 0.001$) [6].

- However, an observation 7-year follow-up of the study participants found that systemic treatment was associated with a better mean vision of 7 letters and that uveitis control was no longer superior in the implant treatment eyes. By 7 years, the proportion of patients with legal blindness decreased by 1% in the systemic therapy group but increased by 8% in the implant group [7].
- It is of note that over the extended 7-year follow-up period, the majority of implant assigned eyes (84%) only received 1 implant, which lead to uveitis reactivation and visual decline. It is possible that failure to perform a scheduled replacement of the implant has resulted in this poor outcome. However, the high implant cost, variation in the therapeutic implant duration, and the high rate of ocular side effects are essential barriers for repeat insertion of fluocinolone implants.
- The 7-year extension most likely mirrors what happens in clinical practice, specifically, the difficulty in indicating the time for retreatment with intravitreal implants—should we treat at fixed intervals, for example, 4 months for dexamethasone implant (Ozurdex) or 3 years for Retisert or wait till inflammation flares up (pro re nata).
- Regarding medication safety, as expected, the intravitreal treatment group had a significantly high risk of cataract, glaucoma, and the requirement of glaucoma surgery. Systemic therapy was associated with a greater likelihood of infection requiring treatment.
- The MUST trial also looked at which treatment was better for uveitic cystoid macular edeme (CME). At 2 years, systemic macular edema was controlled better in the intravitreal fluocinolone acetonide group [8].
- In practice, there is a proportion of uveitis where inflammation is controlled on systemic steroids and/or immunosuppression, such as on mycophenolate mofetil (Cellcept) or methotrexate, but the patient still has recalcitrant CME. In this cohort, adding treatment with intravitreal steroids such as Ozurdex or suprachoroidal triamcinolone (Xipere™) is effective. The periocular steroid is worth trying in non-extensive CME, but their efficacy is less than the intravitreal route. Another option is switching to anti-TNF such as adalimumab (Humira™). Adding more systemic steroids or conventional second-line immunosuppressives such as methotrexate or cyclosporine usually does not help CME.
- In noninfectious uveitis entities like VKH disease, which have concomitant extraocular or systemic manifestations, the systemic therapy is obviously preferred over local therapy.
- It is important to rule out the possibility of infective etiology before administering local therapy. Best to "test the water" with systemic and not intravitreal steroids.

7 Does Vitrectomy Improve Posterior Uveitis?

- Scarce literature from single centers mainly in relation to intermediate uveitis suggests a decreased uveitis intensity and a lower need for immunomodulation therapy after PPV.

- This is not universally accepted. A review article by Henry et al. in 2018 [9], looking at the use of PPV for the treatment of uveitis, concluded that it is not possible to suggest that PPV reduces the need for anti-inflammatory medications in uveitis.

8 Diagnostic Indications of Pars Plana Vitrectomy in Uveitis

- When the differential diagnosis of posterior uveitis is wide, diagnostic PPV can be of a great aid.
- PPV in this context provides opportunities for (1) better examination of the posterior segment and (2) obtaining vitreous biopsy or chorioretinal biopsy, particularly when suspecting lymphoma.
- For a vitreous biopsy, we encourage the technique of vitreous biopsy under air infusion (Video 2). Using this technique, we can obtain a sizeable vitreous biopsy (up to 2 ml of neat vitreous) without the collapse of the globe. Vitreous samples can then be sent to (1) microbiology for bacterial and fungal cultures, (2) polymerase chain reaction (PCR) for herpes viruses and toxoplasma, and (3) flow cytometry/histochemistry for lymphoma. Table 2 summarizes the vitreous sample yield in different types of ocular inflammation. For cytology, a low cut rate of 800 cpm is preferred to prevent the degradation of cells.

Table 2 The yield of vitreous biopsy in different types of ocular inflammation

	Yield	Note
(1) Infective		
• Bacterial endophthalmitis culture	50%	
• Fungal endophthalmitis culture	50%	– Yield is more with vitrector > needle – Yield is more with large biopsy (under air infusion)
• Viral polymerase chain reaction (PCR)	>90%	– Negative PCR = unlikely viral retinitis – Aqueous PCR yield is comparable
• Toxoplasma PCR	65%	– Negative PCR = could be toxoplasma still – Aqueous PCR yield is comparable
(2) Lymphoma		
Flow/immunohistochemistry	65%	– Yield is more with vitrector > needle

9 Therapeutic Indications of Pars Plana Vitrectomy in Uveitis

- Table 3 summarizes the therapeutic indications of PPV in uveitis.
- Please refer to Endophthalmitis chapter for a discussion on bacterial endophthalmitis. Video 3 shows a suggested technique for outpatient vitreous tap and intravitreal injection to avoid multiple needle stabs.
- For fungal endophthalmitis, data from current literature indicates that PPV compared to medical treatment alone with systemic and intravitreal antifungal medications does not result in better postoperative VA. Still, it may decrease the risk of subsequent RD. Other indications of PPV in fungal endophthalmitis include treatment of complications such as vitreous opacities and epiretinal membrane (ERM) [10].
- Regarding ERM surgery in uveitis, it is important to note the following: (1) possible absence of a hyaloid separation in young patients; (2) significant adherence of secondary uveitic epiretinal membrane to the retina, so one needs to be gentle while peeling uveitic ERM so as not to induce any retinal tears in the macular area; and (3) if CME coexists, it is best to treat this first, then undertake epiretinal membrane removal later if vision remains compromised or the macular edema fails to resolve with treatment. This is, in a way, like the management of coexisting diabetic macular edema and epiretinal membrane.
- For rhegmatogenous retinal detachment (RRD), treatment is along the same lines as primary RRD including the choice of tamponade. Of note, retinal tears usually happen at the edge of retinal necrosis or retinal scars and more eyes have PVR at the time of primary surgery. The success rate of retinal attachment in uveitis is lower than in primary RRD.
- Chronic hypotony in uveitis usually indicates ciliary body atrophy. In the absence of cyclodialysis or an over-filtering glaucoma surgery (also consider excluding occult wound leaks in trauma cases), chronic hypotony in uveitis is usually irreversible. Important measures include aggressive treatment of uveitis from the

Table 3 Therapeutic indications for pars plana vitrectomy in uveitis

(1) Infection/inflammation
• Bacterial endophthalmitis
• Fungal endophthalmitis
• Retained lens matter
(2) Treatment of complications
• Vitreous opacities
• Vitreoretinal traction/epiretinal membrane
• Rhegmatogenous retinal detachment
• Hypotony
(3) Drug reservoir

Table 4 Commonly used intravitreal antimicrobials

Class	Drug	Dose (typically in 0.1 mL)
Anti-bacterial	Vancomycin	1–2 mg
	Ceftazidime	2 mg
	Amikacin	0.4 mg
Anti-fungal	Amphotericin B	5–15 ug
	Voriconazole	100 ug
Anti-viral	Foscarnet	2.4 mg
	Ganciclovir	3–6 mg
Anti-protozoal	Clindamycin	1 mg

Table 5 Intravitreal medications in noninfectious uveitis

Class	Drug	Dose
Corticosteroids	Triamcinolone	2 mg/0.05 mL, 4 mg/0.1 mL
	Dexamethasone implant	0. 7 mg implant (Ozurdex™)
	Fluocinolone acetonide	0.59 (Retisert™)
		0.18 mg (Yutiq™)
Antimetabolite	Methotrexate	400 ug/0.1 mL
	Sirolimus	440 ug/0.1 mL
Anti-VEGF	Ranibizumab	0.05 mg /0.05 mL
	Bevacizumab	1.25 mg/0.05 mL
Biologics	Rituximab (off-license)	1 mg/0.1 mL

beginning to prevent this complication. Peeling of cyclitic membranes could be attempted in eyes with chronic hypotony [11]. In our experience usually this does not result in improving the intraocular pressure. However, most cases we attempted were chronic. PPV and SO tamponade has been suggested as a possible solution for hypotony [11]. However, the presence of hypotony results in SO movement to the anterior chamber and the IOP usually does not increase much. The eye would now be suffering two problems: hypotony + silicone oil in the anterior chamber. Intraoperative injection of OVD has been suggested [12]. It is our experience the effect of OVD is temporary and not of tangible benefit. Unfortunately, chronic hypotony in uveitis is a very poor sign for visual outcome, and most if not all eyes go into phthisis eventually.

– The vitreous can be a sustained reservoir for medications for noninfectious uveitis and infectious uveitis (Tables 4 and 5). Please note the following: (1) If the vitreous cavity is filled with SO, the dose of most antimicrobials needs to be reduced (usually halved) to avoid retinal toxicity. (2) Most of the steroid implants (dexamethasone, 0.7 mg, Ozurdex™) and fluocinolone acetonide (0.18 mg, Iluvien™ and 0.56 mg, Retisert™) may be used during the time of vitrectomy. Unlike medications such as anti-vascular endothelial growth factor (anti-VEGF) and triamcinolone acetonide, the change in environment caused by the PPV surgery does not appear to negatively influence those implants, and their duration is not significantly shortened in vitrectomized eyes [13, 14]. (3) Intravitreal anti-VEGF use is of limited benefit in uveitis or uveitic CME treatment except for the treatment of inflammatory choroidal neovascular membrane.

10 Other Uveitis Topics that Are Relevant for the Retina Surgeon

10.1 Control of Inflammation before Cataract Surgery in Uveitic Eyes

It is important to aggressively control inflammation before elective intraocular surgery. Patients should have no active inflammation in the 3 months prior. Operating on inflamed eyes is associated with a higher risk of complications, including severe postoperative inflammation and hypotony. Intravitreal steroids can be used during or before surgery to avoid postoperative exacerbation of uveitis and macular thickening [14].

10.2 Exudative Vs. Rhegmatogenous Retinal Detachment

It is important for the retina surgeon to be aware of the causes and presentation of exudative retinal detachment, particularly in the context of a retinal detachment and no detectable retinal tears.

Differential diagnosis of serous retinal detachment:

(1) Congenital optic nerve anomaly including optic nerve pit, morning glory syndrome, and advanced glaucomatous cupping; (2) vascular conditions including malignant hypertension, disseminated intravascular coagulopathy, pregnancy, age-related macular degeneration, and idiopathic polypoidal choroidal vasculopathy (IPCV) disease; (3) infection/inflammation uveitis, most importantly, VKH and posterior scleritis; (4) neoplastic causes such as choroidal metastasis, choroidal hemangioma, and choroidal melanoma; and (5) miscellaneous causes including uveal effusion syndrome and central serous retinopathy.

Points that help favor the diagnosis of RRD over serous detachment:

1. Presence of PVD and vitreous pigments in RRD.
2. Presence of retina tears in RRD. In 5% or more of RRD, there may not be an obvious retinal tear.
3. Absence of fluid shifting in RRD.
4. B scan ruling out conditions such as choroidal tumors or scleritis.

5. PVR occurrence is suggestive of RRD.
6. Negative therapeutic test with anti-inflammatory medications such as oral steroids and detachment progression.

Note: hypotony and choroidal detachment may occur in both exudative and RRD (Video 11, Chap. 8).

10.3 Unusual Features of Intermediate Uveitis that Are of Surgical Importance

(a) Vitreous hemorrhage can occur in intermediate uveitis, particularly in children. This results from retinal neovascularization or traction.
(b) Retinoschisis (Fig. 6a). Not uncommon in children and indicates the need for more aggressive treatment of uveitis [15].
(c) Vasoproliferative tumor (Fig. 6b). Presence also indicates the need for more aggressive treatment of uveitis [16].

Key Points
– Always consider the causes of uveitis under three categories: inflammation, infection, and masquerade.
– Never treat new cases of presumed noninfectious uveitis with intravitreal steroids. These cannot be easily reversed if things get worse and the uveitis happens to be due to an infection. Oral steroids are safer in this context.
– Apart from retained lens fragments, PPV generally does not impact uveitis positively in the long term as a therapeutic modality.
– PPV has an important role in treating uveitis complications such ERM and CME.
– Best to refer cases of uveitis affecting the posterior segment to fellowship-trained uveitis specialists.

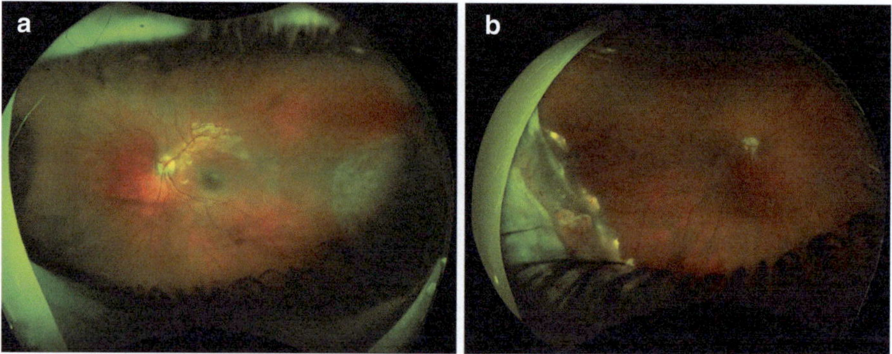

Fig. 6 Color fundus photographs of retinoschisis (**a**) and vasoproliferative tumor in two different patients with intermediate uveitis

References

1. Whitcup SM, Stark-Vancs V, Wittes RE, Solomon D, Podgor MJ, Nussenblatt RB, Chan CC. Association of interleukin 10 in the vitreous and cerebrospinal fluid and primary central nervous system lymphoma. Arch Ophthalmol. 1997;115(9):1157–60.
2. Cole CJ, Kwan AS, Laidlaw DA, Aylward GW. A new technique of combined retinal and choroidal biopsy. Br J Ophthalmol. 2008;92(10):1357–60. Epub 2008 Jul 29. PMID: 18664500.
3. Mastropasqua R, Thaung C, Pavesio C, Lightman S, Westcott M, Okhravi N, Aylward W, Charteris D, da Cruz L. The role of chorioretinal biopsy in the diagnosis of intraocular lymphoma. Am J Ophthalmol. 2015;160(6):1127–32.e1.
4. Rice JC, Liebenberg L, Scholtz RP, Torr G. Fatal air embolism during endoresection of choroidal melanoma. Retin Cases Brief Rep. 2014;8:127–9.
5. Ruschen H, Romano MR, Ferrara M, Loh GK, Wickham L, Damato BE, da Cruz L. Perfluorocarbon syndrome—a possible, overlooked source of fatal gas embolism following uveal-melanoma endoresection. Eye (Lond). 2022;36(12):2348–9.
6. Multicenter Uveitis Steroid Treatment (MUST) Trial Research Group, Kempen JH, Altaweel MM, Holbrook JT, Jabs DA, Louis TA, Sugar EA, Thorne JE. Randomized comparison of systemic anti-inflammatory therapy versus fluocinolone acetonide implant for intermediate, posterior, and panuveitis: the multicenter uveitis steroid treatment trial. Ophthalmology. 2011;118(10):1916–26.
7. Writing Committee for the Multicenter Uveitis Steroid Treatment (MUST) Trial and Follow-up Study Research Group. Association between long-lasting intravitreous fluocinolone acetonide implant vs systemic anti-inflammatory therapy and visual acuity at 7 years among patients with intermediate, posterior, or panuveitis. JAMA. 2017;317(19):1993–2005.
8. Tomkins-Netzer O, Lightman S, Drye L, Kempen J, Holland GN, Rao NA, Stawell RJ, Vitale A, Jabs DA, Multicenter Uveitis Steroid Treatment Trial Research Group. Outcome of treatment of uveitic macular edema: the multicenter uveitis steroid treatment trial 2-year results. Ophthalmology. 2015;122(11):2351–9.
9. Henry CR, Becker MD, Yang Y, Davis JL. Pars plana vitrectomy for the treatment of uveitis. Am J Ophthalmol. 2018;190:142–9.
10. Haseeb AA, Elhusseiny AM, Siddiqui MZ, Ahmad KT, Sallam AB. Fungal endophthalmitis: a comprehensive review. J Fungi (Basel). 2021;7(11):996.
11. Yu YZ, Zou XL, Chen XG, Zhang C, Yu YY, Zhang MY, Zou YP. Chronic hypotony management using endoscopy-assisted vitrectomy after severe ocular trauma or vitrectomy. Int J Ophthalmol. 2023;16(6):947–54.
12. Tosi GM, Schiff W, Barile G, Yoshida N, Chang S. Management of severe hypotony with intravitreal injection of viscoelastic. Am J Ophthalmol. 2005;140(5):952–4.
13. Jaffe GJ, Lin P, Keenan RT, Ashton P, Skalak C, Stinnett SS. Injectable fluocinolone acetonide long-acting implant for noninfectious intermediate uveitis, posterior uveitis and panuveitis: two-year results. Ophthalmology. 2016;123:1940–8.
14. Kirkland KA, Uwaydat SH, Siddiqui MZ, Chancellor JR, Soliman MK, Kurup S, Sallam AB. Outcome of intravitreal dexamethasone implant use in uveitic eyes undergoing pars plana vitrectomy surgery. Ocul Immunol Inflamm. 2021;29(6):1126–31.
15. Pichi F, Srivastava SK, Nucci P, Baynes K, Neri P, Lowder CY. Peripheral retinoschisis in intermediate uveitis. Retina. 2017;37(11):2167–74.
16. Pichi F, Neri P, Agarwal A, Invernizzi A, Choudhry N, Amer R, Lembo A, Nucci P, Thompson I, Sen HN, Shields CL. Vasoproliferative tumors in intermediate uveitis. Retina. 2020;40(9):1765–73.

Endophthalmitis

Ferenc Kuhn, Robert Morris, and Giampaolo Gini

1 Definition

Endophthalmitis is a severe, purulent infection of the intraocular contents; the toxic, tissue-destructive effects of the infecting organism's endo- and exotoxins and enzymes are exacerbated by the body's immune reaction [1]. The condition qualifies as an *abscess*: pus contained in a closed cavity.

Supplementary Information The online version contains supplementary material available at https://doi.org/10.1007/978-3-031-47827-7_27.

F. Kuhn (✉)
Helen Keller Foundation for Research and Education, Birmingham, AL, USA

Department of Ophthalmology, University of Pécs Medical School, Pécs, Hungary

Department of Ophthalmology, University of Halle, Halle, Germany

R. Morris
Helen Keller Foundation for Research and Education, Birmingham, AL, USA

Retina Specialists of Alabama, Birmingham, AL, USA

G. Gini
Department of Ophthalmology, University Hospitals Sussex NHS Foundation Trust, Worthing, West Sussex, UK

A. B. Sallam et al. (eds.), *Practical Manual of Vitreoretinal Surgery*, https://doi.org/10.1007/978-3-031-47827-7_27

2 Classification

It is typical to classify endophthalmitis as mild, moderate, or severe. This, however, gives the impression of a static condition, which endophthalmitis is certainly not. It is therefore advised to describe the condition as *early* vs. *advanced*: [2] this signals that even if the ophthalmologist makes the diagnosis at an early stage, an infection that is not treated promptly and properly can rapidly lead to widespread, severe, and irreversible tissue damage.

3 Etiology

Endophthalmitis may be:

- Exogenous:

    - Postoperative including post intravitreal injection and bleb-related endophthalmitis.
    - Posttraumatic.
    - Corneal ulcer-related.

- Endogenous.

- The causative organism is usually a bacterium (bacteria) but may also be a fungus or virus. The vast majority of the cases are acute (hours or a few days after surgery, intraocular injection, or injury). The chronic cases occur weeks after cataract surgery, typically by *Propionibacterium acnes* or fungi.

4 Incidence

- Cataract surgery: 0.04% [3]. The rate increase by 1.5-fold if patient is diabetic, 3-fold if cataract surgery is combined with pars plana vitrectomy or in eyes that had previous vitrectomy, and 7-fold if posterior capsule rupture occured during surgery [4, 5].
- Pars plana vitrectomy: 0.05– 0.157% [5, 6].
- Intravitreal injection: 0.017–0.025% [7].
- Keratoprosthesis implantation: rates are high at 5% and infection can present late and without pain [8].
- Posttraumatic endophthalmitis: 3%. The risk is higher with intraocular foreign body, wounds contaminated with organic lens matter, and lens capsule disruption [9].

5 Clinical Diagnosis

The following are the typical signs and symptoms (for a differential diagnosis regarding toxic anterior segment syndrome [TASS], see Table 1).

- Reduced visual acuity.
- Pain. Of note pain may be absent in endophthalmitis in about 20% of cases [8].
- Corneal edema.
- Hypopyon, cells, and fibrin in the anterior chamber (Fig. 1).
- Small pupil.
- Reduction, or complete loss, of the red reflex.
- Vitreous opacities ranging from cells to a massive yellow-white cloud.
- Endophthalmitis retinopathy: tortuous and sheathed blood vessels, stress hemorrhages, edema, and, in advanced cases, necrosis.
- Endophthalmitis maculopathy: like in endophthalmitis retinopathy, hypopyon.

Table 1 Toxic anterior segment syndrome (TASS) vs. acute postoperative endophthalmitis: differential diagnosis[a]

Variable	TASS	Endophthalmitis
Time of onset	Rapidly after surgery (<24 h)	1–7 days after surgery
Pain	Usually none to mild	Mild to significant
Vision	Blurred/slight reduction	Significant reduction
Scleroconjunctival injection	None to mild	Severe
Lid swelling	None to minimal	Significant
Corneal edema	Significant	Mild, especially initially
Pupil	Typically wide	Constricted
Intraocular pressure	Low-normal-high-very high	Normal
Vitreous cavity	Normal	Infiltrated

[a]These are, obviously, general rules; in any individual case, the diagnosis may be more difficult than the table might suggest

Fig. 1 The anterior segment in an eye with acute endophthalmitis. Note the edema in the cornea, the relatively small pupil, and the accumulation of pus inferiorly; the picture was taken at the slit lamp. This hypopyon may become invisible if this patient is in the supine position

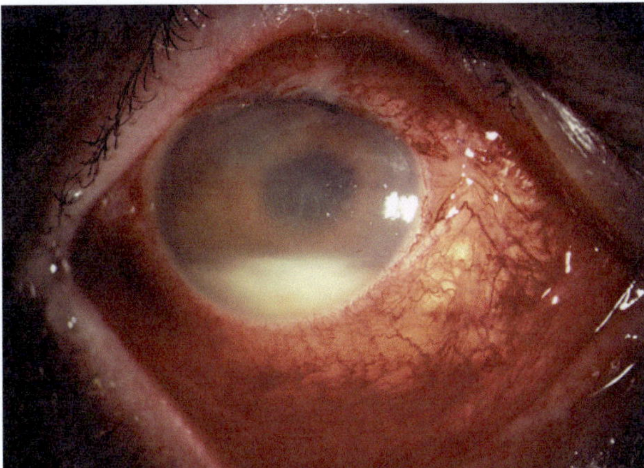

Endophthalmitis in a trauma setting is unique: the typical signs described above are often masked by other pathologies caused by the injury (corneal or iris trauma, vitreous hemorrhage, etc., Fig. 2), which can make the diagnosis very challenging. The organism is also often more virulent, making it even more important to intervene on an emergency basis and attempt to perform a complete surgery in the posterior segment (CEVE, see below).

The initial diagnosis of the infection should be a clinical one so that the treatment is not delayed; laboratory confirmation of the diagnosis comes hours to days later, based on the yield of the specimen. The material to be cultured is ideally taken from both the anterior chamber and the vitreous cavity before the antibiotic therapy has been initiated.

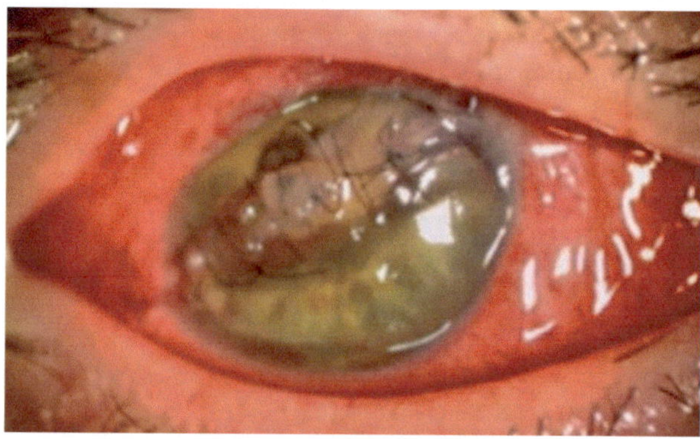

Fig. 2 Posttraumatic endophthalmitis (image taken from intraoperative video). This 18-year-old patient had a car accident. The cornea was sutured (very poorly), but no further intervention was performed for 3 weeks; the visual acuity remained light perception. There was no sign of endophthalmitis, nor did the patient have any pain. During the unnecessarily delayed vitrectomy, very advanced endophthalmitis was found; the culture grew three different bacteria. Despite an anatomically successful surgery, the visual acuity did not improve

6   Management Philosophy

6.1   Timing

Endophthalmitis is an emergency condition. While the type of treatment to be employed may be the subject of an argument (see below), the question of how soon to start the treatment is a universally accepted fact: immediately. Both medically and legally, it is impossible to justify delaying the onset of at least the initial treatment.

6.2   Treatment

The primary goals are:

- To stop the active infection.
- To remove, if possible, in its entirety, the toxic brew from wherever it is residing inside the eye (completeness of the intervention).

  The secondary goals include the following:

- Minimization of the damage inflicted by the toxic brew (speed of the initiation of the intervention).
- Dealing with the complications already present.
- Prevention of subsequent complications.

6.3   Decision-Making

Other factors, such as the patient's general condition, must also be considered. Only strictly eye-related issues are discussed here.

The "evidence-based" recommendation (Endophthalmitis Vitrectomy Study, EVS) [10] is to employ intravitreal injections rather than surgery unless the visual acuity drops to light perception. Every ophthalmologist must, in every case, make an individual decision whether to accept this recommendation or perform a vitrectomy based on the clinical picture and the consequences of a purulent intraocular infection; here are a few selected points to consider when making that decision.

- It has been known for two millennia that "what is not there, cannot hurt" (*Ubi pus, ibi evacua;* Hippocrates).
- Even if the antibiotics (originally chosen "blindly" based on assumptions rather than on the actual culture yield) are effective and kill off the organisms, the toxic intraocular brew will remain inside the eye for some time, worsening the prognosis [1].
- The surgical technique the EVS described erred on the cautious side: 50% of the vitreous was to be removed (obviously, the anterior and not the posterior vitreous), and detachment of the posterior vitreous cortex was not to be induced intraoperatively. Therefore, the study's surgical arm was an enlarged biopsy, *not* a true vitrectomy.

- The main reason why the EVS instructed against a complete vitrectomy was to avoid causing an iatrogenic retinal detachment. It has always been arguable whether the greater enemy is retinal detachment, a condition that surgeons routinely treat with a high success rate, or an infection that can cause irreversible and widespread tissue damage.
- The technology of vitrectomy has changed dramatically since the publication of the EVS (1995): the risk of iatrogenic complications has been significantly reduced, and the treatment of almost any potential intraoperative complication is more successful nowadays.
- *Complete* vitrectomy is thus possible in most cases, including the detachment of the posterior hyaloid (see below, under "Surgical Technique").
- Performing vitrectomy *early* (before the view of the posterior retina gets compromised, see Chap. 31) further reduces the risk of an intraoperative, iatrogenic complication. Furthermore, technically, it is much easier to operate on a still-rather-healthy eye than on one with extensive and advanced tissue pathologies.

For all these reasons, the authors have employed complete and early vitrectomy for endophthalmitis (*CEVE*) for decades [11, 12]. This treatment philosophy relies on the fundamentals of the clinical condition, rather than the presenting visual acuity, to drive the decision-making. CEVE allows sample-taking and medical therapy (see below) as long as the posterior retina can be visually monitored (such monitoring in the first 24 h involves hospitalization with the nurse checking on the patient [pain, vision, eye appearance] every hour). If despite medical therapy, the view is worsening, vitrectomy is recommended after 24 hours; in fact, during counseling, CEVE is always offered as a treatment option to all patients, regardless of the presenting VA.

6.4 Management

The description here concerns postoperative endophthalmitis. Cases with different etiology (bleb-related, traumatic, endogenous) are managed similarly but should be considered potentially more devastating because of the increased virulence of the suspected organism.

6.5 Patient Instructions

Patients with endophthalmitis feel sick and act accordingly: they typically lie in bed. This allows the heavy purulent material to settle on the posterior pole, which then presents as a macular hypopyon, explaining the deterioration of central vision and limited visual recovery if the pus is not removed surgically. The patients, therefore, should be advised to remain upright (sit in a chair) for as long as possible (the process of this "asking" is part of counseling: the dialogue in which the ophthalmologist describes the condition—as opposed to the normal—and makes all management decisions based on a mutual agreement with the patient; ideally, supportive family members are also present).

7   Treatment Options

7.1   Medical

Antibiotics in the form of an intravitreal injection are mandatory; systemic antibiotics are highly recommended and can be complemented by peribulbar, subconjunctival, or topical (fortified) administration. Topical and intravitreal corticosteroids should be considered seriously to lessen the harmful effects of the body's immune reaction. Table 2 shows a regimen that can be considered as the initial therapy; based on the results of the culture, this is to be modified accordingly.

Before antibiotic use, the material should be collected for culturing ("tap and inject"). The vitrectomy probe should be used to take an adequately sized sample from the vitreous cavity; either no infusion should be utilized or air should be employed to avoid diluting the specimen.

Table 2 Recommended medical therapy of endophthalmitis[a]

Route of administration	Drug and its dose (volume)	Frequency
Intravitreal injection	Antibiotics: Vancomycin 2 mg (0.1 ml) *and* Ceftazidime 2.25 mg (0.1 ml) Corticosteroids: Dexamethasone 0.4 mg (0.1 ml)	Repeat the next day if necessary; also to be used at the conclusion of vitrectomy[b]
Oral[c]	Ciprofloxacin 750 mg *or* Gatifloxacin 400	Every 12 h Every 6 h
Subconjunctival	Antibiotics: Vancomycin 25 mg (0.5 ml) *and* Ceftazidime 0.1 g (0.5 ml) Corticosteroids: Dexamethasone 12 mg (3 ml)	Daily or as needed
Parabulbar	Identical to the subconjunctival route	
Topical	Moxifloxacin 0.5% *and/or* Ofloxacin 0.3% *and/or* Tobramycin 0.3% Corticosteroids: Prednisolone 1% Cycloplegics: Atropine 1%	Typically: Hourly for all, except the cycloplegic (every 12–24 h)

[a]Listed in order of importance per route of administration. The use of the options other than the intravitreal injection is to be decided on an individual case basis
[b]If injected into silicone oil, 1/2–2/3 of the regular dose should be used
[c]Fighting a blinding condition, adding oral antibiotics is not an "overkill"

7.2 Surgical

The benefits of surgery (which is not instead of but in addition to medical treatment) include:

- Allowing the taking of adequate specimens for culturing.
- Clearing, or as a minimum, reducing, the media opacity (Fig. 3).
- Allowing direct visual inspection of the retina and ciliary body.
- Removing the toxic brew from the vitreous cavity.
- In pseudo- or aphakic eyes, the [at least partial] cleaning of the ciliary body and vitreous base.
- Removing the posterior vitreous cortex to allow vacuuming of the retinal surface.
- Providing direct access of the intravitreally injected medications to the retina itself.
- Treating existing pathologies (e.g., retinal detachment).
- Preventing late complications (e.g., retinal detachment, phthisis) to the extent possible.

As mentioned above, the vitrectomy should be complete and early (CEVE), [10] which means that the posterior hyaloid should be surgically detached if this can be done safely; alternatively, it should be "fenestrated" to allow the vacuuming of the macular surface and the intravitreal medications to "lubricate" it.

If a vitrectomy cannot be performed for any reason, full medical therapy should be initiated and continued until surgery becomes possible. If there is a recurrence of the infection or the initial surgery could not have been a complete one, the vitrectomy must be repeated (CEVE+) [13].

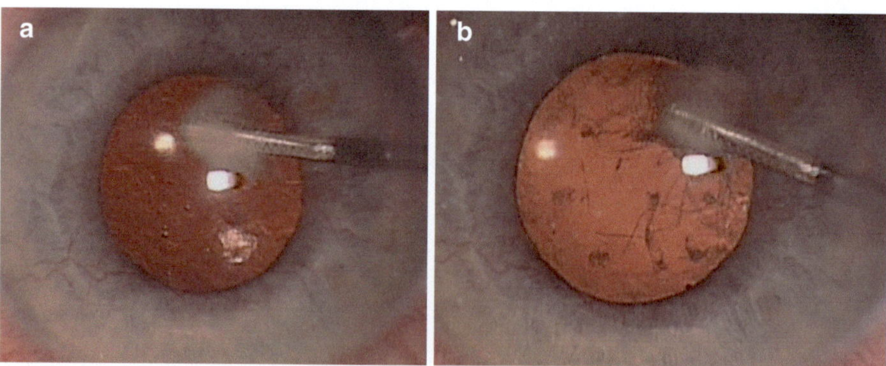

Fig. 3 Cleaning the anterior surface of the intraocular lens (images taken from intraoperative video). (**a**) A miniature piece of cotton is grabbed using intraocular forceps with a firm grasp. There are many deposits on the anterior lens surface. (**b**) Most of the debris has been dislocated (pushed to the periphery of the lens or into the anterior chamber from where it is then irrigated out), and the view is much improved. Deeper into the operation, the same maneuvers are to be repeated to clean the posterior surface of the intraocular lens

7.3 *Surgical Technique*

The typical vitrectomy technique for postoperative endophthalmitis is described in Table 3, Video 1. Vitrectomy for other etiologies is very similar; for chronic endophthalmitis, it is very important to make a large capsulectomy and irrigate the capsular bag copiously; if this is not possible, the capsular bag and intraocular lens are to be removed. A meticulous anteroposterior approach is needed; skipping any step results in suboptimal intraoperative conditions and, thus, a worse prognosis.

Table 3 Vitrectomy for endophthalmitis

Step	Comment
Preparation	In addition to the "routine" equipment/s, instruments, and materials, prepare for taking (care of) samples from the anterior chamber and the vitreous cavity.
	Select the gauge that you are confident using without compromise. Place the pars plana infusion cannula but do not open it unless you are certain the tip is in the vitreous cavity. If unsure, use an anterior-chamber maintainer until the tip is visibly past all layers of the eyewall
Infusion fluid	The irrigation fluid ideally contains the effective dose of antibiotics and corticosteroids; i.e., the concentration should be the same as with an intraocular injection—Lower concentrations are not bactericidal
Cornea	The epithelium is always edematous, and its removal significantly improves visualization. Scrape the epithelium, even in a diabetic patient, but the area of scraping should be kept to the minimum and avoid injuring the Bowman layer
	If the stroma is also edematous, press a dry sponge against it for a few seconds or use high-concentration glucose topically
	If Descemet's membrane is folded, clean the anterior chamber, and fill it tightly with cohesive viscoelastic (obviously impossible in an aphakic eye) If the cornea is completely opacified, a temporary keratoprosthesis or endoscope could be used, as described in Chap. 29
Anterior chamber	Even if a true hypopyon is not visible (a small hypopyon seen at the slit lamp "disappears" with the patient lying down), there are always cells and flare, and very often, a fibrinous membrane. Cleaning the anterior chamber, which may have to be repeatedly done during surgery, especially in young children, significantly improves visualization The irrigation of the anterior chamber may be done through one or two paracenteses. The latter is preferred because certain manipulations may require increased chamber depth. The "working" paracentesis is ideally in the superotemporal quadrant, even if it is on the side of the surgeon's nondominant hand Following copious irrigation, use serrated or large-platform vitrectomy forceps (e.g., FC23R06, Vitreq, Vierpolders, the Netherlands) to carefully engage any fibrous membrane present. Grab it over on the nasal side of the anterior chamber, and avoid damaging the iris, which can easily bleed. Slowly withdraw the forceps; a "spaghetti" maneuver may be necessary to remove the entire membrane in a single grab. The membrane is elastic and, if moved slowly, will be extracted without breaking up

(continued)

Table 3 (continued)

Step	Comment
Pupil	It must be made as wide as possible, whether using medications (adrenaline, cycloplegics), viscoelastics, or some kind of mechanical iris dilatator (e.g., retractor)
Crystalline lens	Remove the lens if it interferes with the success of the surgery (visualization of the posterior segment or cleaning of the vitreous base, should the latter be possible). As a general rule, do not implant an intraocular lens (IOL) if the lens is removed
IOL	Thoroughly clean the IOL's anterior (and later the posterior) surface. This can be done by taking a tiny piece of cotton (from an applicator), wetting it, and using the forceps to sweep the IOL surface/s with it (Fig. 3). An IOL rarely needs to be removed; in eyes with chronic endophthalmitis, it may be necessary to remove both it and the capsules if the bag cannot be adequately irrigated
Posterior capsule	Make a large capsulectomy and irrigate the capsular bag, so no organism is left inside
Vitreous cavity if the retina is visible	Proceed as in a normal case, preferably in a posterior to anterior direction. Mark the posterior hyaloid with triamcinolone (if "nature" did not do it before, Fig. 4) and carefully create a posterior vitreous detachment (never assume one is already present). Vacuum the macular surface with the flute needle (Fig. 5) and complete the vitrectomy, consistent with safety: As a general rule, be more "aggressive" posteriorly than at the vitreous base (Fig. 6). If the posterior hyaloid cannot be (safely) detached, at least open it to allow vacuuming of the retinal surface and for the medications to irrigate the surface (fenestration, see the text for details)
Vitreous cavity if the retina is not or only barely visible	Proceed in an anterior-posterior direction: Clean the area behind the lens (IOL) first, then the central vitreous, and do the creation of this "well" on the nasal side; if the retina is detached and necrotic (i.e., no bleeding even if bitten into), only a small area would be damaged before the retina is recognized. Deal with the posterior vitreous as described above, and try to vacuum the macular surface. The retina may be fragile and easily damaged; if (some of) the vitreous is extremely adherent to the surface, abandon its detachment At the vitreous base, do not attempt the usual "as much as possible" vitreous removal. If present, the yellowish-white, nontransparent ring of purulent vitreous (Fig. 4) makes it impossible to see where this ends and where the underlying retina begins. This ring may be thinned a little but should be left behind If there is necrotic retina, do not attempt detachment of the overlying posterior vitreous cortex. Instead, try to wall it off with a laser barrier in the adjacent (relatively) healthy retina
Ciliary body	Phthisis being one of the main postoperative complications, in aphakic or pseudophakic eyes, the ciliary processes must be cleaned, using scleral (preferably self-) indentation, as much as this is consistent with safety

Step	Comment
Tamponade	Typically, balanced salt solution (BSS) is left behind. However, if a retinal break is found or has been created, large areas of the retina are necrotic, or a retinal detachment is already present, it is best to use silicone oil as tamponade. The oil has additional advantages: It is transparent and does not interfere with early postoperative visualization of the retina; organisms do not live in it, and it does not preclude the intravitreal injection of medications Some surgeons leave behind air/gas; the problem with this option is that it makes early postoperative inspection of the retina impossible
Completion of the surgery	Close all wounds and inject antibiotics and corticosteroids into the vitreous cavity (see Table 2 for the doses) once the ports have been closed. If silicone oil has been used, inject 2/3 of the conventional doses of antibiotics and corticosteroid into the oil
Postoperatively	Depending on the intraoperative findings and course, repeat the vitrectomy (CEVE+); laser treatment may also become necessary

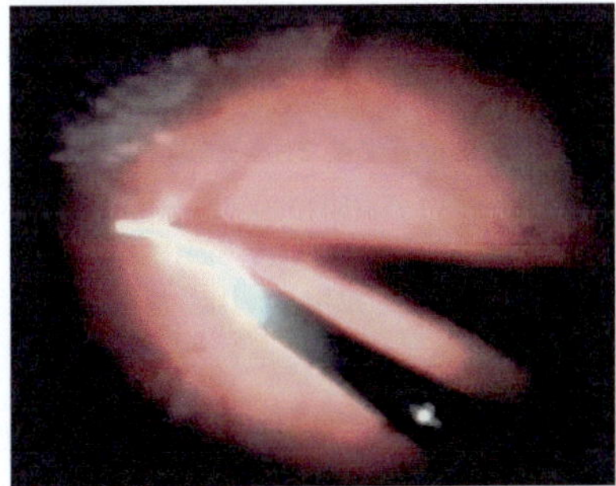

Fig. 4 Elevation of the nondetached posterior hyaloid (image taken from intraoperative video). In this 71-year-old woman, there is still no posterior vitreous detachment despite the 2-week-old endophthalmitis and a previous vitrectomy surgery (the image is hazy due to long-standing corneal edema). The posterior hyaloid is finally detached using forceps; it is marked not by triamcinolone but by the colonies of bacteria ("nature's stain")

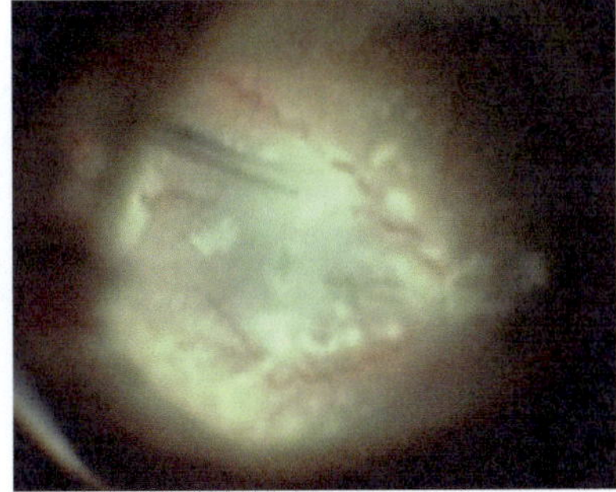

Fig. 5 Vacuuming the macular surface (image taken from intraoperative video). Once the posterior hyaloid has been removed, the surface of the posterior retina is gently cleaned by passive suction using the flute needle. The typical image of endophthalmitis retinopathy is seen (tortuous, engorged vessels, edema)

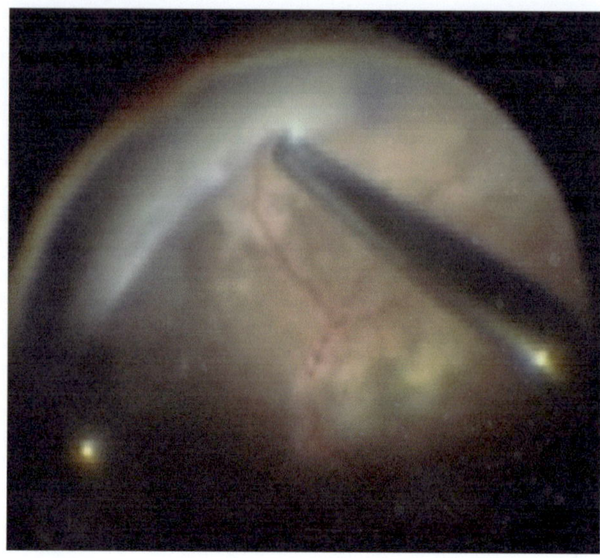

Fig. 6 Vitrectomy at the vitreous base (image taken from intraoperative video). A ring of yellow-white vitreous covers the retinal periphery; the central vitreous has been removed, allowing a clear view of the posterior pole with the typical signs of endophthalmitis retinopathy. The vitreous is carefully trimmed at the base, with no attempt to remove all of the tissue here

In summary, endophthalmitis is an emergency condition; the delaying of the proper intervention can do more damage to the eye than choosing a suboptimal treatment option. The definite intervention, offering the best possible prognosis, is timely and complete vitrectomy (CEVE), supported by the maximum antimicrobial regimen.

Key Points

- Endophthalmitis qualifies as an abscess: pus in a closed cavity.
- The damage to the thin tissue—the retina—lining the closed cavity is done not by the organisms themselves but by the toxins and enzymes the organisms produce and by the body's immune reaction.
- Even if the antibiotic therapy—chosen based on statistics rather than specific noxa—is successful in neutralizing the organisms, the toxic brew inside the eye continues to damage the intraocular tissues.
- Early and complete vitrectomy, combined with intravitreal antibiotic therapy, offers the best chance to restore the anatomy and function of the eye.

References

1. Han P. Intravitreal human immune globulin in a rabbit model of staphylococcus aureus toxin-mediated endophthalmitis: a potential adjunct in the treatment of endophthalmitis. Trans Am Ophthalmol Soc. 2004;102:305–20.
2. Morris R, Witherspoon CD, Kuhn F, Byrne J. Endophthalmitis. In: Roy H, editor. Master techniques in ophthalmic surgery. Baltimore: Williams and Wilkins; 1995. p. 560–72.

3. Pershing S, Lum F, Hsu S, Kelly S, Chiang MF, Rich WL 3rd, Parke DW 2nd. Endophthalmitis after cataract surgery in the United States: a report from the intelligent research in sight registry, 2013-2017. Ophthalmology. 2020;127(2):151–8.

4. Low L, Shah V, Norridge CFE, Donachie PHJ, Buchan JC. Royal College of Ophthalmologists' National Ophthalmology Database, Report 10: Risk Factors for Post-Cataract Surgery Endophthalmitis. Ophthalmology. 2023;130(11):1228–30.

5. Baudin F, Benzenine E, Mariet AS, Ben Ghezala I, Bron AM, Daien V, Korobelnik JF, Quantin C, Creuzot-Garcher C. Epidemiology of acute endophthalmitis after intraocular procedures: a national database study. Ophthalmol Retina. 2022;6(6):442–49.

6. Chen G, Tzekov R, Li W, Jiang F, Mao S, Tong Y. Incidence of endophthalmitis after vitrectomy: a systematic review and meta-analysis. Retina. 2019;39(5):844–52.

7. VanderBeek BL, Bonaffini SG, Ma L. Association of compounded bevacizumab with postinjection endophthalmitis. JAMA Ophthalmol. 2015;133(10):1159–64.

8. Lee T, Robbins CB, Wisely CE, Grewal DS, Daluvoy MB, Fekrat S. Clinical characteristics and visual outcomes in endophthalmitis after keratoprosthesis implantation. Retina. 2022;42(2):321–7.

9. Bhagat N, Nagori S, Zarbin MA. Traumatic endophthalmitis. Surv Ophthalmol. 2011;56(3):214–51.

10. Doft B, et al. Results of the endophthalmitis vitrectomy study. A randomized trial of immediate vitrectomy and of intravenous antibiotics for the treatment of postoperative bacterial endophthalmitis. Endophthalmitis Vitrectomy Study Group. Arch Ophthalmol. 1995;113:1479–96.

11. Kuhn F, Gini G. Vitrectomy for endophthalmitis. Ophthalmology. 2006;113:714.

12. Dib B, Morris RE, Oltmanns MH, Sapp RS, Glover JP, Kuhn F. Complete and early vitrectomy for endophthalmitis after cataract surgery: an alternative treatment paradigm. Clin Ophthalmol. 2020;14:1945–54.

13. Morris R, Kuhn F. Complete and early vitrectomy for endophthalmitis. Eur J Ophthalmol. 2021;31:2794–5.

Vitreoretinal Surgery in Ocular Trauma

Ferenc Kuhn, Robert Morris, and Giampaolo Gini

This chapter discusses the treatment of an eye with a serious injury (defined by the United States Eye Injury Registry as *trauma potentially resulting in permanent and significant, structural, or functional change*). Only such trauma to the eyeball is included here; other ophthalmic injuries or insignificant globe traumas such as a superficial corneal foreign body are not addressed in this chapter. This chapter is restricted to *selected* surgical indications for which vitrectomy is employed; the pathologies are listed in an anteroposterior order.

1 Who Should Treat the Severely Injured Eye?

The treatment of these eyes does not recognize artificial boundaries; unless the tissue damage is clearly limited to the anterior part of the eye wall (cornea and zone I in the sclera) [1], it is preferable for the vitreoretinal, rather than an anterior

Supplementary Information The online version contains supplementary material available at https://doi.org/10.1007/978-3-031-47827-7_28.

F. Kuhn (✉)
Helen Keller Foundation for Research and Education, Birmingham, AL, USA

Department of Ophthalmology, University of Pécs Medical School, Pécs, Hungary

Department of Ophthalmology, University of Halle, Halle, Germany

R. Morris
Helen Keller Foundation for Research and Education, Birmingham, AL, USA

Retina Specialists of Alabama, Birmingham, AL, USA

G. Gini
Department of Ophthalmology, University Hospitals Sussex NHS Foundation Trust, Worthing, West Sussex, UK

© The Author(s), under exclusive license to Springer Nature Switzerland AG 2024
A. B. Sallam et al. (eds.), *Practical Manual of Vitreoretinal Surgery*,
https://doi.org/10.1007/978-3-031-47827-7_28

segment, surgeon to be the leading force. A vitreoretinal surgeon should be well trained to treat any and all consequences of a globe injury (Fig. 1). What is absolutely unacceptable is for the surgeon to start an operation only to discover intraoperatively that there are (t)issues that must be addressed but which are beyond his expertise: don't start what you cannot finish.

2 Surgery Vs. Abandoning the Eye Vs. (Primary) Enucleation

The question of *whether to operate on an eye*, which has lost light perception and has severe intraocular disorganization due to the injury, is often raised [2].

- While sympathetic ophthalmia does represent a real risk, that risk is extremely small (one in a few thousand cases of serious injury) and should neither be the primary factor in determining this question nor serve as justification for primary enucleation or the abandonment of reconstruction.
- Abandoning the eye has similar consequences to enucleation, except sparing the patient the psychological trauma of an amputation.
- The patient must decide, after extensive and objective counseling.

3 The Primary Focus of Surgery

The two intraocular tissues that primarily determine the outcome of a severe trauma are the *ciliary body* and the *(central) retina*. The surgeon's most important task is to save these; while several other tissues also play a role in the final

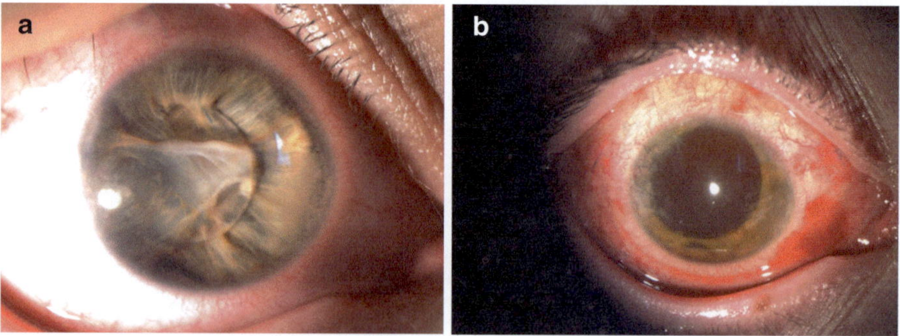

Fig. 1 Anterior segment reconstruction (images taken from intraoperative video). (**a**) Complete disorganization of the anterior segment, months following a severe open-globe injury. (**b**) The prolapsed vitreous has been removed, along with the opacified capsules and subluxated intraocular lens

outcome, these tissues are either less important or easier to deal with, both in terms of the "how" and the "when."

4 Timing

The general rule is: the sooner the better. Obviously, an open-globe injury requires surgery much sooner than a contusion; however, postponing any surgery ("let's see what happens if we wait" or "perhaps nature will take care of it") that has been deemed necessary makes no sense medically and will be very difficult to justify legally. If the attending ophthalmologist is unable, for whatever reason, to do timely surgery, urgent referral is needed to one who is both able and willing.

"Early surgery" offers two options.

- Primary comprehensive intraocular reconstruction: everything that needs to be done is performed during the initial surgery, from the eye wall (wound closure) to the subretinal space (e.g., irrigation of blood).
- Vitrectomy as a second procedure, performed within 4 days after the injury.

5 Endophthalmitis

It is discussed in Chap. 27.

6 Corneal Wound

The technique of suturing in trauma is discussed in Video 1. Emphasis is put on placing the sutures full thickness with minimal handling of the wound edges to achieve water tight closure with minimal corneal edema.

7 Hyphema

While a moderate amount of liquid blood in the anterior chamber can be addressed via nonsurgical methods or irrigation, a clotted, complete ("eight- or black-ball") hyphema requires rapid and complete removal. Such an intervention will prevent corneal blood staining (Fig. 2), synechia formation, and the development of secondary glaucoma; it will also result in instant visual rehabilitation – provided no other pathology is present—and allow visual inspection of the eye's deeper structures as about half of these eyes need surgery for a trauma-related posterior segment pathology.

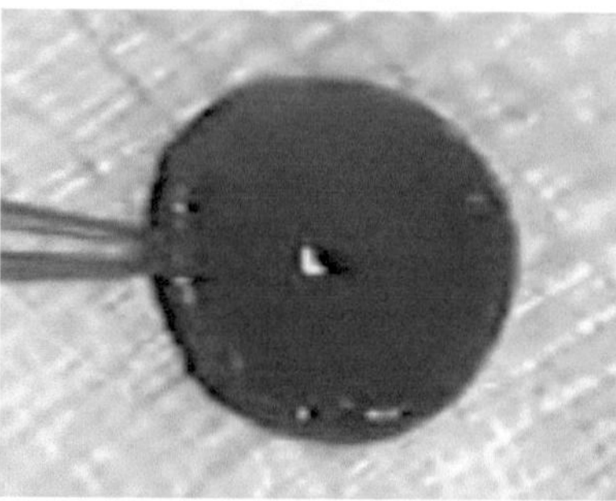

Fig. 2 Corneal imbibition (image taken from intraoperative video). The original attending ophthalmologist decided against removing the clotted hyphema, accepting some artificially recommended guidelines regarding the intraocular pressure "never exceeding 30 mmHg" and duration of the hemorrhage "barely 5 days". The eye required vitreoretinal surgery due to the vitreous hemorrhage and retinal detachment; a temporary keratoprosthesis vitrectomy had to be performed. The removed corneal button is shown against white gauze as contrast to highlight its high blood content

7.1 Surgical Technique of Clot Removal

- As in vitreoretinal surgery in general, an infusion line is the first one in (and the last one out). Either a bent 23- or 25-gauge needle (bimanual technique) or an anterior-chamber maintainer is used (monomanual technique). The advantage of the former is that the surgeon can manipulate the eye more easily and orient the incoming fluid's jet stream to where it is really needed; the disadvantage is that with the surgeon's focus on the tip/port of the vitrectomy probe, the needle can inadvertently damage the cornea, angle, iris, or crystalline lens. If a maintainer is used and the eye is phakic, it is safest to place the cannula so that its entirety is over the iris (Fig. 3). If a bimanual technique is selected, the surgeon must ask the assistant to continually monitor the position of the needle and literally scream if the needle's tip is approaching any tissue or is about to be pulled out.
- The infusion pressure is kept rather high (~ 40 mmHg), and the cut rate is set at ~600 cycles per minute. The paracenteses should be created so that no leakage occurs. It is therefore best to use a MVR (microvitrectomy) blade rather than a 15-degree blade: the internal aperture of the wound should be larger than the external aperture.
- The port of the vitrectomy probe is held sideways or upward, never downward; the cutting is briefly activated in the center and creates a small space free of clot. This central "empty" space is then enlarged by careful probe movement. When the aspiration/cutting are activated, the port must be kept occluded so as to never let the anterior chamber collapse.
- Any peripheral clot is pulled, using only a suction, to the center where the anterior chamber is deep, and removed there.
- Finally, the anterior and posterior chambers are copiously irrigated. If liquid blood is resupplied from behind the iris, it signals the presence of a nonclotted,

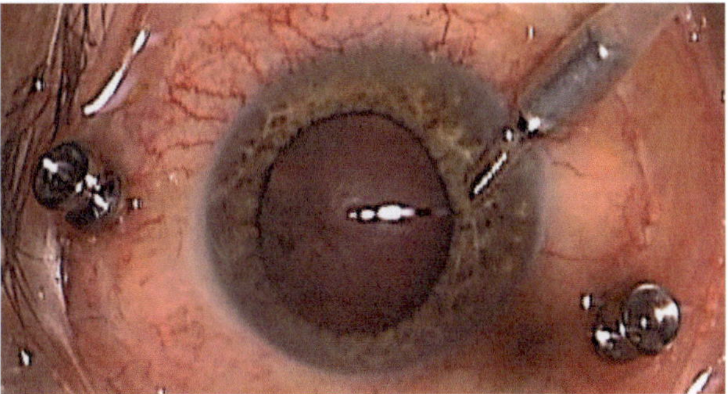

Fig. 3 Placement of the anterior-chamber maintainer (image taken from intraoperative video). The tip of the maintainer is kept over the iris. If the pupil were wider, the maintainer would still be inserted at 7 o'clock, but would point toward 5 o'clock

nonbound vitreous hemorrhage, which is pushed anteriorly by the infusion that is flowing posteriorly. If the lens is clear and there is no blood in the vitreous cavity, the red reflex should by now be restored.

If the bleeding source can be identified, endodiathermy can be applied to coagulate it. Balanced salt solution or air can be injected after all instruments have been removed and the wounds closed (hydration or sutures) to ensure that the intraocular pressure (IOP) is slightly higher than normal.

8 Anterior-Chamber Intraocular Foreign Body (IOFB)

Even if inert, these are better not be left behind: if mobile, they can cause damage to any tissue that constitutes the chamber's wall, and ferrous ones can cause siderosis.

8.1 Surgical Technique

There are three cardinal rules to keep in mind.

- The anterior chamber must never be allowed to collapse. All iatrogenic injuries caused by such an event can be prevented by using an anterior-chamber maintainer or injecting a cohesive viscoelastic. In the former case, the entire anterior-chamber depth is controlled; in the latter case, the material must cover not only the area where the IOFB is located but also the "channel" connecting it with the removal incision.
- The wound architecture is of crucial importance. The paracentesis must be long enough to accommodate both the IOFB and the jaws of the forceps that holds the IOFB and oriented so that it, on the one hand, allows keeping the anterior chamber closed to the extent possible and, on the other hand, prevents wrinkling of the cornea throughout the entire procedure.

- As a general principle, it is better to access the area where the IOFB is located from a paracentesis that is 90–180 degrees away, rather than using the intuitive "direct cut-down" location, just above the IOFB. This allows the surgeon to carry out any manipulation that may be required, even if the IOFB gets dislocated during the grabbing attempts or in the process of withdrawal.

Depending on the size, surface, shape, and material of the IOFB, there is a wide selection of potential tools to use for the extraction: vitrectomy probe, flute needle, lasso (snare), and various types of forceps.

9 Lens: Subluxation, Luxation

- A crystalline lens that is mostly *in place* (Fig. 4) may not need any treatment if it does not cause visual symptoms, elevation of the IOP by swelling and a pupillary block, and the lens remains clear.
- A *subluxated* lens may be left in situ if the patient is symptomless.
- A completely *dislocated* (luxated) lens requires intervention. An anteriorly luxated lens needs rapid removal to limit the damage to the endothelium; a lens luxated into the vitreous cavity, suprachoroidally or subretinally, requires timely but typically nonemergency removal, unless a phacoanaphylactic reaction or pupillary block with high IOP is present.
- With either subluxation or luxation, there may be *vitreous prolapse* into the anterior chamber (this is readily visible at the slit lamp but may become unrecognizable under the surgical microscope; injecting triamcinolone is a great diagnostic tool; Fig. 5). Surgical treatment should be considered for anterior vitreous pro-

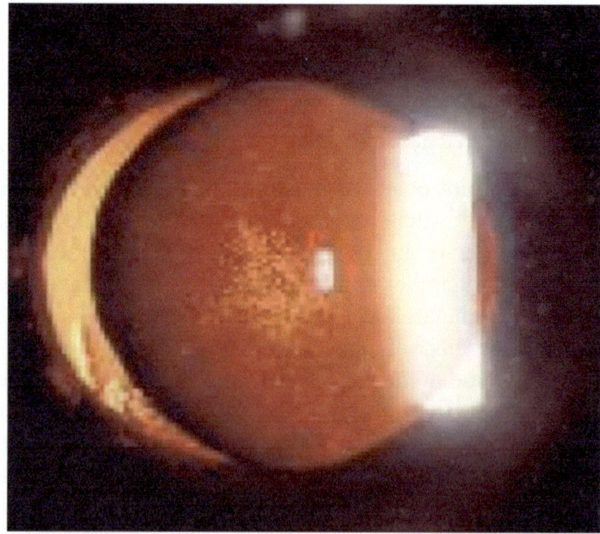

Fig. 4 Subluxated crystalline lens (image taken from intraoperative video). An individual decision must be made whether such a slight dislocation requires surgical intervention (see the text for more details)

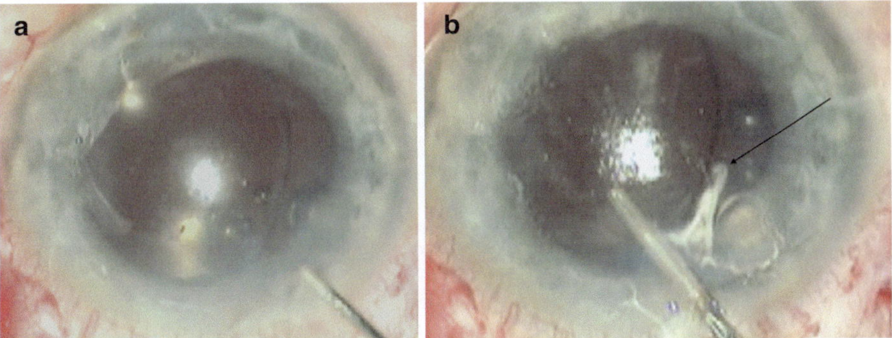

Fig. 5 Subluxated crystalline lens (images taken from intraoperative video). (**a**) The dislocated IOL is clearly visible; the prolapse into the anterior chamber of the vitreous is not. (**b**) After injecting triamcinolone, the vitreous is readily recognizable (black arrow)

lapse since it causes permanent traction on the vitreous base and may lead to retinal detachment (RD) with time.

9.1 Surgical Technique

Vitreous Prolapse

The anterior (limbal) approach appears to be the obvious choice; however, this always leaves the prolapsed vitreous adherent to the back surface of the iris and the posterior lens capsule. In experienced hands, therefore, it is preferable to do the anterior vitrectomy through the pars plana. To maintain crystalline-lens integrity, small air bubbles can be injected (Fig. 6): this will indicate to the surgeon the exact location of the posterior lens capsule. The goal is less the removal of the prolapsed vitreous in toto than severing the connection between the vitreous proper and vitreous prolapsed.

Lens Subluxation

- If it can be definitely confirmed that there is no vitreous prolapse into the anterior chamber (see above), a "standard" phacoemulsification is acceptable.
- If, however, vitreous prolapse is present or its presence cannot be excluded, phacoemulsification is contraindicated: the aspiration will exert traction on the vitreous base and retinal detachment (RD) will ultimately develop. The RD is not instantaneous; the surgeon will therefore blame it on the injury, rather than his own incompetence.
- In such cases *lensectomy* is the safest option, performed through the pars plana: the MVR blade or a needle is used to slice the lens capsule open at its equator to

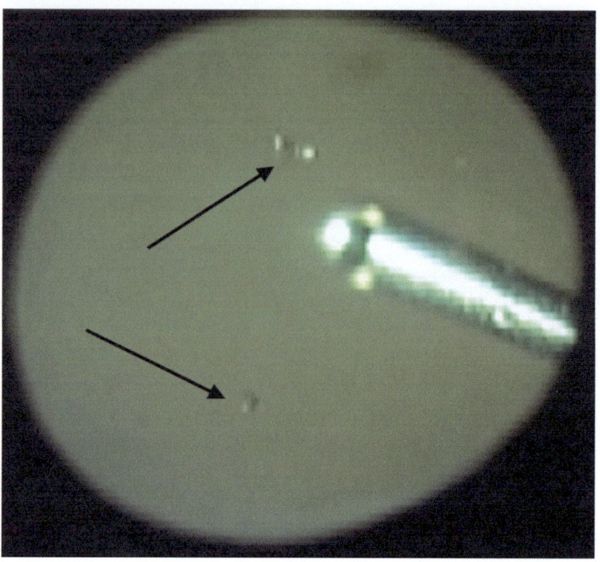

Fig. 6 Vitrectomy behind a clear lens (image taken from intraoperative video). After small air bubbles (black arrows) have been injected behind the lens, the anterior vitreous can safely be removed. Once there is a fluid pocket (no vitreous) just posterior the lens capsule, the bubbles rapidly migrate toward the equator of the lens

allow resistance-free entry of the vitrectomy probe through the slice into the lens proper (thus preventing undue traction on the remaining, unbroken zonules).

The initial step is to perform an anterior vitrectomy, just behind the lens (see above), trying to avoid cutting into the posterior capsule (see below).

The vitrectomy machine's settings are then changed: maximum aspiration (flow) and reduced cutting: the harder the lens (the older the patient), the lower the cut rate (depending on the type of vitrectomy machine, the cut-off age is typically 65–70 years; above this age, the anterior vitrectomy can be followed by a loop-assisted lens removal or phacoemulsification).

Ideally, the port is always occluded and never turned upward and rarely downward: on the one hand, it is not possible to preserve the posterior capsule; on the other hand, if a large opening is made in the posterior capsule too early, lens particles can fall into the vitreous. (Conversely, a small opening facilitates infusion fluid entering the lens, thereby reducing the risk of a collapse of the capsules. If this is happening, the surgeon may switch to a hand-held infusion: a bent needle is connected to the line. The needle is then forwarded into the lens and keeps the bag irrigated at a low pressure.)

Once the nucleus is removed, the cortex is pulled centrally and aspirated (occasional cutting is also necessary to prevent a blockage in the shaft of the probe) and removed; finally, a large anterior capsulectomy is made. In certain cases the entire capsule is taken, if:

- The patient is young (under ~18 years (see below)).
- Severe proliferative vitreoretinopathy [PVR] is present or expected.
- The capsule is not considered secure enough to hold an intraocular lens (IOL).

The issue of primary IOL implantation is beyond the scope of this chapter, but it needs to be emphasized that the use of capsular tension rings in the context of trauma is a risky endeavor: as the remaining zonules may or may not survive the extra tension they will be exposed to (Fig. 7).

Lens Luxation

- If the lens is in the *anterior chamber*, a loop is the best tool for removal (Fig. 8); as much as possible, the endothelium should be protected using viscoelastics. The most common error in this maneuver is to make the limbal incision too small. As described above, the lens removal should be preceded by an anterior vitrectomy through the pars plana.
- A *suprachoroidal* lens may also be removed with the loop, once it has been brought anteriorly or via a direct scleral cut-down.

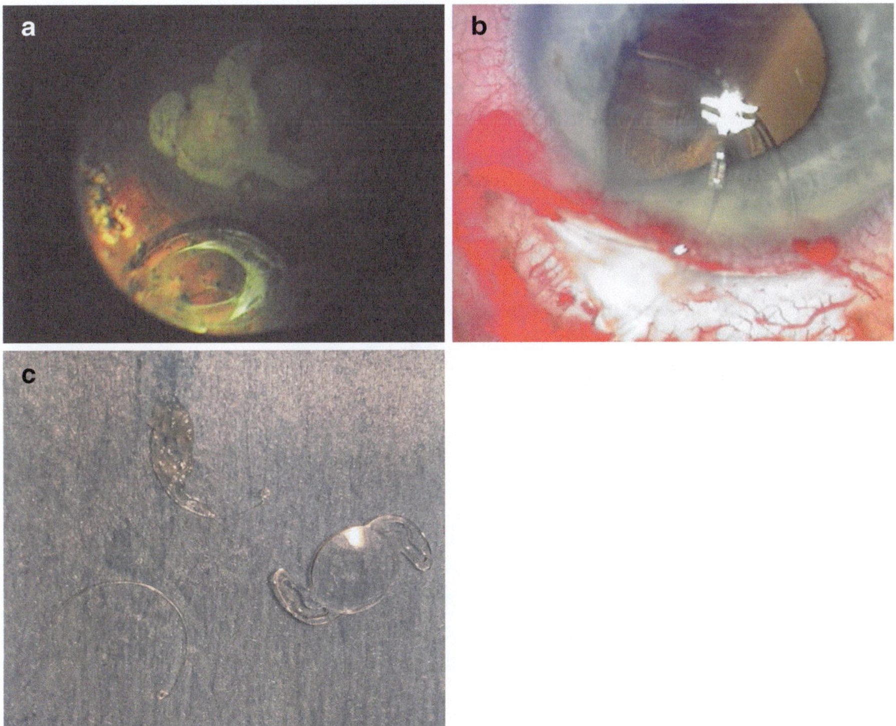

Fig. 7 Capsular tension rings in an injured eye (images taken from intraoperative video). (**a**) Following a contusion injury that resulted in lens subluxation, the original surgeon implanted an IOL. Months later, the patient experienced a sudden deterioration of vision; no second injury occurred. Intraoperatively, a posteriorly dislocated IOL was found, still in the bag. (**b**) During removal, three capsular tension rings were found. (**c**) Two of the rings (one still inside the bag) and the IOL, external view

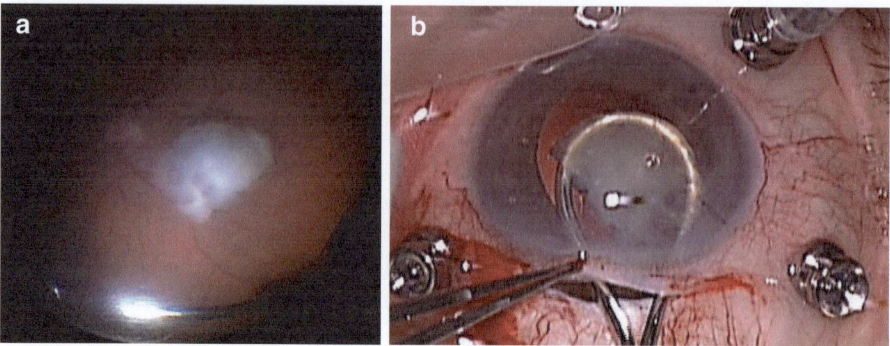

Fig. 8 Removal of a luxated lens using a loop (images taken from intraoperative video). (**a**) Lens particles lying on the posterior retina. (**b**) The corneal endothelium should be protected by viscoelastic; the wound should be sufficiently long

- A *posteriorly* luxated lens, which is by far the most common occurrence, requires a complete vitrectomy—detachment and removal of the posterior hyaloid included. If the lens is soft, lensectomy, as described above, is a safe choice; the light pipe helps feeding (crushing) lens particles into the port of the vitrectomy probe. If the nucleus is hard, this technique may still work, or phacofragmentation is chosen.

10 IOL: Subluxation

What can/should be done depends on how severe the subluxation is, what caused it, whether it is progressing, and if yes, how fast.

10.1 *Surgical Technique*

In an ideal situation, the IOL can simply be observed or repositioned, typically using some type of a hook. Many surgeons choose implanting a capsular tension ring to stretch the capsule if the zonules are broken in a limited area (see above).

The easiest permanent solution is to use a long (preferably curved) needle, armed with a Prolene suture, to fix the haptic to the iris (using a McCannel suture or a sliding knot).

An IOL that is severely dislocated or being flipped (inverted) by an ongoing capsular contraction or scarring (i.e., anterior PVR) process represents another dilemma where the surgeon must make an individual decision. It may be best to remove the IOL (a soft IOL can be cut almost-in-half or folded inside the anterior chamber and removed through a smaller incision, or an incision slightly larger than the optic is made for the extraction).

11 Lens Capsules

In children, the surgeon should seriously consider removing the capsule of a lens that must be removed anyway. It undoubtably makes (subsequent) IOL implantation less straightforward, but it is never the IOL that determines the outcome of a serious injury. The capsules may contract with time and induce traction on the ciliary processes. These in turn may lead to ciliary body atrophy and phthisis develops [3].

11.1 Surgical Technique

The easiest method is to create a capsulectomy and use a large-platform intraocular forceps to grab the capsule, followed by a "spaghetti" maneuver to slowly disconnect the zonular fibers from the ciliary processes, then remove the capsule. It almost never comes out in one piece so the maneuver must be repeated several times. In young patients the ciliary processes can be torn off before the zonules break; either chemical zonulolysis (alpha chymotrypsin 1:5000) must be used, or the zonules be mildly stretched and then cut with the vitrectomy probe or scissors.

12 IOL: Luxation

An IOL that is completely out of its normal position not only becomes useless but may cause additional complications.

12.1 Surgical Technique

In the extremely rare case of an anteriorly dislocated IOL, it is usually best removed as described above. If the IOL is in the vitreous cavity, a complete vitrectomy is the initial step. If the posterior capsule is still firmly in place, a sufficiently large capsulectomy should be created first. The surgeon then takes a forceps and, ideally, carefully grabs the IOL by the distal haptic, replaces the light pipe with a spatula, and guides the proximal haptic into the anterior chamber superiorly; finally, the distal haptic is positioned in front of the iris inferiorly. The IOL is then either repositioned into the bag or onto the capsule (sulcus) or removed.

It is difficult to justify leaving the posteriorly luxated IOL in place and simply implanting another one.

13 Ciliary Body Cleaning

Unless the eye is phakic, it is a grave sin to leave material (vitreous, fibrin, blood) over the ciliary processes; this material can rapidly turn into a white scar over the ciliary body—if this happens, it is "game over": the tissue is irreversibly lost. The risk of subsequent phthisis is almost eliminated if the cleansing has been timely and thorough, although it is still possible for the eye to become phthisical if the trauma, typically a contusion, causes necrosis of the ciliary body or if anterior PVR develops postoperatively.

13.1 *Surgical Technique*

The best approach is self-indentation for precise control: the ciliary processes need only mild trauma to result in profuse bleeding, whose exact location is very difficult to identify and cauterize. The surgeon uses various instruments (spatula, scissors, hooked needle, vitrectomy probe, etc., Fig. 9) in the working hand to liberate the surface of the processes until they are all visible and clean. These maneuvers are carried out 360 degrees; it thus may take 15–20 minutes to complete the procedure.

If either the injury or the cleansing results in ciliary body detachment (cyclodialysis), the tissue should be reattached. Cryopexy or diathermy is sufficient if the lesion is very small (~less than 2 clock hours); otherwise suturing (direct, after a scleral cut-down, or indirect, using a McCannel suture) is required.

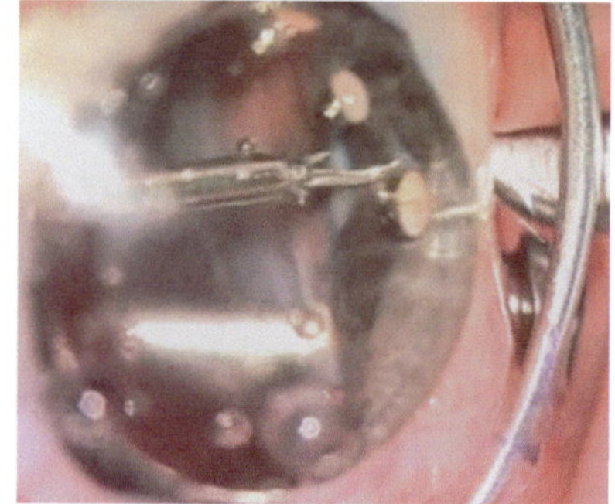

Fig. 9 Ciliary body cleansing (image taken from intraoperative video). The surgeon indents the sclera so that the ciliary processes are in view and uses various tools, such as scissors shown here, to remove any tissue or material covering the processes

14   Vitreous Hemorrhage

Blood in the vitreous cavity in the context of trauma has two major implications: it is usually severe enough to interfere with the view (the ophthalmologist cannot examine the retina) and vision (for the patient); and it is a crucial risk factor in PVR development.

Vitrectomy for traumatic vitreous hemorrhage can be challenging. Even if done by an experienced clinician, ultrasonography may not allow recognition of an RD behind the blood. Intraoperatively, the formed vitreous in young patients shows onion-like layers with blood streaks on them; these resemble the appearance of the retina. Conversely, the retina may be necrotic and attached to the vitreous; if the vitrectomy probe cuts into it, the retina will not bleed, and the surgeon can inadvertently remove large parts of the retina without realizing it. The surgeon should therefore always proceed as if an RD were present.

14.1   Surgical Technique

- Introduce the infusion cannula but do not turn it on unless the tip is clearly visible and not covered by the pars plana epithelium. Until certain, use an anterior-chamber maintainer.
- Proceed with the vitrectomy in an anteroposterior sequence. Start behind the lens if it is to be preserved or remove it if it hinders the success of the operation in any way (see above).
- Gradually extend the vitreous removal toward the periphery so as to visualize the infusion cannula; turn it on once its proper position is confirmed (as just described).
- Move the vitrectomy probe to the nasal side (even if the retina has not been recognized in time and part of it got removed, it is the nasal, not the temporal, retina that has been cut into) and start "digging" in a mostly vertical fashion. The goal is to create a tunnel so as to eventually visualize the retina. Once the retina is identified, the rest of the operation becomes a lot easier and less stressful.
- It is a crucial part of the surgery to detach and remove the posterior hyaloid (Fig. 10). Obviously, it may be very difficult, occasionally impossible, to detach it in these typically young patients, especially if the retina is detached; nevertheless, an honest attempt must be made. Many postoperative complications can be prevented by doing so (keep in mind the most basic law of vitrectomy: future problems arise from vitreous still present, not from vitreous already removed).
- Extend the vitreous removal to the base (shaving) and make sure the surface of the ciliary body is cleansed (see above).

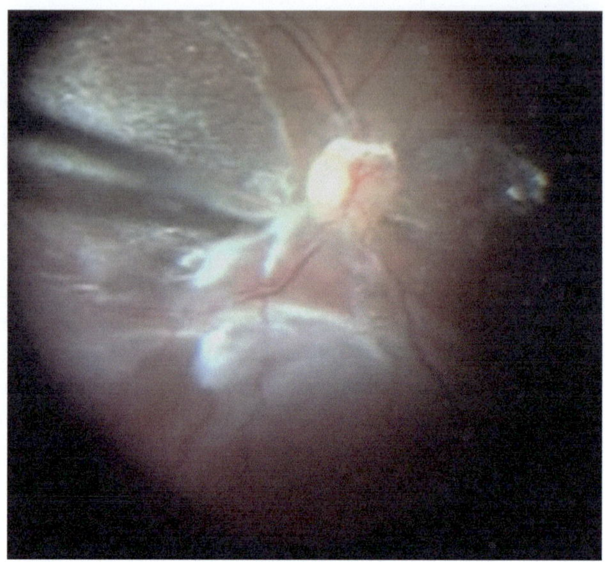

Fig. 10 Lack of posterior vitreous detachment (PVD) in traumatic RD (image taken from intraoperative video). In this eye with a postcontusion RD, triamcinolone has been injected to demonstrate the lack of PVD. Without triamcinolone use, the surgeon assumes that PVD exists; any left-behind vitreous poses a significant complication risk postoperatively

15 Retinal Detachment

In most cases, a traumatic RD does not substantially differ from one of nontraumatic origin (see Chap. 6); the treatment does not differ either. The exceptions include the following.

- Vitreous hemorrhage is much more common than in other types of RD.
- *Dialysis is usually the cause particularly when trauma is in* young patients with healthy vitreous; consequently, the detachment follows the trauma by several months or even years.
- *The frequency of an accompanying subretinal hemorrhage.* Blood under the detached retina is much more common than with a nontraumatic etiology.
- *The likelihood of the posterior hyaloid still being attached.* Even though the lack of posterior vitreous detachment (PVD) is rather common in idiopathic RDs, in the trauma setting spontaneous (already existing) PVD is an exception.
- *The risk of pre- and postoperative scarring.* Proliferative vitreoretinopathy is more likely to be associated with an RD in the trauma setting. In young people, a closed-funnel, complete RD may present as early as 1 week postinjury.
- *The timing of intervention.* As should be obvious from the list above, it is very important to perform early surgery to treat or, preferably, prevent RD after an injury.
- *The staging of intervention.* If feasible, the initial operation for an open-globe injury (wound closure) is combined with comprehensive intraocular reconstruction, i.e., scleral buckling and/or vitrectomy in the same session (while the risk of an intraoperative ["expulsive"] hemorrhage is increased during such a com-

prehensive surgery, the benefits are numerous). If such a comprehensive primary surgery is not feasible (the personnel, facility, surgical infrastructure, etc. are not available), the initial surgery should be a prompt wound closure, followed by intense topical corticosteroid treatment, and the ultimate intraocular reconstruction within 4 days (see above).

- Endolaser cerclage is recommended to help prevent postoperative RD development due to break formation and/or mild traction.

15.1 Surgical Technique

The actual surgical technique does not differ from that employed for RD of nontraumatic etiology. The technique is discussed in Chap. 8; here we list some additional considerations.

- *Pneumatic retinopexy.* This is almost never used in a trauma setting.
- *Scleral buckling* vs. *vitrectomy.* Because of the high probability of existing comorbidities, it is uncommon to choose scleral buckling over vitrectomy; it may be reasonable, though, to supplement the vitrectomy with an additional scleral buckle. Crucially, the vitrectomy must be complete, not relying on the buckle to compensate for the lack of completeness.
- *Prophylactic chorioretinectomy.* In certain types of trauma (large posterior scleral wound, perforating wound with an exit wound beneath the sclera, deep [choroideo-scleral] impact site in an IOFB injury), the risk of scarring originating at the wound/impact site (even if PVR does not develop, the retina may get caught in the local scar, and full-thickness retinal folds will develop; these folds can be more than a centimeter long, thereby reaching into the fovea even from quite a distance) is very high. This site should be treated properly and promptly, before the PVR process starts [4].

  - Complete the vitreous removal, including the creation of a PVD.
  - Set the diathermy power to the maximum.
  - Create a barrier around the site by applying a contiguous row of spots with the endodiathermy probe. This maneuver is intended not to deal with bleeding (although it does that, too) but to burn both the retina and the choroid around the site so that in the end only bare sclera remains. The probe should be kept at each application spot long enough to achieve tissue destruction. Bubbles emerge from each application site as the retina and choroid get vaporized.
  - Vacuum the entire area to remove any tissue debris; make sure there is no tissue bridge left behind, which would connect the wound/impact site with the remaining retinal edge.
  - Apply endolaser around the site only if the lesion is anterior, where the removal of the vitreous is questionable or impossible. Endolaser posteriorly is not necessary; it just enlarges the scotoma.

- If the lesion is close to the fovea or a major blood vessel would be incorporated posteriorly, there is a risk of late foveal involvement in the pigmentary reaction that may follow the chorioretinectomy or the closure of the vessel. In such cases an individual decision must be made whether to proceed; one option is to do an incomplete chorioretinectomy, sparing the macular side of the lesion and the vessel.
- If no chorioretinectomy has been performed prophylactically and retinal folds develop in the postoperative period, the procedure can still be done, and the folds should disappear [5].

16 Proliferative Vitreoretinopathy

The scarring process may start much earlier than in a nontraumatic setting; it may also be more aggressive, and more prone to recur. All of these argue in favor of an earlier (prophylactic) vitrectomy as well as for a more complete one. The *surgical technique*, however, is no different from a postoperative PVR and is discussed in Chap. 11. We just emphasize the usefulness of a hooked needle in searching for, and removing, epiretinal proliferative tissue (Fig. 11).

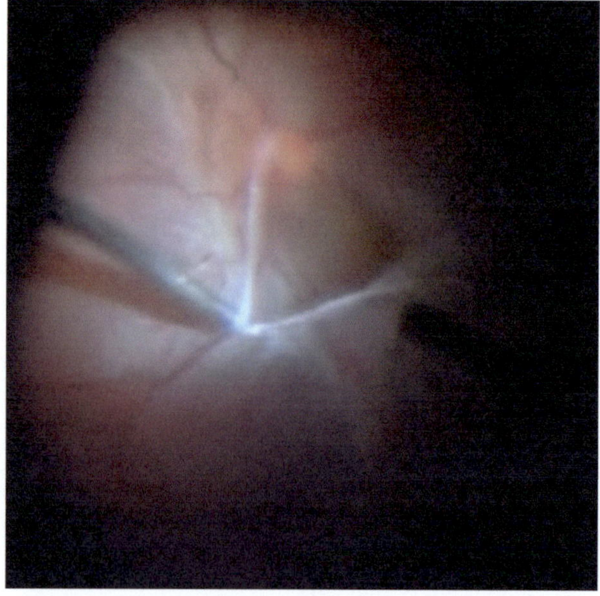

Fig. 11 Use of a hooked needle in PVR surgery (image taken from intraoperative video). The needle has a small hook at the tip, which can be turned toward the retina and carefully dragged over the surface to identify membranes or turned away from the retina to lift the membrane

17   Intraocular Foreign Body

Leaving behind a ferrous IOFB always poses the risk of siderosis; an intralenticular or encapsulated IOFB is no exception. This risk must always be kept in mind if the surgeon decides not to remove the IOFB. The only exceptions are IOFBs that are inert, free of endophthalmitis risk, and without sharp edges; in addition, no serious additional pathology is present (even then, it is psychologically difficult for many people to accept harboring foreign material in their eye, and they may push to have it removed). Not recognizing that an injury involves an IOFB is the most common cause of malpractice litigation; the ophthalmologist should therefore always take a careful history and err on the side of caution (i.e., the word "hammer" should always sound the alarm) (Fig. 12).

The goal of surgery is *not* the removal of the IOFB; it is to restore the normal anatomy so that function can follow. IOFB extraction is only a *part* of treatment, however important a part it is.

17.1   Surgical Technique [6]

- Complete the vitrectomy before IOFB removal is attempted. This is true even if the IOFB is in the vitreous, with no retinal involvement.
- If the IOFB is already encapsulated, the capsule must be fully opened with sharp instruments so that the IOFB is completely free of any tissue connections.
- The extraction instrument must be carefully chosen, based on the IOFB's size (3-dimensional, not just its length), surface texture (slippery?), shape (spherical?), and material (ferrous?). A strong permanent intraocular magnet should be used for IOFBs that are magnetic, and a proper forceps or lasso for all others.
- The extraction incision must never be too small. Calculate the 3-dimensional size of the IOFB (compare it to a precisely known object such as the intraocular instrument, not to a guessed-only entity such as the optic disk or a retinal blood vessel) plus the removal tool's size (i.e., forceps jaws) before cutting the sclera. If transconjunctival surgery is performed, make a fourth incision rather than take out a cannula. Once the sclera is incised, use Vannas scissors to cut the choroid at each wound end (the choroid is elastic; without the extra cuts, its opening will always be smaller than the one in the sclera, and the IOFB may get stuck/lost here.). Always remember: a wound that is a little too large is never a problem; one that is a little too small surely is.
- Engage the IOFB and remove it slowly; when it is in the midvitreous cavity, switch out the light pipe for a toothed forceps and slightly open the scleral wound to further reduce the risk of IOFB loss.
- Suture the incision and complete the vitrectomy as needed.
- In aphakic eyes and eyes rendered aphakic at the time of surgery, IOFB can be removed through the anterior segment (Video 2).
- Always finish surgery with endolaser cerclage (Fig. 12).

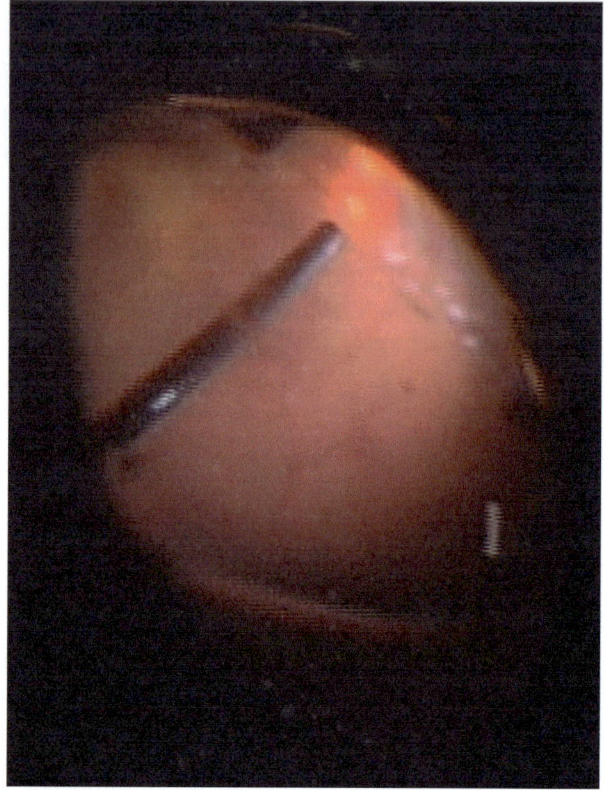

Fig. 12 Laser cerclage (image taken from intraoperative video). The endolaser probe is used to create a new ora serrata to reduce the risk of a postoperative RD, either from a break or mild traction from a developing proliferative tissue. The area to be lasered includes all the retina peripheral to the equator

18 Submacular Hemorrhage

A thick layer of blood, sandwiched between the retinal pigment epithelium and the photoreceptors, can inflict damage on the latter as early as 1 day postinjury. Early removal or at least dislocation from under the fovea is therefore essential; if the macular area is spared, the decision whether to intervene or observe is an individual one.

If intervention is selected, there are many options, including:

- Intravitreal injection of tPA and an air bubble.
- Subretinal injection of tPA and an air bubble plus a subretinal air bubble.
- Surgical removal—this is described below (see Chap. 21 for further details).

18.1   Surgical Technique

Following a complete vitrectomy, a decision must be made whether the blood is to be removed through a relatively small paramacular retinotomy (Fig. 13) or a large peripheral one. The latter has the advantage of giving much better access to the blood but the disadvantage of posing a higher PVR risk.

Inject tPA (0.4 ml of fluid, containing 0.125 mg of tPA in 0.1 ml), wait ~30 min, and irrigate out the liquefied blood. If a clot remains, it can be removed with suction or with forceps. If tPA has not been used or was ineffective, remember: the clot is elastic and will require a retinotomy smaller than the size of the clot itself.

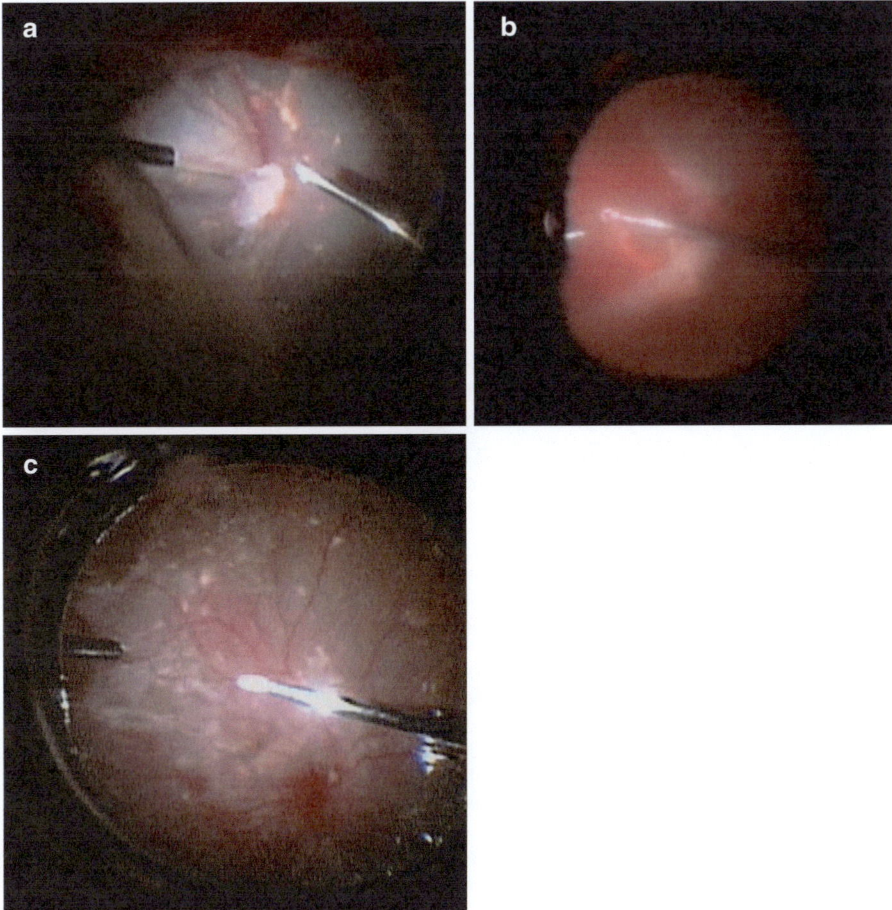

Fig. 13 Removal of subretinal blood (images taken from intraoperative video). (**a**) The posterior retina is detached over a large bleed. Triamcinolone is still seen on the disc; it was used to confirm that the posterior hyaloid had been detached and removed. (**b**) A paramacular retinotomy has been created and the subretinal blood is being irrigated out. (**c**) The subretinal blood has been removed and the retina is now reattached

19 Macular Hole

There is controversy whether surgical intervention should be performed early, or observation is warranted since these holes have a presumably higher chance of spontaneous closure compared to idiopathic macular holes. This and the duration of observation require an individual decision, based on the patient's decision after proper counseling.

Obviously, comorbidities such as a choroidal rupture can limit the visual prognosis.

The *surgical technique*, should this be the chosen option, is no different from that for an idiopathic hole and is discussed in Chap. 15.

Key Points
- More eyes than not have tissue damage not only anteriorly but posteriorly as well; hence, it is usually preferable for the vitreoretinal, rather than the anterior segment, surgeon to treat the patient.
- The typical approach to a severely injured eye is the staged management: wound closure as the first intervention, followed by the intraocular reconstruction weeks later. This philosophy should be abandoned and replaced by one in which the comprehensive intraocular reconstruction is done primarily – in the same setting as the wound closure – or no later than within 4 days of the trauma.
- Eyes that lost light perception after the injury should not be given up on but, after careful counseling of the patient, managed no differently from an identical injury where light perception is still present.
- The removal of a vitreous hemorrhage is typically straightforward, regardless of etiology – except if the bleeding occurs in the context of trauma. The surgery is especially difficult if the patient is young.

References

1. Pieramici DJ, Sternberg P Jr, Aaberg TM Sr, Bridges WZ Jr, Capone A Jr, Cardillo JA, DeJuan E Jr, Kuhn F, Meredith TA, Mieler WF, Olsen TW, Rubsamen P, Stout T. A system for classifying mechanical injuries of the eye (globe). Am J Ophthalmol. 1997;123:820–31.
2. Agrawal R, Wei HS, Teoh S. Predictive factors for final outcome of severely traumatized eyes with no light perception. BMC Ophthalmol. 2012;19:12–6.
3. Kuhn F, Mester V. Anterior chamber abnormalities and cataract. Ophthalmol Clin N Am. 2002;15:195–203.
4. Kuhn F, Schrader W. Prophylactic chorioretinectomy for eye injuries with high proliferative-vitreoretinopathy risk. Clin Anat. 2018;31:28–38.
5. Kuhn F, Teixeira S, Pelayes D. Late versus prophylactic chorioretinectomy for the prevention of trauma-related proliferative vitreoretinopathy. Ophthalmic Res. 2012;48(S1):331–7.
6. Loporchio D, Mukkamala L, Gorukanti K, Zarbin M, Langer P, Bhagat N. Intraocular foreign bodies: a review. Surv Ophthalmol. 2016;61:582–96.

Vitreoretinal Surgery in Pediatrics

Şengül Özdek and Hüseyin Baran Özdemir

1 Introduction

This chapter discusses the philosophy of pediatric vitreoretinal surgery (VRS) with its features, highlights, and differences from adult VRS.

1.1 *Differences in Pediatric VRS*

VRS in pediatric eyes has a different philosophy than in adult eyes. It has its own rules and unique complications, does not forgive faults, and does not accept apologies. So, before starting with pediatric VRS, the surgeon should have had enough practice with adult VRS.

Anatomical Differences

- Limited surgical space: Interpalpebral rim is very narrow, which limits eye movements for surgical maneuvers in premature babies and neonates. This can be widened with a small canthotomy, and it can be sutured with a U-shaped subcutaneous 7/0 vicryl suture at the end of the surgery.

Supplementary Information The online version contains supplementary material available at https://doi.org/10.1007/978-3-031-47827-7_29.

Ş. Özdek (✉) · H. B. Özdemir
Department of Ophthalmology, Gazi University School of Medicine, Ankara, Turkey
e-mail: sozdek@gazi.edu.tr

A. B. Sallam et al. (eds.), *Practical Manual of Vitreoretinal Surgery*,
https://doi.org/10.1007/978-3-031-47827-7_29

359

- Small eye: The globe is small, but it is not a smaller model of the adult eye. The crystalline lens is relatively large and spherical, the pars plana has not fully developed yet (till 8–9 months of age), and the sclera is thin and elastic. Pediatric eyes have a very formed vitreous, which is usually strongly adherent to the retina [1, 2].

Philosophical Differences

- Iatrogenic retinal breaks should be avoided for any purpose. Retinal breaks usually end up with surgical failure in stages 4–5 retinopathy of prematurity (ROP), familial exudative retinopathy (FEVR), and posterior persistent fetal vasculature (PFV) if it is in a proliferative area like around the ridge or transition area [3].
- Proliferative vitreoretinopathy (PVR) is frequent and severe. Wound healing is more aggressive in children. Retinectomy and posterior drainage retinotomy should be avoided, especially in tractional retinal detachment (TRD) cases [3].
- Perfluorocarbon liquids (PFCL) and silicone oil (SO) are rarely used, especially for TRDs [4].
- Small children do not obey instructions for head positioning!
- The functional outcome may be limited because of amblyopia in children ≤7 years of age. So, the surgeon should take into account the amblyopia problem.

Surgical Considerations

- Limbal versus pars plana/plicata approach: This is one of the most important and decisive steps of the surgery, and it deserves special attention in children, especially under 3 years of age. The eye should be examined again just before the surgery to assess the peripheral retina to determine for any dragged retina anteriorly through the ciliary body toward the back of the lens. These parts should be avoided as an entry site for sclerotomy which may lead to retinal break formation at the beginning of the surgery. The safest place for the entry sites can be determined by using transscleral illumination, which is another useful method to determine the location of the pars plana. This is especially important in eyes with significant anterior segment abnormalities like microphthalmos and PFV, where peripheral retinal (anterior retinal elongation through the ciliary body) and ciliary body abnormalities are common. At this point, the surgeon should decide whether it is possible to enter the eye through pars plicata safely (to preserve the lens). If the peripheral retina and pars plicata look safe, then sclerotomy through pars plicata/pars plana is the first choice. If not, a limbal approach with a lensectomy should be used [5].
- The limbal approach means that the surgeon has to sacrifice the lens, which is the major disadvantage in children. The other disadvantages are the risk of iris injury and induced miosis, endothelial damage and corneal edema induction, limited view of the posterior segment because of the corneal distortion caused by limbal

entry sites, and limited access of instruments to the posterior retina hitting the indirect viewing systems. Additionally, the limbal incisions must be sutured with 10/0 vicryl or monofilament nylon sutures, which may need to be removed in another examination under general anesthesia (EUGA) session. This approach's most important advantage is avoiding peripheral retinal damage during entry. Other advantages are as follows: there is no need for canthotomy and this approach protects the conjunctiva [6].

- Trans-iris root approach, where the trocars are entered just posterior to the limbus through the iris root to reach the back of the iris, is another alternative for the entry site. Lens has to be sacrificed. However, it is possible to avoid corneal distortion problems caused by limbal entry sites to some extent and still avoid peripheral retinal damage. Complications of this approach are bleeding from the iris root into the anterior chamber, iris root damage, and iridodialysis.
- Sclerotomy step: In prematures and neonates (till 6 months old), the distance of the sclerotomy site from the limbus should be 1.5 mm, and the distance should be increased accordingly with age, which reaches 3.5 mm after 3 years of age like in adults (Table 1) [7].
- Trocars: Trocars should be placed perpendicularly without angulation in contrast to adults. Oblique entry may increase the risk of lens or peripheral retinal damage. The length of the regular adult trocars is not appropriate for the babies, and total insertion of the cannulas may cause damage to the structures, like retinal folds within the vitreous cavity. Therefore, using a piece of silicone band or buckle at the bottom of the trocar to shorten its intraocular length may be a good solution (Fig. 1). The tip of the infusion cannula should be secured and watched carefully throughout the surgery to prevent lens and peripheral retinal damage with inadvertent movement of the cannula [8].
- A conjunctival peritomy at the sites of sclerotomies should be done at the beginning, and all the sclerotomies sutured in pediatric cases. It is sometimes difficult to have watertight closure of the sclerotomies in pediatric cases. This is extremely important, especially in eyes with active neovascularization, because leakage through the sclerotomies may end up with hypotony causing postoperative hemorrhages and failure. A preplaced suture for the infusion cannula may prevent hypotony during sclerotomy closure (Fig. 1).
- Gauge: Any gauge (20–27 G) vitrectomy settings can be used during pediatric VRS. The most commonly used ones are 23 G and 25 G. Although there are vitrectomy settings with short vitrectomy and illumination probes, we do not

Table 1 Preferred limbus to sclerotomy distances for children

Age	Limbus to sclerotomy distance
0–6 months	1.5 mm
6–12 months	2 mm
1–2 years	2.5 mm
2–3 years	3.0 mm
>3 years	3.5 mm

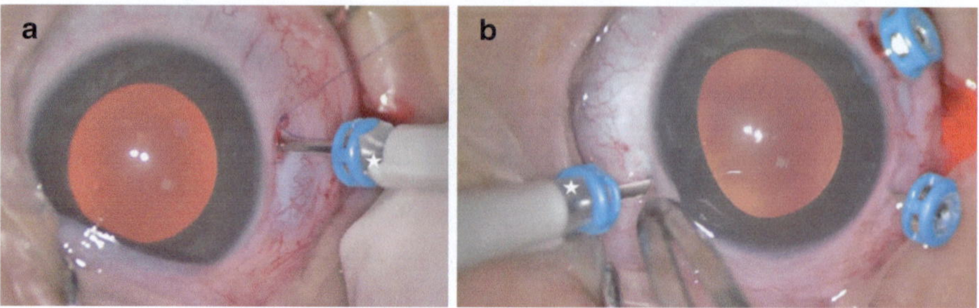

Fig. 1 (a) Insertion of the shortened 25-gauge trocar for the infusion cannula after placement of a piece of silicone band (white star) before the cannula through the preplaced 8/0 vicryl sutured sclerotomy area. (b) Pars plana insertion of other shortened trocars after peritomy

believe that this has any advantage over regular adult probes since the surgeon can insert only the needed length of the instrument, unlike the trocars. However, shorter trocars and cannulas may avoid peripheral retinal and lens problems during entry to some extent.

- Two- vs. three-port entries: Two-port vitrectomy needs different surgical instrumentation setups like infused forceps and scissors and endoillumination probes, etc., since there is no separate infusion port in this setting. There are only superior two ports which give the advantage of enough space to move the eye during surgery which is normally limited with the third trocar in the inferotemporal quadrant so there is no need for canthotomy in neonates and prematures. However, one hand has to be within the eye all the time to avoid hypotony, which may be tiring for the surgeon, and there may be more risk of hypotony during the closure of sclerotomies. Three-port vitrectomy, on the other hand, has the advantage of using the same instrumentation as in adults, which all surgeons are familiar with. There is no need for a different setup and instruments. Another advantage is less risk of hypotony because of the use of a separate infusion cannula. However, the third entry means an additional risk for peripheral retina or lens damage, and there is less space for maneuvers within the narrow interpalpebral rim, especially in babies.
- Use of cannulas in entry sites: It is possible to do the surgery with or without a cannula. Valved cannulas are useful to prevent vitreous herniation and leakage through the entry sites. However, it may prevent visualization and access to the peripheral retina, where you need to retract the cannula outward. In very small eyes (microphthalmia) and eyes with predominantly anterior retinal pathologies, the risk of damage to the lens or peripheral retina with trocars and cannulas is higher, and the cannulas may restrict the extent of maneuvers of microforceps and scissors in the peripheral retina by restricting the opening of the tips of the forceps squeezed in the tight cannula. In such cases, scleral or limbal entry can be done directly without a cannula. However, this approach has risks of vitreous herniation, leakage through the entry sites in the pars plana/plicata approach, iris damage and herniation together with pupillary problems, and increased incidence of corneal edema in the limbal approach.

- Lensectomy: When lensectomy is planned, a total capsulectomy has to be performed since the residual capsule serves as a scaffold for membrane proliferation and secondary circumferential vitreoretinal contraction. This may result in ciliary body detachment and hypotony. It may be impossible to peel this membrane when it turns into a contractile anterior ring. In cases with lenticular-retinal apposition, it is usually easy to dissect the capsular material with forceps without causing retinal breaks. However, one should be cautious about not causing retinal dialysis [9].
- Lensectomy complications: Secondary glaucoma, aphakia-related problems, and amblyopia are the main concerns in lensectomized eyes. Aphakia correction and amblyopia treatment are the main additional concerns in such eyes.
- Perfusion pressure of the retina is lower in children since they have lower systolic blood pressure. The infusion pressure should be kept lower than the adults during surgery, and prolonged scleral depression should be avoided to prevent central retinal artery occlusion [10].
- Posterior hyaloid removal: This is essential for cases with a retinal break, like in rhegmatogenous retinal detachment (RRD) and trauma. It is not essential for TRD cases like in ROP, FEVR, and PFV. In these conditions we always attempt to remove the posterior hyaloid from the posterior pole area only to decrease the risk of future posterior hyaloid contractions leading to visual loss. Triamcinolone is important for this purpose. The posterior vitreous detachment (PVD) can be induced easily with the vacuum of the vitrector in approximately half of the cases. If this is not possible, microforceps can be used to grasp the hyaloid at the edge of the disc together with a piece of the inner limiting membrane (ILM) in some occasions. When a small opening is made, it is easy to detach the remaining hyaloid with hydrodissection by the circulating balanced salt solution (BSS) in the vitreous cavity. PVD separation should be done in a limited area, especially in eyes like ROP, avoiding the ridge area, which may cause hemorrhage and iatrogenic retinal breaks. If it is impossible to detach the hyaloid, one should forego this step, avoid iatrogenic break, and trim the vitreous as much as possible by using the triamcinolone again and again to see the remaining vitreous. However, if a retinal break already exists, PFCL can be used as a third hand both to stabilize the retina and to dissect the hyaloid from the retina once it is initiated at one point [11, 12].
- The main aim of the surgery is to relieve the tractions as much as possible without inducing an iatrogenic break in TRD cases like ROP, PFV, and FEVR. Perioperative attachment of the retina should not be expected in these cases. Total peeling of all membranes or removal of all the hyaloid is never aimed. They may be left in place if the surgeon feels further peeling is associated with a high risk of retinal break or hemorrhage.
- Tamponade and iatrogenic retinal break: Air is our first choice in pediatric VRS if there is no retinal break. Air helps to seal the entry sites, to decrease the risk of postoperative hypotony and hemorrhage, and to decrease inflammation. If there is a retinal break in TRD cases like PFV, ROP, and FEVR, this will change the choice of tamponade. If the retinal break is in a silent area, try to clear the vitreous and any residual membrane, at least locally, around the break area, and continue with argon laser photocoagulation (ALP) to the break and place a C3F8 gas tamponade. If it is in the most proliferative area, like the vicinity of a ridge or transition zone where

there is quite a lot of membrane and tissue which has a very high contraction capacity, recurrent PVR may be unavoidable, and it may be logical to abandon the surgery. It is almost impossible to get rid of all the membranes in such conditions. Another option may be the use of a segmental scleral buckle if the break is not in a too posterior location and is suitable for a local buckle placement. The tamponade of choice is C3F8 gas in such situations. SO is not preferred since there are always residual membranes in these diseases which may contract and cause subretinal migration of SO. However, it can be used effectively in eyes with RRD and ocular trauma in pediatric eyes where it is possible to clear all the vitreous and the membranes. High viscosity SO should be preferred in pediatric VRS to try to prevent early emulsification, which is supposed to occur earlier in pediatric cases [9].

- Scleral buckling (SB): SB is a very effective surgical tool for pediatric RRD, which preserves the vitreous and the lens. It can also be used for other cases like ROP, FEVR, and Coats diseases to counteract the peripheral traction caused by residual membranes, as an adjunct to pars plana vitrectomy (PPV). It supports the vitreous base and peripheral retina. However, when the patient is too young (less than 3 years of age), the encircling band has to be removed 6 months after the surgery [13].

- Same-day bilateral surgery: It is normally avoided in adults because of the risk of endophthalmitis. However, in pediatric cases, like ROP and FEVR, where both eyes show similar findings and need immediate surgery, waiting for days or weeks might lead to blindness in the later operated eye. Amblyopia risk and transport difficulties may add to other factors. Furthermore, general anesthesia-related complications in a small baby increase when anesthesia is repeated in a short interval. These benefits outweigh the small risk of endophthalmitis and supports performing bilateral surgery in the same session (i.e., immediate sequential bilateral vitrectomy surgery).

2   Pediatric Vitreoretinal Surgery in Featured Cases

Pediatric VRS techniques are mainly needed for ROP stages 4 and 5 and cicatricial stage, PFV, FEVR, advanced Coats disease, CXLR, shaken baby, and other pediatric ocular trauma and pediatric RRD.

2.1   Vitreoretinal Surgery for ROP

Surgery for Stage 4 ROP (Video 1)

- This is the most typical surgery where the surgeon should know when to stop. The proverb "Perfection is the enemy of good" by Voltaire fits very well to this condition. The surgeon should avoid any iatrogenic retinal break formation. Stage 4A is the last chance for the baby to get a useful good vision (Fig. 2) [14].

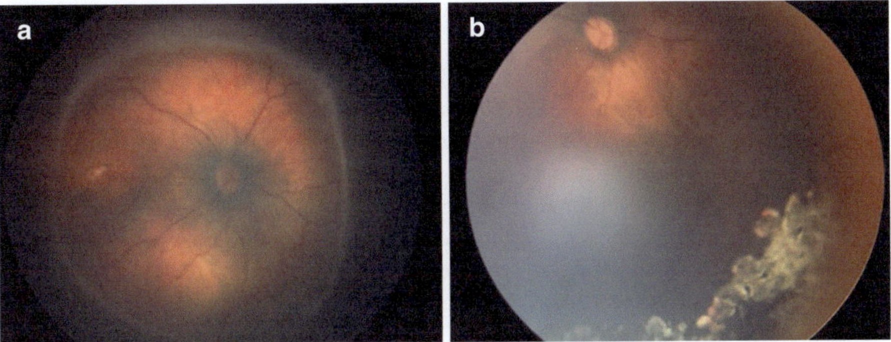

Fig. 2 Stage 4A retinopathy of prematurity (ROP). (**a**) Preoperative 360° peripheral retinal detachment. (**b**) Postoperative fully attached retina with laser scars at the peripheral retina of the same eye

- We prefer a 3-port entry with a 25- gauge (g) vitrectomy setting with shortened trocars after canthotomy, and peritomy in most of the pars plana surgeries.
- The main aim is to cut the fibrotic membranous connections from the ridge to the peripheral retina/pars plana and the back of the lens anteriorly and to the optic nerve head posteriorly. This will release the traction and let the retina go backward during follow-up. Perioperative attachment of the retina is not expected. PVD induction in a limited area in the posterior pole is advised but not a must. When PVD is induced, it should never be done all of a sudden till the periphery, as done in adults, but one should be very cautious to avoid induction of retinal breaks by the traction of the posterior hyaloid. Membrane peeling is not a must in stage 4A cases, but it has to be done in most of the stage 4B cases very cautiously. Air-fluid exchange at the end of the surgery is a rule in our practice for all ROP cases [15].
- VRS should be performed as soon as possible when RD is detected. If the retina is vascularly very active with plus disease, anti-VEGF injection the day before the surgery may help to prevent preop and postop hemorrhages. However, if the interval between the injection and the surgery gets longer, detachment may get converted into a crunch-type total RD.
- Early argon laser photocoagulation (ALP) usually stabilizes the peripheral retina, which makes lens-sparing vitrectomy (LSV) more likely and the surgery easier.
- The major factors negatively affecting the success rate of the surgery were the advanced stage of the disease, absence of preoperative treatment, presence of preoperative plus disease, postoperative vitreous hemorrhage, inability to induce PVD, lensectomy, and iatrogenic tear formation [16–19].

Surgery for Stage 5 ROP

- VRS is questionable, especially in unilateral cases. Anatomical and functional results are very poor at stage 5. However, not all stage 5 cases are the same. Eyes with total RD where the posterior pole can be seen ophthalmoscopically do better with surgery than those with total leukocoria where there is closed funnel RD. Visual expectations are very low. We can expect preservation of light perception or some ambulatory vision (if fortunately) at most. Some surgeons do not operate stage 5 eyes when the fellow eye is good. However, these eyes usually become deformed over time with the development of phthisis bulbi and/or corneal opacification. That is why VRS may even be done for only cosmetic purposes to preserve the globe and to prevent the development of a deformed and unacceptable appearance for such eyes. Lensectomy-vitrectomy (LV) surgery with a limbal entry is the preferred method for eyes with leukocoria (Fig. 3); however, LSV with pars plana entry may still be used in eyes where the peripheral retina is not dragged to the back of the lens or ciliary body (Fig. 4).

- A "staged surgery" is a good option in leukocoric stage 5 cases. The main fibrotic bands causing tractions are usually removed during the first surgery. The retina is given time to settle down and go backward to attach at least partially within a few months. Then, a second surgery can be planned to remove smaller membranes and relieve the retinal tractions further.
- Advanced late-stage 5 cases usually come with anterior segment changes like very shallow anterior chamber and irido-corneo-lenticular adhesions leading to corneal opacification (Fig. 5). We do not prefer to do surgery after corneal opacification.

Surgery for Cicatricial ROP

It is well known that low vision, high myopia/astigmatism, amblyopia, strabismus, glaucoma, cataract, vitreous hemorrhage, late reactivation of fibrovascular proliferation and exudation (3.6%), RRD, and TRD are more prevalent in previously regressed ROP during their whole life.

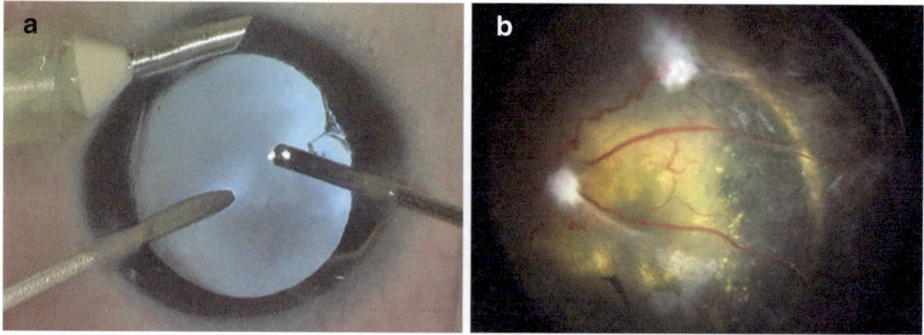

Fig. 3 (**a**) Leukocoric stage 5 retinopathy of prematurity (ROP) treated with limbal lensectomy vitrectomy. (**b**) Postoperative fourth-year fundus picture with total shallow detachment and some residual membranes over the disc and arcuate vessels. Visual acuity is hand motion

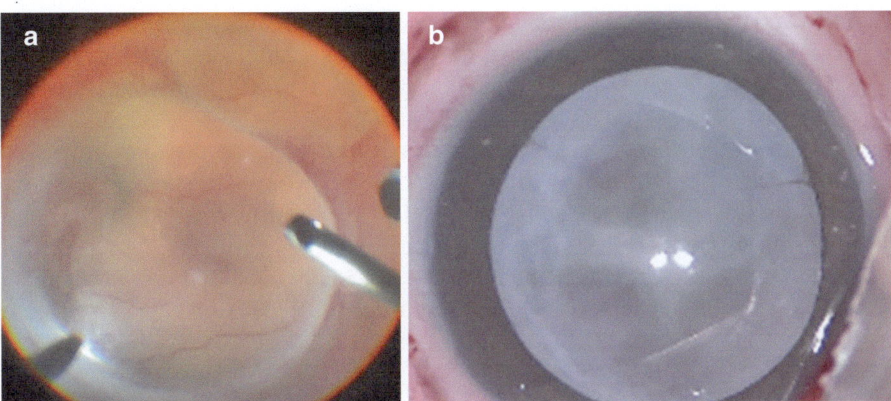

Fig. 4 Stage 5 retinopathy of prematurity (ROP). (**a**) Retinal detachment (RD) with an open funnel where lens sparing vitrectomy is still possible. (**b**) Closed funnel RD with leukocoric presentation where a limbal lensectomy vitrectomy is the preferred technique for surgery

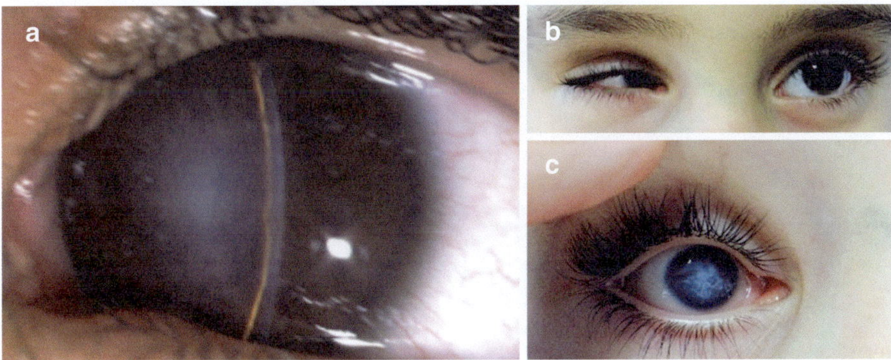

Fig. 5 (**a**) Corneal opacification with irido-corneo-lenticular adhesions in a late cicatricial stage 5 ROP. (**b**) Another bilateral stage 5 ROP. Right eye (RE) was unoperated; Left eye was operated. Note that RE has bad cosmesis with pre-phthisis bulbi and corneal opacification within several years (**c**) [20]

- TRD in cicatricial ROP: VRS may lead to good anatomical and functional results in selected cicatricial ROP cases. Case selection is important and one should keep in mind the risk of losing present vision after the surgery because of surgical complications. Sometimes no surgery is a better decision. Factors that should be considered in this context include the following: Is the retina detached since the neonatal period, or has the detachment developed later in life with the growth of the globe? Is there severe amblyopia? Is it possible to get a useful vision if anatomical success is achieved? If the history reveals that the vision was better previously but got worse over time, it may be possible to get a good functional result after surgery. Another clue for operability is the nature of the membrane and the direction of the traction. If the membranes are too tightly attached to the retina and the traction is tangential, then it may be better not to operate such eyes. However, if there is anteroposterior traction by the membrane and if this traction could easily and safely be relieved with dissection of this membrane, then the surgery would most probably be a success (Fig. 6).

- It is known that the eye grows with age, but fibrotic tissue does not grow, and during this period, retinal traction may get worse, causing progressive TRD. Relieving these tractions may lead to good anatomical and visual outcomes in selected late cicatricial ROP cases.
- Anatomical success was achieved in 91%, and improvement in VA was noted in 82% of cases in our series of TRD in cicatricial ROP [21].

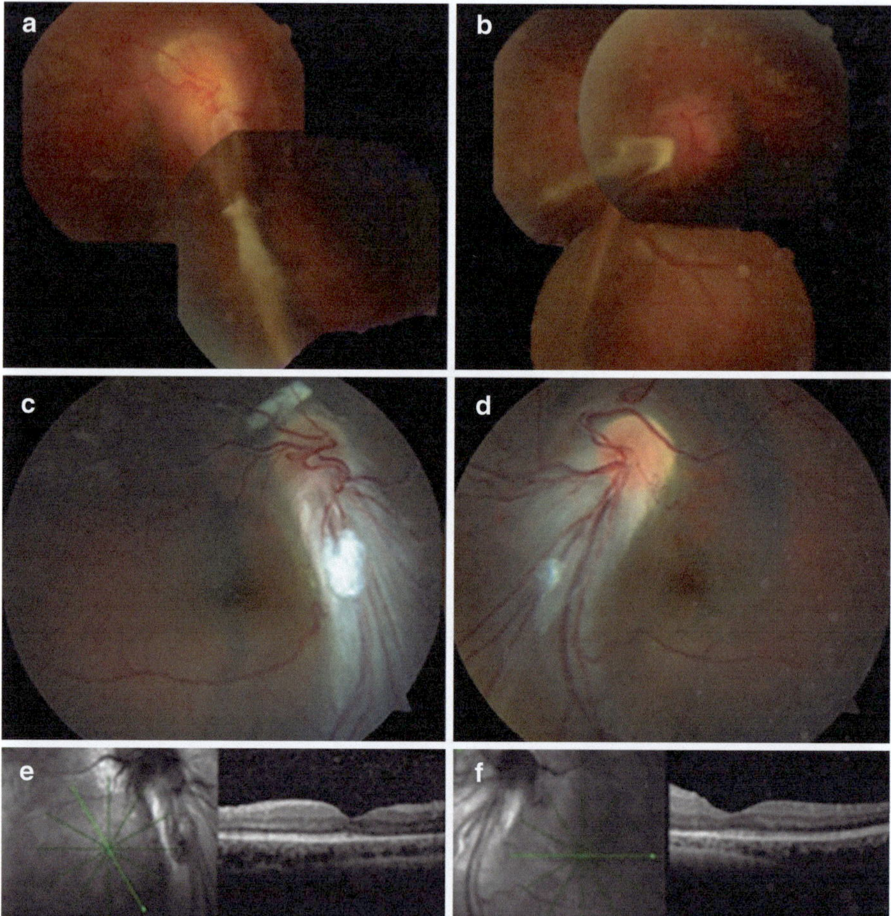

Fig. 6 Cicatricial retinopathy of prematurity (ROP). (**a, b**) A 6-year-old boy with a premature birth history. He did not have any treatment for ROP during the neonatal period. Preoperative tractional retinal detachment in both eyes where the retina is dragged to the inferonasal periphery with a VA of 0.1 (OD) and 0.15 (OS). (**c–f**) Postoperative third-year colored picture and optical coherence tomography (OCT) of the same case following lens-sparing vitrectomy with a VA of 0.3 (OD) and 0.7 (OS)

- RRD in cicatricial adult ROP is frequently misdiagnosed as Stickler-like disease because of the high frequency of high myopia and lattice degeneration in these eyes. Adolescents or young adults with RRD associated with high myopia and shallow foveal contour should be asked about premature birth history for differential diagnosis.
- RRD in cicatricial ROP is usually a more complex detachment, and it is more likely to require multiple procedures with lower visual and anatomical outcomes. Two-thirds of the patients who underwent PPV had poor postoperative visual acuity in this group.
- RRD should be tried to be treated with scleral buckling procedures without PPV if possible. Vitreoretinal and membrane adhesion may be very strong, and may not be possible to peel the membranes in these cases during PPV, which leads to the failure of the surgery.
- High myopia, lattice degenerations, vitreoretinal interface disorders, retinoschisis, late reactivation of proliferation and exudation, and vitreous hemorrhage are the other common problems during adolescence or adulthood in addition to complex RRD and TRD.
- Even cataract surgery has some peculiarities and is associated with a high rate (23%) of retinal complications in cicatricial ROP cases [21].

2.2   Familial Exudative Vitreoretinopathy

Familial exudative vitreoretinopathy (FEVR) is a hereditary retinal vascular disease in which the peripheral retinal vessels fail to develop, resulting in a peripheral avascular retina resembling ROP in full-term babies. The main difference from ROP is the life-long progressive nature of the disease. It may have variable periods of quiescence. The most common pattern of inheritance is autosomal dominant. A positive family history (present in 45% of the cases) is helpful but not mandatory for the differential diagnosis. Family screening may yield a high rate of asymptomatic disease in family members. Retinal angiogenesis is defective, leading to insufficient vascular differentiation and incomplete peripheral retinal vascularization. This may lead to the formation of vascular buds in the junction of the vascular-avascular retina, which may result in fibrovascular membranes, dragged retinal vessels, and retinal folds pulling the retina to the periphery till the back of the lens. Exudation may accompany all these processes. There is tractional or exudative RD in 21– 64% of the cases [22, 23].

Differential Diagnosis of FEVR

- ROP: Fluorescein angiography (FA) is important for differential diagnosis. There is a classical regular homogeneous vascularization pattern at the ridge in ROP in contrast to irregular vascularization and sprouting beyond the transition zone, vascular pruning, and pinpoint hyperfluorescent dots in FEVR cases.

- FEVR in premature babies is called ROPER. These babies are usually bigger with milder prematurity, who develop ROP-like disease. FA again gives important clues for the differential. It is important to differentiate ROP and FEVR because their prognosis is different. FEVR has a lifelong progression that needs treatments during the whole life in contrast to ROP [24].
- Incontinentia pigmenti (IP) is an inherited retinal disease with X-linked dominant inheritance. Only the female gender is affected since it is fatal in male fetuses. The disease can be differentiated from FEVR by the characteristic skin abnormalities as well as dental and neurological problems.
- Norrie disease affects almost entirely males with an X-linked recessive pattern of inheritance. The majority of patients suffer from progressive hearing loss starting mostly in their second decade of life and learning difficulties. It almost always leads to blindness. Genetic testing is important for differential diagnosis [25].
- Coats disease is an important differential diagnosis. Differentiating features are unilaterality, absence of family history, exudation is more prominent than the TRD, male predominance, and typical telangiectatic vessels.
- Diseases causing TRD: Posterior PFV (unilaterality, microphthalmia), *Toxocara* and *Toxoplasma* (unilaterality, serological tests).
- Diseases with neovascularization: IRVAN and Eales diseases should be concerned.

Clinical Findings

- Bilateral but mostly asymmetric findings.
- Peripheral avascular areas (more in temporal), straightening of vessels, and macular ectopia.
- Peripheral vascular loops, hard exudates, and neovascularization (NV).
- Fibrovascular proliferation: Macular fold, exudative retinal detachment (ExRD), and TRD.
- Dysgenic vitreous (also in Norrie, PFV, ROP): Vitreoretinal adhesion is very strong. The hyaloid membrane is multilaminar, like onion rings. Posterior hyaloid may contract following ALP or anti-VEGF treatment.

Classification

- Stage 1: Peripheral avascular retina.
- Stage 2: Retinal NVE (2a, without exudation; 2b, with exudation).
- Stage 3: Macula on RD (macula ectopic) (3a, without exudation; 3b, with exudation).
- Stage 4: Macula off RD (macular fold) (4a, without exudation; 4b, with exudation).
- Stage 5: Total RD-leukocoria (5a, open funnel; 5b, closed funnel).

Treatment (Video 2)

- ALP can be used in the early stages. We usually prefer ALP in stage 1 (peripheral avascular retina) and stage 2 (retinal neovascularization) if the patient is less than 3 years of age. In older children, however, we perform ALP to the avascular retina only if there is neovascularization (stage 2). It is well known that the early presentation of the disease is a sign of a worse prognosis for FEVR.
- VRS is useful for eyes with vitreous hemorrhage secondary to retinal NVE and TRD with epiretinal membrane (ERM). In advanced cases, staged surgery may be a good option where a step-by-step removal of membranes was done with consecutive surgeries, decreasing the risk of retinal breaks (Fig. 7). FEVR may be complicated with RRD, especially in adolescence or adulthood. In such conditions encircling band should be added to PPV, which increases the success rate.
- Anti-VEGFs or steroids may be used as a last option in persistent exudation or cystoid macular edema (CME) associated with LAPPEL (LAte-Phase angiographic posterior and PEripheral vascular Leakage in FA), which is considered to be a retinal endothelial cell inflammation marker and capillary dropout precursor [26, 27].

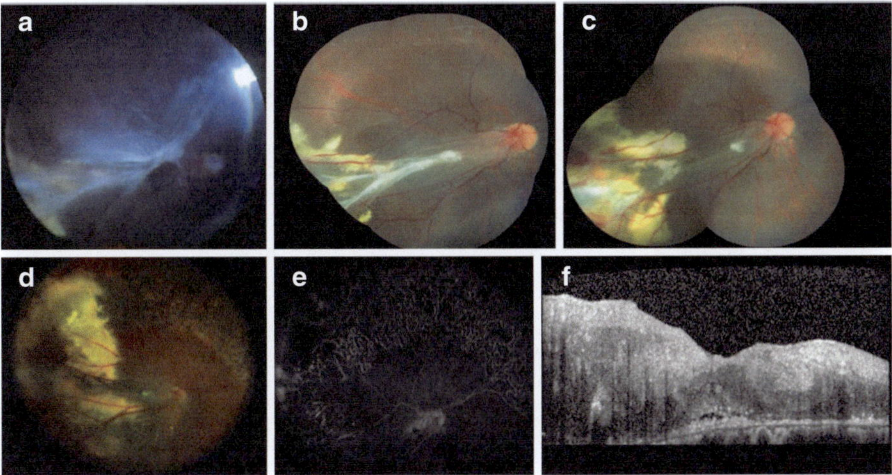

Fig. 7 Staged surgery for a familial exudative vitreoretinopathycase with only one functioning eye; left eye was lost during early childhood. (**a**) Preoperative tractional and exudative retinal detachment. The optic nerve head is barely visible. (**b**) Fundus picture 12 months following the first surgery. Note the residual membrane in the macular area and the exudation in the temporal retina. (**c**) Fundus picture after the second vitreoretinal surgery where only a very small part of the residual membrane is left. Macula became visible, which was ectopic temporally. (**d-f**) Fundus picture, flourescein angiogram and optical coherence tomography scan during a 5-year follow-up time

2.3 *Coats Disease*

Coats disease is an endothelium and pericyte disease leading to inner blood-retina barrier defect, exudation, and ischemia in early stages with a resultant ExRD and TRD in later stages. The cause is still unknown. It is seen mostly in boys during the first decade of life. Since it is unilateral in 90% of the cases, it is usually discovered late after the development of strabismus, xanthocoria/leukocoria, or painful red eye in children. The disease is more severe and aggressive in younger children, especially those under 3–4 years of age.

Classification

The current classification of Coats disease has been suggested by Shields and colleagues and updated recently to add foveal changes: [28].

- Stage 1: Only retinal telangiectasia.
- Stage 2: Telangiectasia and exudation.

  - 2a: Extrafoveal exudation.
  - 2b: Foveal exudation.

    2b1: No subfoveal nodule.
    2b2: With subfoveal nodule.

- Stage 3: ExRD.

  - 3a: Subtotal RD.

    3a1: Extrafoveal RD.
    3a2: Foveal RD.

  - 3b: Total RD.

- Stage 4: Total ExRD + neovascular glaucoma (NVG).
- Stage 5: End-stage disease (painful red eye).

Treatment

- Primary treatment: ALP (stage 1, 2, 3a) +/− intravitreal anti-VEGF, steroids.
- Cryotherapy: Stage 1, 2, 3a.
- Surgery: Stage 3–4:

  - Transscleral drainage of subretinal fluid (TSDSRF), cryo/ALP, intravitreal anti-VEGF, or steroids.
  - PPV with TSDSRF, cryo/ALP, intravitreal anti-VEGF: PPV is added when there is vitreous hemorrhage, opacity, ERM, or TRD (Fig. 8).

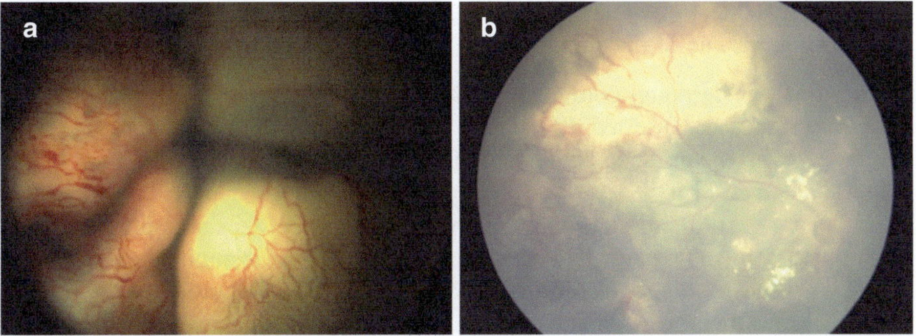

Fig. 8 (**a**) Stage 3B Coats disease with total bullous retinal detachment presenting with unilateral xanthocoria in a 1.5-year-old girl. Note the telangiectatic vessels and pathological new vessels all over the retina. Postoperative fundus picture following the external drainage, pars plana vitrectomy, endolaser, cryotherapy, fluid-air exchange, and intravitreal anti-vascular endothelial growth factor injection. (**b**) Retina was totally attached within 2 months with some residual subretinal exudates

Visual expectations are very low, and surgery is usually performed to preserve the globe to prevent progression to NVG and painful red eye in advanced cases (for cosmesis and comfort).

16% of the eyes with Coats disease are enucleated because of the painful eye. This is even higher in advanced Coats disease reaching up to 80%. Poor visual outcome (20/200 or worse) was found in 53% with stage 2, 74% with stage 3, and 100% of stages 4 and 5 of Coats disease. Spontaneous resolution of ExRD in advanced cases is extremely rare [28–31].

Surgical Steps for TSDSRF (Video 3)

1. Performing a scleral incision in the area corresponding to the most massive SRF and exudate.
2. Drainage of the SRF and exudate using a cotton bud.
3. Maintaining IOP by using a valved 25-g trocar placed at the pars plana (if the retina is not located behind the lens, in order to enable safe entry through the pars plana) or by using a limbal incision (if the detached retina is located behind the lens), as applicable.
4. Placement of a 25-g trocar at the pars plana in patients; it was not previously placed when the detached retina behind the lens moves posteriorly after drainage of SRF.
5. ALP of abnormal dilated telangiectatic vessels with a lighted endolaser probe through the trocar.
6. Application of cryotherapy in areas of peripheral telangiectasia and adjacent avascularity under indirect ophthalmoscopy (not more than two quadrants). This can also be performed using an operating microscope with indirect viewing systems by placing a chandelier light on the pre-existing trocar.

7. Intravitreal injection of bevacizumab (1.25 mg/0.05 mL, Avastin; Genentech and Roche) at the end of the surgery.

In patients undergoing combined TSDSRF and PPV, after the first three steps, three 25-g trocars are inserted through the pars plana, and a central core lens-sparing vitrectomy with membrane peeling is performed. PVD is attempted in the posterior pole till just anterior to arcuate vessels if possible. Complete separation of PVD till the periphery is not required. Following that, the last three steps are performed with the addition to air-fluid exchange before the intravitreal bevacizumab injection.

We have shown that the addition of PPV to the TSDSRF decreased the need for additional treatments in the long term as an adjunct to ablative treatments for advanced Coats disease [32].

2.4 Persistent Fetal Vasculature Syndrome

Persistent fetal vasculature (PFV), previously known as the persistent hyperplastic primary vitreous, is a rare congenital developmental abnormality caused by the failure of involution of the primary vitreous and hyaloid vasculature. PFV is a spectrum of disease that includes the remnants of the fetal hyaloid system, extending from the optic disc to the lens to varying degrees. It can be classified as anterior, posterior, and combined forms. Anterior PFV includes the presence of microphthalmia, the retrolental fibrovascular membrane, elongated ciliary processes, or cataract (Fig. 9). In contrast, the posterior subtype consists of an elevated vitreous membrane and a stalk from the optic nerve, retinal fold, or tractional detachment (Fig. 10). Nevertheless, most cases exhibit features of both, and the variety of presentations makes PFV challenging for surgical management. PFV may be together with other ocular pathologies like Peters syndrome and coloboma of the uvea [33].

The main goals of surgery for PFV are to clear the media to prevent amblyopia and relieve tractional forces to prevent RD, glaucoma, and phthisis. By releasing the

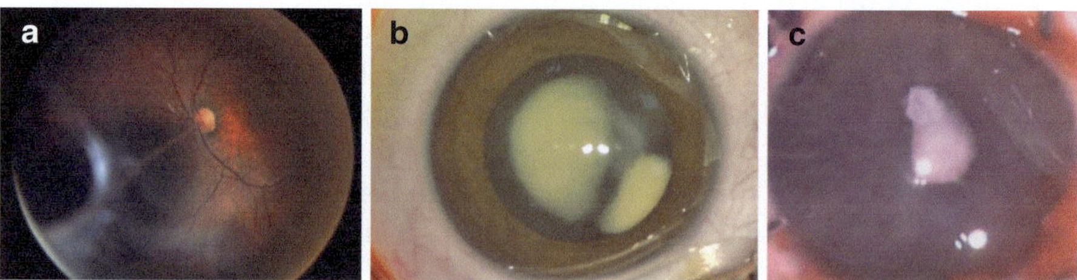

Fig. 9 Anterior PFV spectrum. (**a**) Mild anterior PFV with a thin and eccentric hyaloid artery connection to the back of the lens. (**b**) Moderate anterior PFV. Note that the periphery of the lens is mostly clear. (**c**) Severe anterior PFV with significant microphthalmia, posterior synechia, and a totally white opaque lens including vascular elements in it

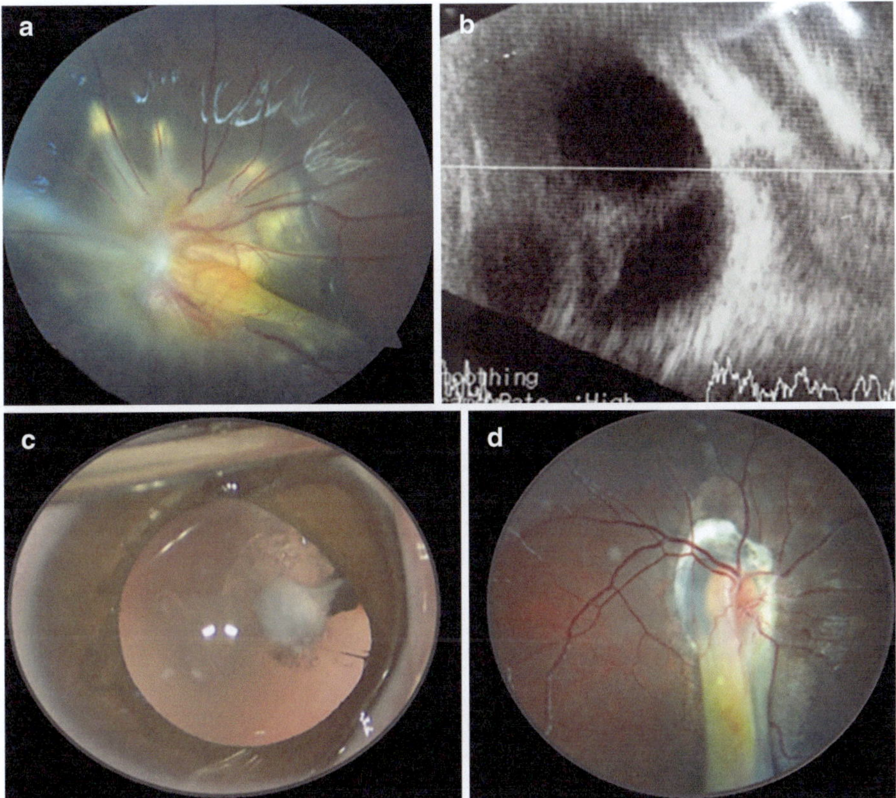

Fig. 10 A spectrum of posterior persistent fetal vasculature. (**a**) Dome- or tent-shaped tractional retinal detachment (TRD). (**b**) Closed funnel detachment on ultrasonography. (**c**, **d**) Mixed (combined) persistent fetal vasculature having both significant lens opacity and TRD

connections of the rigid hyaloidal stalk, the eye has the opportunity to grow with acceptable functional and anatomic results. Determinants of the functional result of the surgery are severity and type of the disease, complications like glaucoma, retinal break, RD, vitreous hemorrhage, pupillary re-obliterations, degree of retinal dysplasia, and amblyopia management. However, the development of complications may compromise the success of the surgery. Such complications tend to occur more often in the presence of anatomical anomalies.

Since it is a developmental pathology, pars plana is usually under-developed, there are no zonules, and there are peripheral retinal abnormalities in 80% of the anterior PFV cases, like anterior elongation of the retina toward the fibrovascular tissue at the back of the lens which is continuous with that tissue in severe cases [34]. This pathology is more common in nasal and inferior quadrants. In posterior and mixed PFV, the incidence of peripheral retinal pathologies is less common than anterior PFV.

The lens may have different anomalies: total/partial opacity of the lens, fibrotic/membranous or cartilage-like lens, retro-lenticular hemorrhage sequestered between the lens and the fibrovascular plaque, posterior lenticonus, and complete absence of the posterior capsule.

Surgical Treatment (Video 4)

- Anterior PFV: Limbal entry is the preferred method since the rate of peripheral retinal elongation through pars plana/plicata is very high, and there is a risk of retinal damage during pars plana/plicata entry [34]. However, if the peripheral part of the lens is clear enough to examine the ora serrata, pars plana/plicata entry may be possible by avoiding the peripheral retinal elongation areas. The capsule and the fibrovascular tissue adjacent to the capsule should be totally excised to prevent recurrent obliteration of the pupil with the contraction of this fibrovascular tissue left in the periphery. The peripheral capsule can be left in place for future placement of IOL only in selected mild to moderate cases not associated with fibrovascular component at the back of the lens. In cases with peripheral retinal elongation beyond the ora serrata to become continuous with the retrolental fibrovascular tissue (Fig. 11), there are two options: first, the whole fibrovascular tissue is excised, leaving large retinal break areas behind, which needs to be fixed as standard RRD with posterior hyaloid removal and endolaser and silicone oil/gas tamponade. The second choice may be to leave the most peripheral part of the fibrovascular tissue adjacent to the ciliary processes and do radial cuts in this tissue to prevent future circular contraction. However, leaving part of the fibrovascular tissue still has the risk of later contraction, causing pupillary obliteration, secondary cataract formation, glaucoma, TRD, and iris neovascularization.
- There is usually a very thin hyaloid artery coming through the optic nerve head. This stalk is usually shortened and cauterized with diathermy to prevent postoperative hemorrhage. A central core vitrectomy is usually done to prevent pupil

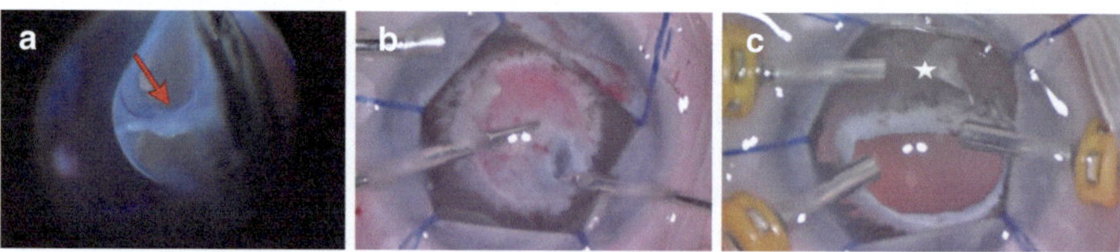

Fig. 11 (**a**) Anterior retinal elongation through nasal pars plana in a mild anterior PFV case. (**b**) 360-degree posterior synechia, released with iris hooks and prominent ciliary processes with thick fibrovascular plaque, became visible afterward in a severe anterior PFV case. (**c**) 360-degree peripheral retinal elongation (white star) continuous with the anterior fibrovascular tissue in the same case

block by the vitreous. Peripheral retina and pars plana should always be checked for peripheral developmental abnormalities. The eye is usually left with air tamponade, and either 10/0 monofilament nylon or a vicryl suture is used to close the entry sites. Attention should be paid to prevent hypotony during suturing, and ocular viscoelastic device (OVD) can be used for this purpose.

- Posterior PFV: The posterior PFV can be either dome-shaped (tent-like) TRD which is a relatively milder form, or closed funnel TRD, which is the severe form of the disease and needs to be differentiated from Norrie disease with genetic analysis, especially when it is bilateral. This severe form of the disease is usually a combined/mixed form associated with total leukocoria, and the prognosis is very poor. Bilaterality is more common in closed funnel posterior PFV [35].

- Dome-shaped posterior PFV: The incidence of peripheral retinal elongation is much less in eyes with mild posterior PFV. Suppose the peripheral retina could be visualized preoperatively to find safe entry places for sclerotomies. In that case, it is possible to do LSV through pars plana entry in most of the dome-shaped posterior PFV cases. The attachment at the back of the lens could easily be cut and trimmed with the vitrector, and the stalk should be shortened as far as the surgeon feels safe. Attention should be paid to avoid retinal damage during the trimming of the stalk because some retinal tissue may have invaginated into this stalk. Releasing this connection will relieve the TRD and let the retina reattach within weeks. The eye is left with air tamponade, and sclerotomies are sutured with 8/0 vicryl. A central little retinal fold may remain at the posterior pole in the long term (Fig. 12).

- *Closed Funnel Posterior PFV:* It is the most severe form of the disease with the most guarded prognosis. A considerable part of these cases is bilateral and associated with microphthalmia. Surgical treatment of such cases is questionable. However, when it is left untreated, phthisis, corneal opacification, or buphthalmos may develop in a short time. Surgery may be considered for cosmetic purposes to preserve the globe with very low visual expectations (light perception) in bilateral cases (Fig. 13).

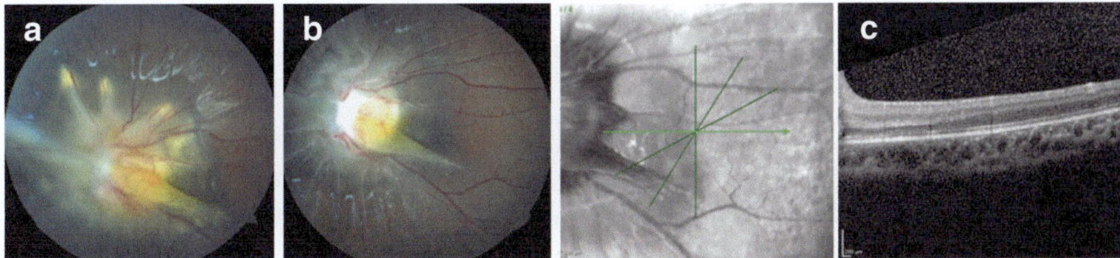

Fig. 12 Dome-shaped posterior persistent fetal vasculature in a newborn baby. (**a**) Preoperative fundus picture. (**b**) Postoperative fifth-year fundus picture. Note there is no exudation; dome-shaped elevation has disappeared, leaving a fibrotic residual membrane over the optic disc and a small macular fold. (**c**) VA is 0.1 with the attached retina in the posterior pole

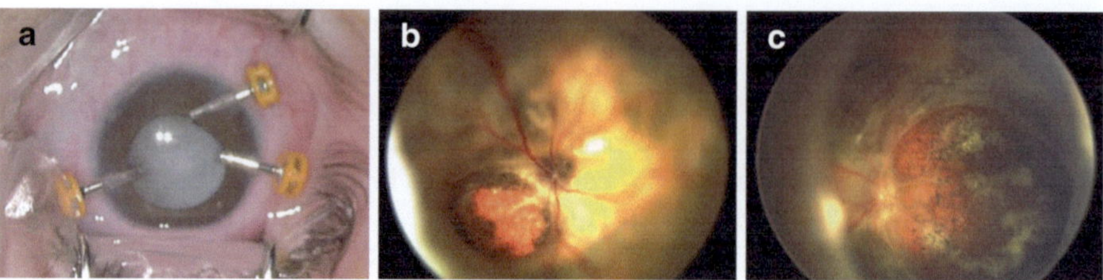

Fig. 13 Closed funnel type; bilateral severe mixed persistent fetal vasculature presenting with leukocoria in a 3-month-old baby. The closed funnel could be opened with limbal lensectomy-vitrectomy surgery. (**a**) At the beginning of the surgery. (**b, c**) Postoperative 4th-month fundus pictures. Note that the closed funnel retinal detachment has opened with a small central area of the attached retina with shallow retinal detachment in the surrounding retina. The baby can move his head toward the light

2.5 Congenital X-Linked Retinoschisis

Congenital X-linked retinoschisis (CXLR) is a relatively common inherited retinal degenerative disease caused by mutations of the retinoschisin 1 (RS1) gene located on Xp22.13. It is an X-linked recessive disease that occurs most commonly in males. RS1 gene encodes retinoschisin which plays an important role in cell-cell adhesion and neuroconduction [36]. There are more than 200 reported mutations of the RS1 gene. The prevalence of CXLR ranges from 1:5000 to 1:20,000.

Clinical Findings [36]

- Clinical features and severity of CXLR vary among the patients, even those with the same RS1 mutation.
- The most characteristic sign of CXLR is foveal schisis present in nearly all patients.
- Peripheral retinoschisis is present in 33–60% of patients and is most commonly located in the inferotemporal quadrant.
- Other peripheral fundus changes are vitreous veils, metallic sheen, white speculations, and pigmentary changes.
- The common sight-threatening complications are RRD/TRD, vitreous hemorrhage, intraschitic hemorrhage within a large schisis cavity, and retinoschisis involving the macula (Fig. 14), which are mostly treated with VRS.
- Subretinal exudation and ExRD with vascular abnormalities mimicking Coats disease and FEVR. Dragging of the macula, bullous retinoschisis, and neovascular glaucoma are the other uncommon complications that can be seen at initial presentation.
- The age of onset of CXLR has a bimodal distribution. Sight-threatening complications such as RRD or vitreous hemorrhage may occur as early as 3 months of life and mostly in patients younger than 10 years old and may present with strabismus and nystagmus (Fig. 15). Therefore, most patients with CXLR are pre-

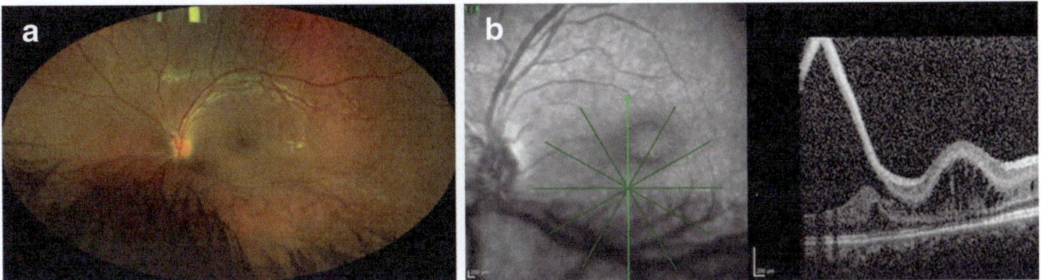

Fig. 14 Widefield fundus image (**a**) and optical coherence tomography (**b**) image of the patient with congenital X-linked retinoschisis and inferior retinoschisis involving the macula. Note that retinoschisis extended to the fovea

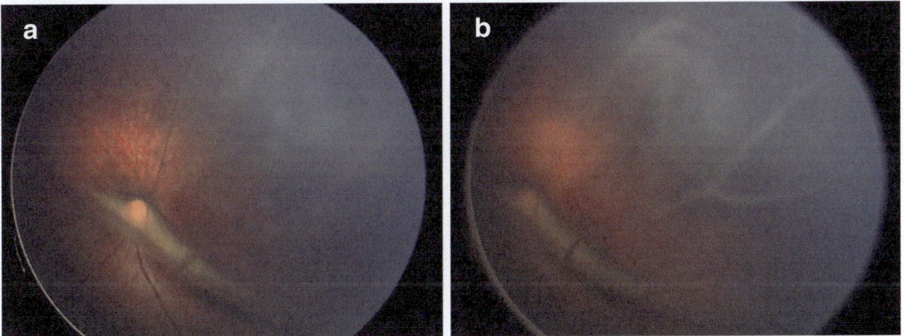

Fig. 15 (**a, b**) A 6-month-old boy whose elder brother has the diagnosis of congenital X-linked retinoschisis was found to have bullous retinoschisis overhanging and involving the macula during screening

sented with vision loss at school age. The most common complaints are low vision and reading difficulties at school. The average visual acuity in young adults is 20/70 ranging from 20/200 to 20/20.

Imaging

- OCT is the best imaging tool for revealing macular pathological changes in CXLR. The schisis may occur in all layers of the retina which can be demonstrated by OCT.
- Fluorescein angiography (FA) may reveal peripheral vascular anomalies such as vascular leakage, retinal non-perfusion areas, and neovascularization (Fig. 16).
- Absence of hyperfluorescence or leakage associated with the cystic-like spaces/retinal splitting in the fovea is typical in FA, unlike classic cystoid macular edema. Foveal hyperfluorescence can be seen if macular atrophy develops.
- Electroretinography (ERG) is another important diagnostic tool for CXLR. Reduced b-wave amplitude with relatively preserved a-wave amplitude and altered b/a ratio (electronegative waveform) are the most significant findings in ERG.

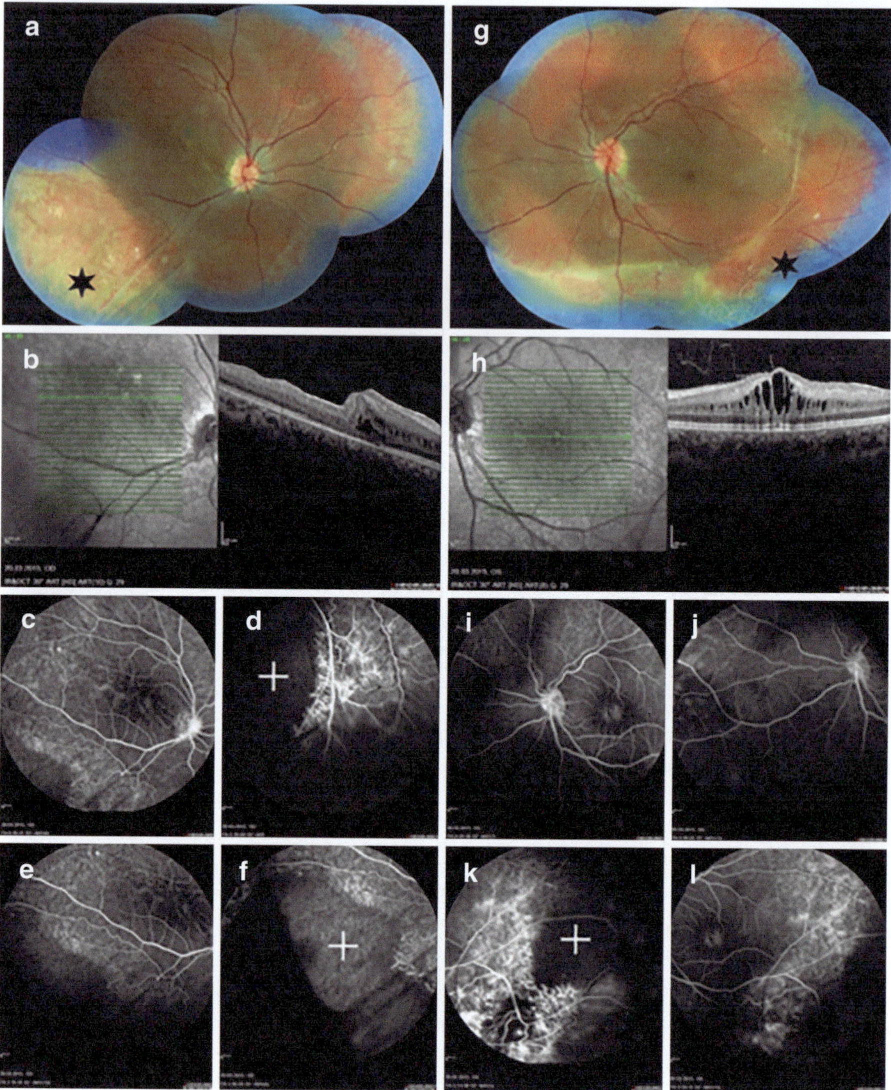

Fig. 16 An 18-year-old male patient was referred to us from another center where he had been followed up for congenital strabismus with a VA of 0.1 in the right eye and 0.4 in the left. Fundus examination (**a**, **g**) revealed retinoschisis in the lower half and temporal of both eyes, and white speculations and avascular areas were noted (black star). Optical coherence tomography showed cysts and retinoschisis mostly in the inner nuclear layer in both eyes (**b**, **h**). On fluorescein angiography, minimal staining of the optic nerve head, inferotemporal retinal vascular leakage, macular staining, and peripheral ischemia were observed in both eyes (**c–f**, **i–l**). Argon laser was applied to the avascular areas and the retinoschisis border as a treatment for this patient

Classification

- The current classification of CXLR is suggested by Trese et al. using OCT and clinical examination (Table 2) [37]. Type 3 CXLR is found to be a risk factor for the development of a combined retinoschisis-RD during follow-up. Change of CXLR type from baseline diagnosis may occur in 17% of patients of CXLR except presented initially with RD.

Differential Diagnosis

- Typical clinical appearance, OCT findings, and ERG abnormalities in a male patient make the diagnosis of CXLR very likely.
- Foveal schisis with peripheral pigmentary changes should be differentiated from conditions with non-leaking macular edema, such as Goldmann-Favre and retinitis pigmentosa.
- Diseases with electronegative ERG, such as congenital stationary night blindness, should be considered.
- Macular atrophy with pigmentary changes or parafoveal white dots can be misdiagnosed as Stargardt disease.
- CXLR may present with exudative changes and may mimic Coats disease, FEVR, uveitis-related exRD, or retinoblastoma (Fig. 17).
- Genetic testing using a multigene panel including RS1 sequences of patient and family members is important to distinguish CXLR from these diseases.

Management [38]

- Patients with slowly progressive disease and stable visual acuity can be observed conservatively. Topical or oral carbonic anhydrase inhibitors may be effective in reducing foveal cysts. The incidence of sight-threatening complications is reported to be about 50%. The most common cause of surgery in patients with CXLR is RRD which has been reported in up to 20% of patients. The occurrence

Table 2 Congenital X-linked retinoschisis types

CXLR type	Clinical findings
1: Foveal	Foveal cystic schisis without macular lamellar schisis or peripheral schisis
2: Foveo-lamellar	Foveal cystic schisis and macular lamellar schisis without peripheral schisis
3: Complex	Foveal cystic schisis, macular lamellar schisis, and peripheral schisis
4: Foveo-peripheral	Foveal cystic schisis, no macular lamellar schisis, but with peripheral schisis

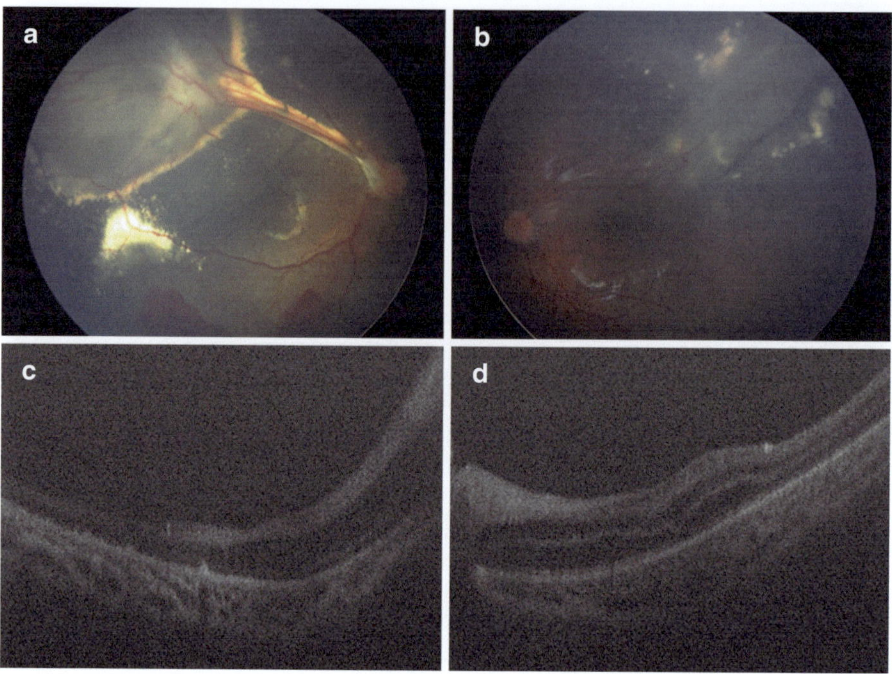

Fig. 17 This 2-year-old boy presented with strabismus. FEVR and Coats disease were considered in the differential diagnosis due to macular dragging and retinal exudation in both eyes (**a**, **b**). OCT revealed typical foveal schisis (**c**, **d**). During the surgery of right eye, the hemorrhage (**a**), which was thought to be subretinal, was found to be intraschitic. With all the findings, the patient was diagnosed with congenital X-linked retinoschisis

of vitreous hemorrhage was reported in 40% of patients. Other sight-threatening complications that needed surgery are retinoschisis involving/threatening macula, traction RD, macular dragging, intraretinal hemorrhage spilled over the vitreous, and bullous retinoschisis. Due to the bimodal age distribution of the disease, surgery is often required before the age of 10 for bullous retinoschisis and vitreous hemorrhage, while RRDs secondary to inner and outer layer tears are seen in the 2nd–third decades of life.

- ALP, SB, and vitrectomy can be performed to treat severe complications of CXLR.
- *Peripheral retinoschisis without involving macula and traction:* ALP to the borders of peripheral retinoschisis should be considered as a preventive treatment.
- *RRD/TRD with peripheral retinoschisis:* The causes of RRD in CXLR are breaks in both inner and outer retinal layers and anteroposterior or tangential traction forces over the retina.

  - SB is a good option, especially in young, phakic patients and can be performed alone or combined with PPV (Fig. 18). SB should be considered a primary surgical intervention if an outer retinal break can be seen in the

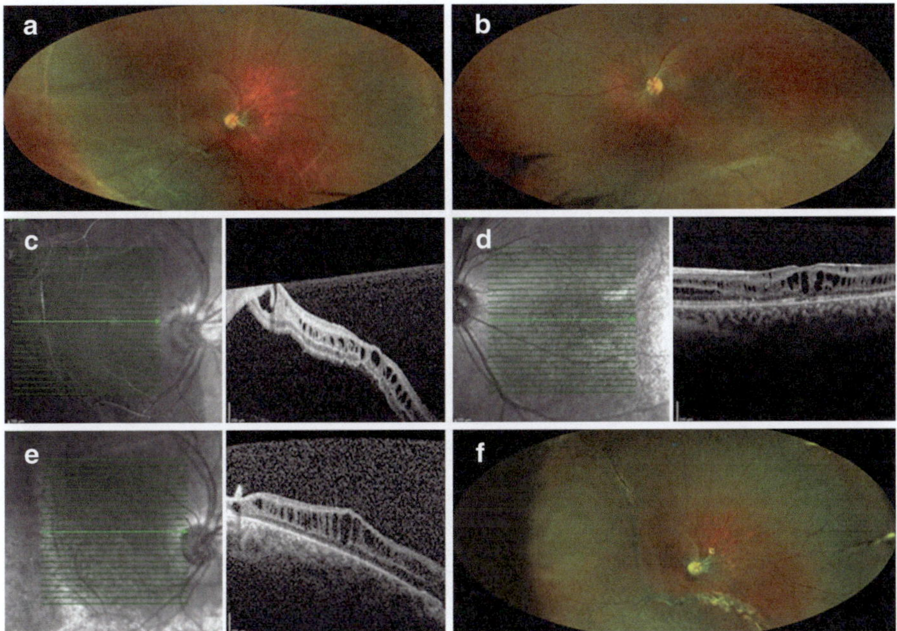

Fig. 18 A 10-year-old male patient with congenital X-linked retinoschisis had rhegmatogenous retinal detachment in the right eye (**a, c**). In the left eye, there was foveal and peripheral schisis without detachment (**b, d**). Scleral buckle, vitrectomy, inner wall retinectomy, and ALP were performed, and 5000 cs silicone oil was used as a tamponade. The retina was attached after surgery (**e, f**). Note the laser scars at the border of the inner retinectomy

peripheral retina and there is no significant traction. Reattachment rates in patients with CXLR were reported to be up to 90% with SB. The most common causes of failure with SB are missed outer retinal breaks and PVR.

- PPV should be performed in the presence of PVR, significant vitreous traction, vitreous hemorrhage, or if the outer retinal break cannot be seen. PPV is the preferred method also for patients with bullous retinoschisis or macular dragging.
- One of the important steps during PPV is the complete induction of PVD. The posterior hyaloid should be separated from the retina, at least in the posterior pole. Hyaloid remnants and poorly cleared cortical vitreous may cause PVR. In some patients with peripheral retinoschisis, there is no effective way to remove the posterior hyaloid. Inner wall retinectomy is a good option in these patients to clear all cortical vitreous and relieve traction on outer retinal layers.
- Inner wall retinectomy does not have a negative effect on vision because patients already have an absolute scotoma in peripheral retinoschisis areas. However, the inner retina may be tried to be preserved for possible future treatments. Fluid drainage from schisis through a small retinotomy with a 38/41-gauge cannula instead of inner wall retinectomy may be tried to reattach the retina [39].

- Adjuvant use of autologous plasmin is another option to ease the induction of PVD [40].
- PFCL is used to stabilize the retina during vitreous base removal and internal drainage of subretinal fluid.
- ILM peeling should be avoided due to the risk of macular hole development and should be performed only in selected cases.
- Endolaser should be performed around the breaks, retinotomy holes, and periphery of schisis cavities.
- 5000 cs should be the choice of SO in patients with RRD. SF6 and C3F8 gas tamponades could be used only in selected cooperative cases.

- *Vitreous hemorrhage:* Rupture of a strained retinal vessel in the schitic retina and neovascularization are the causes of vitreous hemorrhage in CXLR. Intraretinal (intraschisis) hemorrhage may also occur with a ruptured retinal vessel, and this hemorrhage may spill over the vitreous through an inner retinal break.

  - Vitreous hemorrhage may spontaneously resolve, so observation should be considered at the initial presentation.
  - Dense and non-resolving hemorrhages should be treated with vitrectomy. It is important to perform ALP to the non-perfusion areas to reduce the risk of neovascularization.
  - ALP should also be performed around the borders of peripheral retinoschisis for prophylaxis of RRD or extending retinoschisis.

- Flattening of foveal schisis and decrease in foveal cysts after vitrectomy have been reported by many authors. Some authors reported a recurrence of foveal schisis after silicone oil removal.
- Gene therapy through intraocular and subretinal injections is a promising treatment option for CXLR.

2.6 *Pediatric Rhegmatogenous Retinal Detachment*

Pediatric RRD accounts for only 3.2–5.6% of all RRD.

- The most common causes of RRD in children are:

  - Trauma (40%).
  - Nonsyndromic pathological myopia.
  - Prematurity.
  - Hereditary conditions: Marfan syndrome, Stickler-Wagner syndrome, and CXLR.
  - Developmental anomalies: Choroidal coloboma.
  - Previous ocular surgeries: Congenital cataract surgery, vitrectomy, and glaucoma surgery [41, 42].

- Buphthalmic eyes are also prone to develop RRD since these eyes are big eyes with thin retinas and associated developmental abnormalities.
- It is common to find retinal dialysis mostly located in the inferotemporal quadrant together with a macular hole in severe contusion-related RD in children.
- *RRD in children has many differences compared to adults* [43]. Late presentation already complicated with proliferative vitreoretinopathy (PVR), high rate of systemic comorbidities (prematurity, Marfan, Stickler, etc.), poor cooperation for examinations, difficulty in postoperative positioning, bilateral involvements, high rate of attached vitreous and difficult to induce PVD, and high rate of postoperative PVR and recurrences. Functional success is limited further with amblyopia in the amblyopic age group.

Surgical Tips

- Pediatric RRD should be primarily treated with scleral buckle without PPV, as discussed in Chap. 9 "Scleral Buckle Surgery."
- Pediatric RRD may present with inferior chronic RD with subretinal fibrotic bands, and it is usually discovered by chance. In such cases, SB without PPV is still a good option despite the subretinal PVR (Fig. 19). Chandelier-assisted SB provides good visualization and may decrease the risk of missed tears [44].
- In children less than 3 years of age, SB should be removed or cut 6–9 months after the primary surgery to allow the normal growth of the globe and reduce the myopic shift.
- Even if a PPV is planned because of the severe PVR, an encircling buckle (240 band) should be added to the surgery to support the vitreous base and peripheral retina, particularly that complete PVD may not be always possible. We always

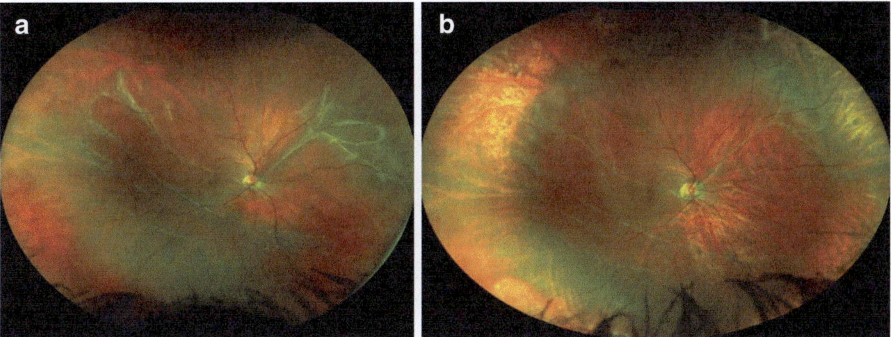

Fig. 19 Preoperative fundus picture of a 16-year-old girl with Stickler syndrome associated with chronic almost total rhegmatogenous retinal detachment with lots of subretinal bands due to proliferative vitreoretinopathy and inferior small retinal holes. She was treated successfully with encircling scleral buckle without vitrectomy

try to preserve the clear lens in pediatric RRD. This makes removing the vitreous base even more difficult in such small eyes.

- Stickler syndrome, which is a dominantly inherited disorder, has typical features of generalized arthropathy, cleft palate, flat face, hearing loss, and spondyloepiphyseal dysplasia in addition to ocular features. Patients usually have early-onset cataracts and high myopia with peripheral retinal thinning and retinal breaks, including giant retinal tears. Membranous or fibrillar vitreous can be found in most eyes with Stickler syndrome, which extends toward the retinal periphery. Lattice degenerations are common, and small retinal holes within the lattice degenerations may cause slowly progressive RD, which usually present late as chronic RDs [41].

- PPV is needed for RRD associated with severe PVR and giant retinal tears. When PPV is planned, the posterior hyaloid is usually attached and is difficult to detach from the detached retina. Triamcinolone staining the vitreous is helpful and so is the use of PFCL to hold the retina in place and detach the posterior hyaloid using bimanual maneuvers with microforceps. Induction of PVD is a "sine qua non" of the surgery. When neglected, a very early recurrence is common, with the thickening of the posterior hyaloid forming severe PVR. Detachment of the hyaloid should be done cautiously to avoid forming new retinal breaks. If it is not possible to detach it to the periphery, the remaining hyaloid can be shaved as much as possible. It is still important to remove all vitreous traction in areas of retinal tears. SO is preferred as a tamponade in PVR cases. However, the surgeon should be aware of the higher rate of emulsification of SO, especially in active children. 5000 cs SO is usually the author's choice of SO tamponade in children.

- Marfan syndrome is a dominantly inherited disorder involving ocular, cardiovascular (aortic dilatation, dissecting aneurysms, and mitral valve prolapse in 65% of patients), as well as the musculoskeletal system (tall stature, hyperextensible joints, arachnodactyly, etc.). RRD occurs in 5–11% of cases and increases to 8–38% in those with ectopia lentis or who have undergone cataract surgery. Special considerations for RD in Marfan syndrome include a poorly dilating pupil and subluxated lens that may limit visualization and assessment of the retina. In eyes with minimal lens subluxation and well-dilated pupils, RD can be successfully repaired using SB. However, complex RDs (mostly associated with giant retinal breaks) with severe lens subluxation are better managed with PPV, lensectomy, and endotamponade using long-acting gas or silicone oil with SB. Careful preoperative assessment and plannning of these cases for general anesthesia is important because prophylaxis for infective endocarditis may be needed [41, 42].

- Choroidal coloboma is a rare condition, and the prevalence of RRDs is between 23%–40%. It may be associated with other ocular anomalies, such as microphthalmia, cataract, or lens coloboma. Coloboma may involve the optic nerve head and macula, which limits both anatomical and functional success. RRD associated with choroidal coloboma may be related to a peripheral retinal break (Fig. 20) or, more commonly, to a break in the intercalating membrane (ICM) in the coloboma area [45]. When a peripheral retinal break is identified, SB surgery can be performed with success; however, if a peripheral break cannot be identified, RD is

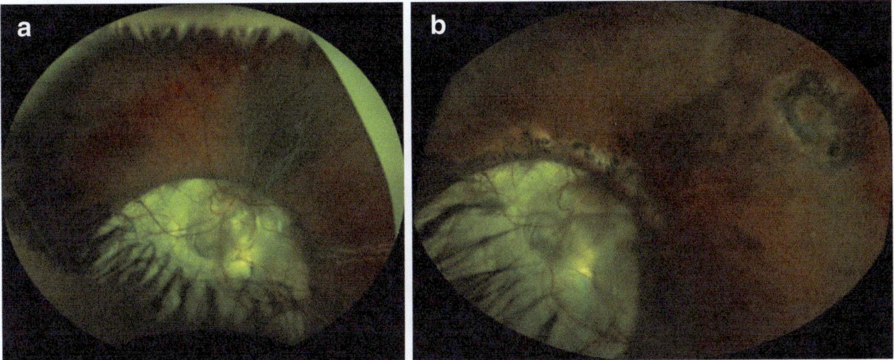

Fig. 20 Pre- and postoperative pictures of a rhegmatogenous retinal detachment associated with choroidal coloboma secondary to a peripheral retinal break in the superotemporal quadrant of the left eye treated with pars plana vitrectomy and silicone oil tamponade. Laser photocoagulation was applied to the borders of the coloboma area and around the break

usually related to a break in the ICM in the coloboma area and needs to be treated with PPV and SO tamponade. The addition of an encircling band does not seem to affect the final anatomical outcome for such eyes. Removal of vitreous attachments and incision of the ICM to weaken it are important steps to relieve traction on the break within the ICM. Laser around the coloboma area is advised (Fig. 20). However, when the coloboma border is in the macular area, we avoid performing laser. We speculate that some of the recurrent RD in choroidal coloboma may be serous RD secondary to subretinal cerebrospinal fluid coming through the optic nerve head in the colobomatous area, similar to optic pit-related detachment. These cases may be observed with caution before deciding on a second surgery since this subretinal fluid may resolve spontaneously within time.

Prognosis

- Anatomical success with single surgery ranges between 50% and 70% and multiple surgeries between 72% and 88%. The mean number of procedures per patient ranges between 1.2 and 2.2 [41, 42].
- Anatomical and functional successes are lower in total RD (as compared to partial RD) and in younger children (<13 y old). RD associated with Stickler syndrome is more common in younger children, and RD associated with trauma is more likely in older cohorts.
- Significantly better anatomical and functional results are obtained with scleral buckling (SB) or SB + PPV, compared to PPV alone, in almost all of the series.
- Successful surgical treatment of RRD in buphthalmic eyes usually leads to reestablishing the IOP. So, the surgeon and the patient should be prepared for an IOP increase following reattachment!

Prophylaxis to the Fellow Eye

- Overall pediatric RRD are bilateral. This risk is higher in Stickler (39% to 51%) and Marfan syndromes (70%) [41, 42].
- Fellow eye examination should be performed in all eyes with RRD. Lattice degeneration, pigmentary retinopathy, retinal holes, or RD may be detected in the fellow eyes.
- Prophylactic treatment in fellow eyes with high-risk peripheral retinal pathology [46, 47] should be considered in the form of 360° ALP or SB prophylaxis.
- Prophylactic ALP around the coloboma area may be done to the fellow eye in bilateral choroidal coloboma cases.

Key Points

- VRS in pediatric eyes has a different philosophy than in adult eyes.
- The rule is to preserve the crystalline (lens-sparing vitrectomy), but if there is a high risk of peripheral retinal damage during sclerotomy, do not hesitate to perform a limbal approach lensectomy-vitrectomy.
- In ROP surgery, the surgeon should avoid iatrogenic retinal break formation.
- In anterior PFV, there is a high incidence of elongation of the retina beyond the ora serrata with incorporation into retrolental fibrovascular tissue in anterior PFV.
- In pediatric RRD, it is best to use SB and not PPV.
- Amblyopia is an important cause of limited vision in pediatric retinal diseases of children younger than 7 years.

References

1. Aiello AL, Tran VT, Rao NA. Postnatal development of the ciliary body and pars plana. A morphometric study in childhood. Arch Ophthalmol. 1992;110(6):802–5. PMID: 1596228
2. Lee JG, Ferrone PJ. Surgical Approaches to Infant and Childhood Retinal Diseases: Intravitreal Surgery. In: Hartnett ME, editor. Pediatric Retina. 3rd edition. Wolters Kluwer Health publisher: 2020. pp: 884–90.
3. Trese MT, Capone A. Surgical approaches to infant and childhood retinal diseases: invasive methods. In: Hartnett ME, editor. Pediatric Retina. Philadelphia, PA: Lippincott Williams & Wilkins; 2005.
4. Turgut B, Demir T, Çatak O. The recommendations for pediatric vitreoretinal surgery. Adv Ophthalmol Vis Syst. 2019;9(6):142–5.
5. Patel CK, Walker NJ, Kam JK. A new, theoretically safer method of intravitreal injection of bevacizumab in progressive retinopathy of prematurity using scleral trans-illumination. Br J Ophthalmol. 2010;94(8):1107–9. Epub 2010 Jun 16. PMID: 20558426
6. Liu X, Zheng T, Zhou X, Lu Y, Zhou P, Fan F, Luo Y. Comparison between limbal and pars plana approaches using microincision vitrectomy for removal of congenital cataracts with primary intraocular lens implantation. J Ophthalmol. 2016;2016:8951053. Epub 2016 May 30. PMID: 27313872; PMCID: PMC4904112

7. Lemley CA, Han DP. An age-based method for planning sclerotomy placement during pediatric vitrectomy: a 12-year experience. Trans Am Ophthalmol Soc. 2007;105:86–9. discussion 89-91. PMID: 18427597; PMCID: PMC2258105

8. Meier P, Wiedemann P. Ryan SJ, editor. Surgery for pediatric vitreoretinal disorders. Surgical considerations and techniques—Posterior segment surgical techniques. *Surgical Retina. Part 1.* (5th ed) 2013;3(Sec. 3. 1936-1939).

9. Gan NY, Lam WC. Special considerations for pediatric vitreoretinal surgery. Taiwan J Ophthalmol. 2018;8(4):237–42. PMID: 30637195; PMCID: PMC6302561

10. Recchia FM, Scott IU, Brown GC, Brown MM, Ho AC, Ip MS, et al. Small-gauge pars plana vitrectomy: a report by the American Academy of Ophthalmology. Ophthalmology. 2010;117:1851–7.

11. Cernichiaro-Espinosa LA, Berrocal AM. Novel surgical technique for inducing posterior vitreous detachment during pars plana vitrectomy for pediatric patients using a flexible loop. Retin Cases Brief Rep. 2020;14(2):137–40. PMID: 29176537

12. Thompson JT. Advantages and limitations of small gauge vitrectomy. Surv Ophthalmol. 2011;56:162–72.

13. Sisk RA, Motley WW 3rd, Yang MB, West CE. Surgical outcomes following repair of traumatic retinal detachments in cognitively impaired adolescents with self-injurious behavior. J Pediatr Ophthalmol Strabismus. 2013;50(1):20–6. Epub 2012 Oct 9. PMID: 23061560

14. Azuma N, Ito M, Yokoi T, Nakayama Y, Nishina S. Visual outcomes after early vitreous surgery for aggressive posterior retinopathy of prematurity. JAMA Ophthalmol. 2013;131(10):1309–13.

15. Lakhanpal RR, Sun RL, Albini TA, Holz ER. Anatomic success rate after 3-port lens-sparing vitrectomy in stage 4A or 4B retinopathy of prematurity. Ophthalmology. 2005;112(9):1569–73. PMID: 16005974

16. Özsaygili C, Ozdek S, Ozmen MC, Atalay HT, Yalinbas YD. Parameters affecting postoperative success of surgery for stage 4A/4B ROP. Br J Ophthalmol. 2019;103(11):1624–32. Epub 2019 Jan 18. PMID: 30658990

17. Yokoi T, Yokoi T, Kobayashi Y, Nishina S, Azuma N. Risk factors for recurrent fibrovascular proliferation in aggressive posterior retinopathy of prematurity after early vitreous surgery. Am J Ophthalmol. 2010;150(1):10-15.e1. PMID: 20609704

18. Singh R, Reddy DM, Barkmeier AJ, Holz ER, Ram R, Carvounis PE. Long-term visual outcomes following lens-sparing vitrectomy for retinopathy of prematurity. Br J Ophthalmol. 2012;96(11):1395–8. Epub 2012 Aug 24. PMID: 22923456

19. Hubbard GB 3rd, Cherwick DH, Burian G. Lens-sparing vitrectomy for stage 4 retinopathy of prematurity. Ophthalmology. 2004;111(12):2274–7.

20. Ozsaygili C, Ozdek S, Ozmen MC, Atalay HT, Yeter DY. Preoperative anatomical features associated with improved surgical outcomes for stage 5 retinopathy of prematurity. Retina. 2021;41(4):718–25. PMID: 32932381

21. Atalay HT, Özdek Ş, Yalınbaş D, Özsaygılı C, Özmen MC. Results of surgery for late sequelae of cicatricial retinopathy of prematurity. Indian J Ophthalmol. 2019;67(6):908–11. PMID: 31124513; PMCID: PMC6552626

22. Benson WE. Familial exudative vitreoretinopathy. Trans Am Ophthalmol Soc. 1995;93:473–521. PMID: 8719692; PMCID: PMC1312071

23. Ranchod TM, Ho LY, Drenser KA, Capone A Jr, Trese MT. Clinical presentation of familial exudative vitreoretinopathy. Ophthalmology. 2011;118(10):2070–5. Epub 2011 Aug 25. PMID: 21868098

24. John VJ, McClintic JI, Hess DJ, Berrocal AM. Retinopathy of prematurity versus familial exudative vitreoretinopathy: report on clinical and angiographic findings. Ophthalmic Surg Lasers Imaging Retina. 2016;47(1):14–9. PMID: 26731204

25. Nikopoulos K, Venselaar H, Collin RW, Riveiro-Alvarez R, Boonstra FN, Hooymans JM, Mukhopadhyay A, Shears D, van Bers M, de Wijs IJ, van Essen AJ, Sijmons RH, Tilanus MA, van Nouhuys CE, Ayuso C, Hoefsloot LH, Cremers FP. Overview of the mutation spectrum in familial exudative vitreoretinopathy and Norrie disease with identification of 21 novel variants in FZD4, LRP5, and NDP. Hum Mutat. 2010;31(6):656–66. PMID: 20340138
26. Pendergast SD, Trese MT. Familial exudative vitreoretinopathy. Results Surg Manag Ophthalmol. 1998;105(6):1015–23. PMID: 9627651
27. Fei P, Yang W, Zhang Q, Jin H, Li J, Zhao P. Surgical management of advanced familial exudative vitreoretinopathy with complications. Retina. 2016;36(8):1480–5. PMID: 26807630
28. Shields JA, Shields CL, Honavar SG, Demirci H, Cater J. Classification and management of coats disease: the 2000 Proctor Lecture. Am J Ophthalmol. 2001;131(5):572–83.
29. Sen M, Shields CL, Honavar SG, Shields JA. Coats disease: an overview of classification, management and outcomes. Indian J Ophthalmol. 2019;67(6):763–71. PMID: 31124484; PMCID: PMC6552590
30. Ong SS, Buckley EG, McCuen BW 2nd, Jaffe GJ, Postel EA, Mahmoud TH, Stinnett SS, Toth CA, Vajzovic L, Mruthyunjaya P. Comparison of visual outcomes in Coats' disease: a 20-year experience. Ophthalmology. 2017;124(9):1368–76. Epub 2017 Apr 28. PMID: 28461016
31. Li AS, Capone A Jr, Trese MT, Sears JE, Kychenthal A, De la Huerta I, Ferrone PJ. Long-term outcomes of total exudative retinal detachments in stage 3B coats disease. Ophthalmology. 2018;125(6):887–93. Epub 2018 Feb 1. PMID: 29361355
32. Ucgul AY, Ozdek S, Ertop M, Atalay HT. External drainage alone versus external drainage with vitrectomy in advanced coats disease [published online ahead of print, 2020 Sep 9]. Am J Ophthalmol. 2020;222:6–14.
33. Haddad R, Font RL, Reeser F. Persistent hyperplastic primary vitreous. A clinicopathologic study of 62 cases and review of the literature. Surv Ophthalmol. 1978;23(2):123–34.
34. Ozdek S, Ozdemir Zeydanli E, Atalay HT, Aktas Z. Anterior elongation of the retina in persistent fetal vasculature: emphasis on retinal complications. Eye (Lond). 2019;33(6):938–47.
35. Sisk RA, Berrocal AM, Feuer WJ, Murray TG. Visual and anatomic outcomes with or without surgery in persistent fetal vasculature. Ophthalmology. 2010;117(11):2178–83.e832
36. Georgiou M, Finocchio L, Fujinami K, Fujinami-Yokokawa Y, Virgili G, Mahroo OA, Webster AR, Michaelides M. X-linked retinoschisis: deep phenotyping and genetic characterization. Ophthalmology. 2022;129(5):542–51.
37. Prenner JL, Capone A Jr, Ciaccia S, Takada Y, Sieving PA, Trese MT. Congenital X-linked retinoschisis classification system. Retina. 2006;26(7 Suppl):S61–4.
38. Ferrone PJ, Trese MT, Lewis H. Vitreoretinal surgery for complications of congenital retinoschisis. Am J Ophthalmol. 1997;123(6):742–7.
39. Trese MT, Ferrone PJ. The role of inner wall retinectomy in the management of juvenile retinoschisis. Graefes Arch Clin Exp Ophthalmol. 1995;233(11):706–8.
40. Wu WC, Drenser KA, Capone A, Williams GA, Trese MT. Plasmin enzyme-assisted vitreoretinal surgery in congenital X-linked retinoschisis: surgical techniques based on a new classification system. Retina. 2007;27(8):1079–85.
41. Smith JM, Ward LT, Townsend JH, et al. Rhegmatogenous retinal detachment in children: clinical factors predictive of successful surgical repair. Ophthalmology. 2019;126(9):1263–70.
42. Gonzales CR, Singh S, Yu F, Kreiger AE, Gupta A, Schwartz SD. Pediatric rhegmatogenous retinal detachment: clinical features and surgical outcomes. Retina. 2008;28(6):847–52.
43. Rumelt S, Sarrazin L, Averbukh E, Halpert M, Hemo I. Paediatric vs adult retinal detachment. Eye (Lond). 2007;21(12):1473–8.
44. Ozdek S, Kiliç A, Gurelik G, Hasanreisoglu B. Scleral buckling technique for longstanding inferior rhegmatogenous retinal detachments with subretinal bands. Ann Ophthalmol (Skokie). 2008;40(1):35–8.
45. Gopal L, Badrinath SS, Sharma T, Parikh SN, Biswas J. Pattern of retinal breaks and retinal detachments in eyes with choroidal coloboma. Ophthalmology. 1995;102:1212–7.

46. Fincham GS, Pasea L, Carroll C, McNinch AM, Poulson AV, Richards AJ, Scott JD, Snead MP. Prevention of retinal detachment in stickler syndrome: the Cambridge prophylactic cryotherapy protocol. Ophthalmology. 2014;121(8):1588–97. Epub 2014 May 1
47. Khanna S, Rodriguez SH, Blair MA, Wroblewski K, Shapiro MJ, Blair MP. Laser prophylaxis in patients with stickler syndrome. Ophthalmol Retina. 2022;6(4):263–7. Epub 2021 Nov 11. PMID: 34774838

Retinal and Choroidal Tumors

Mostafa Hanout, Filiberto Altomare, and Hatem Krema

There is a wide spectrum of choroidal and retinal tumors that can be encountered in a retina clinic and can be detected with dilated fundoscopy. This chapter provides simplified guidelines for diagnosis and briefly discusses differential diagnosis of common lesions with a focus on the tumors of the choroid, retina, and optic nerve. It also highlights key findings in different modalities of diagnostic imaging. We may refer briefly to treatment alternatives where relevant. Lesions of similar pathology in the anterior segment are outside the scope of this chapter and hence are not discussed.

1 Pigmented Uveal Tumors

1.1 Choroidal Nevus

- Choroidal nevus is the most common intraocular tumor that affects up to 8% of the population.

M. Hanout
Ophthalmology, Apex Eye Institute, Corner Brook, NF, Canada

F. Altomare
Department of Ophthalmology and Vision Sciences, Temerty Faculty of Medicine, University of Toronto, Toronto, ON, Canada

Unity Health—St Michael's Hospital, and University Health Network, Princess Margaret Hospital, Toronto, ON, Canada

H. Krema (✉)
Ophthalmology and Vision Sciences, Princess Margaret Cancer Centre, Toronto, ON, Canada
e-mail: hatem.krema@uhn.ca

© The Author(s), under exclusive license to Springer Nature Switzerland AG 2024
A. B. Sallam et al. (eds.), *Practical Manual of Vitreoretinal Surgery*,
https://doi.org/10.1007/978-3-031-47827-7_30

- **Clinical picture:** Choroidal nevus typically presents as asymptomatic slate gray/brown, flat lesion with relatively ill-defined margin, usually discovered accidentally during routine fundus exam. It can grow in thickness and basal diameter at a very slow rate over the course of several years and show signs of chronicity such as surface drusen, retinal pigment epitheluim (RPE) atrophy, RPE hyperplasia, or fibrous metaplasia. Clusters of migrated RPE can also be seen.
- Occasionally, choroidal nevi can be non-pigmented (amelanotic) or may have a non-pigmented halo surrounding a pigmented center (halo nevus). Some choroidal nevi have a large basal diameter (giant nevi) with lack of any other risk factors.
- Long-standing choroidal nevi in macular or subfoveal location can become visually symptomatic due to RPE detachment, photoreceptor degeneration, or subretinal fluid (SRF).
- Choroidal neovascular membranes are rare complications of choroidal nevi and may represent chronicity of the choroidal nevus.
- Choroidal nevus may be a precursor for a choroidal melanoma; therefore, it is important for clinicians to be familiar with clinical features that predict increased risk of malignant transformation. Shields and colleagues [1] reviewed a large series of 3806 choroidal nevi and identified the following risk factors: **t**hickness of >2 mm, **S**RF, **s**ymptoms, **o**range pigments (lipofuscin), **m**elanoma hollowness on B-scan ultrasound, and **d**iam**e**ter > 5 mm. The mnemonic **T**o **F**ind **S**mall **O**cular **M**elanoma **D**oing **IM**aging (TFSOM DIM) can be helpful to recall these factors. The proximity of the nevus margin to the optic disc by <3 mm, absence of drusen, and absence of halo have been previously linked to increased risk of malignant transformation. The 5-year risk of malignant transformation was estimated at 1% if no risk factors are present, 11% with 1 factor, 22% with 2 factors, 34% with 3 factors, 51% with 4 factors, and 55% with 5 factors.
- **Imaging:** assessment of choroidal lesions with multimodal imaging is very helpful in diagnosis and monitoring. Color fundus photographs should be taken at periodic visits for accurate comparison and documentation of basal growth. Fundus autofluorescence (FAF) may show hypofluorescence in chronic lesions due to RPE changes (Fig. 1f). Orange pigments if present appear hyperfluorescent. Optical coherence tomography (OCT) shows slightly elevated dome-shaped subretinal lesion. Chronic long-standing lesions may show overlying retinal cystic changes and/or drusen. Choriocapillaris layer, which is a narrow hyporeflective layer between overlying RPE/Bruch's membrane complex and larger choroidal vessels, is usually preserved due to very slow rate of growth. B-scan ultrasound usually shows flat, acoustically solid lesions with thickness usually <2 mm, although this is not a cutoff for maximum thickness of choroidal lesions.
- **Management:** There is no active treatment required for choroidal nevus. Periodic assessment with thorough documentation of the lesion size and characteristics using multimodal imaging is necessary. Small lesions with no risk factors can be assessed every 12 months, whereas relatively larger lesions and lesions with 1 or more risk factors should be assessed at 6-month interval or less as per discretion of the clinician.

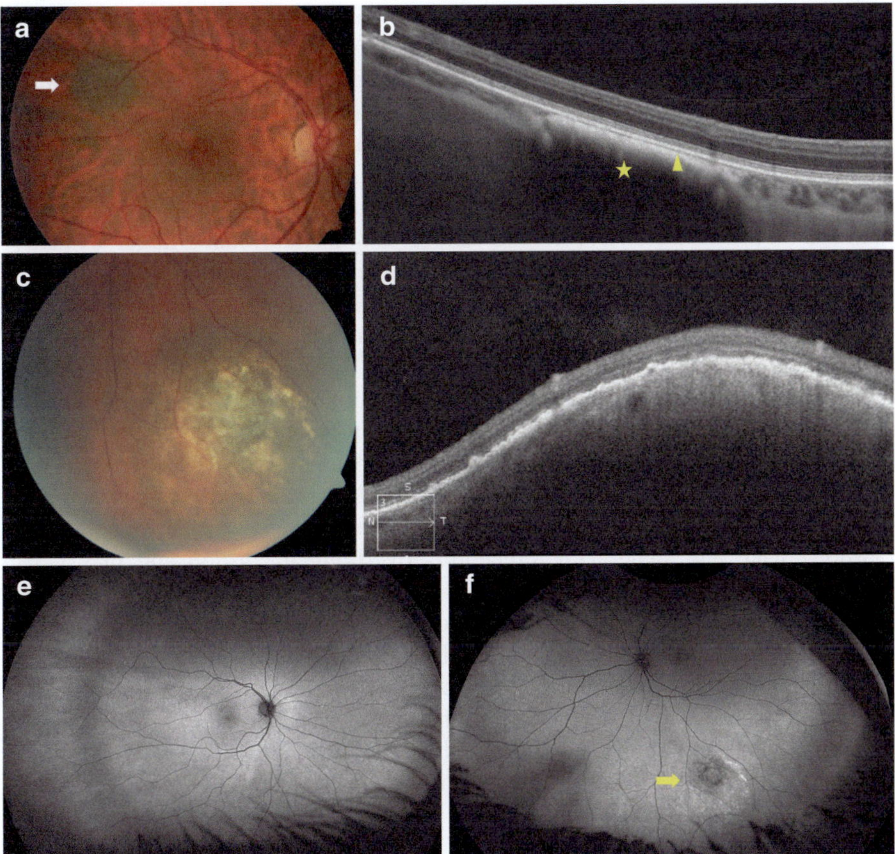

Fig. 1 (**a**) Small flat choroidal nevus along the superotemporal arcade (arrow). (**b**) Optical coherence tomography appearance showing choroidal melanocytic lesion (star) and preserved choriocapillaris (arrow head). (**c**) Chronic choroidal nevus with drusen and RPE metaplastic changes. d) OCT shows overlying drusen and no subretinal fluid. (**e**) Unremarkable fundus autofluorescence of the first lesion. f) Mottled increased and decreased autofluorescence due to chronic retinal pigment epithelium changes (arrow)

1.2 Choroidal Melanoma

- Choroidal melanoma is the most common primary intraocular malignancy and the second most common intraocular malignancy after choroidal metastasis. Approximately 7000 new cases are diagnosed annually worldwide. The incidence ranges from 0.2 to 8.6 per million depending on multiple host and environmental factors.
- Light eye color, fair skin color, older age, preexisting ocular nevus, oculodermal melanocytosis, dysplastic nevus syndrome, and BAP1 germline mutation are all predisposing factors to choroidal melanoma.

- **Clinical picture and diagnosis:** choroidal melanoma is most reliably diagnosed by clinical examination performed by an experienced clinician. Initial symptoms depend on tumor location and may mimic those of posterior vitreous detachment or retinal detachment such as decreased vision, metamorphopsia, or visual field defect either from direct tumor growth or exudative retinal detachment (RD).
- The tumor usually appears as pigmented or occasionally non-pigmented (amelanotic), dome-shaped subretinal mass with orange pigment and serous detachment of the neurosensory retina. Larger tumors likely have larger exudative retinal detachment with fluid shift with change of patient's head position.
- Some ocular melanomas break through Bruch's membrane assuming a mushroom-shaped configuration with higher risk of subretinal or vitreous hemorrhage.
- **Imaging:** color fundus photos are taken for tumor documentation at baseline and subsequent follow-up. Ultra-widefield fundus photographs (x200°) are helpful in identifying the full extent of the tumor and in planning treatment. FAF is the gold standard to detect orange pigment, which appears hyperfluorescent, especially in amelanotic melanoma where orange pigment may not be visible clinically. OCT shows SRF and shaggy photoreceptors overlying the lesion and may detect mushroom-shaped configuration. B-scan ultrasonography shows characteristic acoustic hollowness of the tumor with low internal reflectivity on A-scan (Fig. 2b, c). Intravenous fluorescein angiography (IVFA) may show multiple pinpoint leaks "hot spots." Large tumors may show in early IVFA phase clearly visible intratumor vascular channels deep in the tumor mass underneath overlying retinal vessels, a sign referred to as "double circulation."
- **Ancillary tests:** transillumination test is done using bright light in a completely dark room to measure the full extent of the tumor base that casts a shadow on the sclera. Transillumination is essential for treatment planning and during plaque brachytherapy. Liver function tests, chest CT, and MRI of the liver are ordered at the time of diagnosis for metastatic evaluation.
- **Management:** Several treatment approaches are currently employed to treat choroidal melanoma. Selection of the appropriate treatment approach depends on multiple factors including tumor size and location, status of the affected eye and the fellow eye, age and systemic health of the patient, and patient's preference. For instance, if the tumor affects the better seeing eye, eye-preserving treatment will be favored if possible.
- Plaque brachytherapy is the most widely employed focal radiotherapy. Most common isotopes used are Iodine 125 and Ruthenium 106. High dose of radiation is delivered to the tumor apex (80–100 grays). There is no statistically significant difference in survival in patients treated with enucleation compared with brachytherapy according to the Collaborative Ocular Melanoma Study (COMS) [2], with the advantage of eye preservation with brachytherapy. Tumor response is confirmed by reduction of tumor size and acoustic solidity on ultrasonography. A special notched plaque can be used for juxtapapillary tumors along with adjuvant transpupillary thermotherapy (TTT) to the juxtapapillary margin of the tumor.

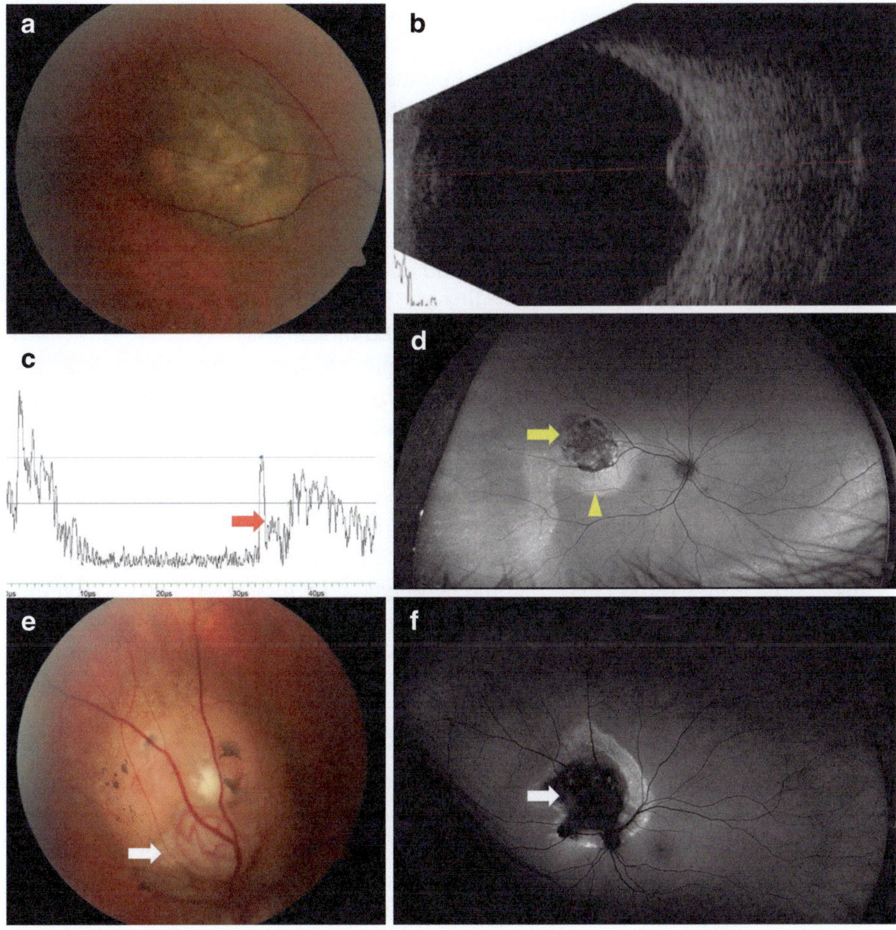

Fig. 2 (**a**) Choroidal melanoma. Note the orange pigment. (**b**) Acoustic hollowness on B-scan. (**c**) Low internal reflectivity on A-scan (arrow). (**d**) Hyperautofluorescent spots characteristic of orange pigment (arrow) and area of hyperautofluorescence (arrow head) highlighting subretinal fluid. (**e**) Amelanotic choroidal melanoma. Part of the tumor broke through Bruch's membrane creating mushroom-shaped configuration (arrow). (**f**) Dense hypofluorescence corresponding to mushroom-shaped area due to absence of the reitnal pigment epithelium (arrow)

- Charged-particle radiation such as proton beam radiotherapy can also deliver focal radiotherapy with less extensive lateral spread. Tumor response is similar to that of plaque brachytherapy.
- Conventional external beam radiotherapy (EBRT) with megavoltage photon irradiation is also effective for control of uveal melanoma with significantly higher complication rates. However, fractionated stereotactic radiotherapy is used in selected cases of juxtapapillary melanoma surrounding large circumference of the nerve that cannot be covered by notched plaques.

- Enucleation is usually reserved for large tumors or in eyes with no useful vision or cannot be adequately covered by focal radiotherapy.
- Some centers consider TTT as solo treatment for small tumors with thickness below 3 mm. The authors, however, do not adopt TTT as monotherapy. It is mainly used as adjuvant with notched plaques or for treatment of marginal recurrence in selected cases.
- **Prognosis:** choroidal melanoma can lead to loss of vision, loss of the eye, metastasis (90% to the liver), and death if left untreated. Radiotherapy can achieve tumor control in up to 98% of cases and earlier intervention reduces mortality. The COMS showed a 5-year mortality of 57% to 62% in large melanomas and 12-year mortality of 41–43% in medium-sized melanomas.
- The risk of metastasis depends on multiple clinical, histopathological, and genetic factors. Clinically, larger tumor size, ciliary body involvement, and extraocular extension are linked to higher risk of metastasis [3]. On histopathological level, epithelioid cell type is associated with higher risk of metastasis. Somatic chromosomal and gene mutations such as monosomy 3 and q8 gain, BAP1 mutation, and absence of SF36B1 and EIF1AX mutations are all associated with increased risk of mutation and poor prognosis. Further, two classes of melanoma (class 1 and class 2) could be detected by using gene expression profiling (GEP) for analysis of mRNA. Therefore, transscleral or transvitreal biopsy for genetic profiling is offered to patients with uveal melanoma for prognostic considerations.
- **Follow-up:** response to treatment is usually assessed using clinical examination and multimodal imaging 3 months after treatment with eye-preserving therapies. Patients are then followed routinely with clinical examination, imaging, and metastatic surveillance (chest CT and MRI of the liver) every 6 months for 5 years then annually for 5 years then discharged at 10-year mark if no recurrence. Patients with unfavorable prognostic factors, such as large tumor size or monosomy 3 mutation, are followed more closely by specialized medical oncology team for metastatic surveillance.
- **Pearl:** patients with treated uveal melanoma commonly present for intravitreal injection of anti-VEGF or steroids for treatment of radiation retinopathy. In eyes with ciliary body involvement injection site should be selected away from tumor site. Further, intervention for radiation-induced cataract should be delayed until there is adequate clinical evidence of tumor control.

1.3 Indeterminate Melanocytic Lesions (IML) of the Choroid

- There is overlap between choroidal nevus and small choroidal melanoma in landmark studies and literature in terms of lesion size and presence of risk factors. Due to this overlap and the lack of consensus on a cutoff tumor thickness that sets the mark between benign and malignant lesions, the term indeterminate melanocytic lesion was coined to describe small lesions that lie on the boundary between a nevus and a small melanoma. These are choroidal melanocytic lesions characterized by relatively small size and the presence of growth risk features such as orange pigment or SRF (Fig. 3) where a definitive diagnosis of a melanoma cannot be established. This is a more accurate term to use to replace misleading terms used by some clinicians such as "suspicious nevus" or "dormant melanoma."

- **MOLES acronym/algorithm:** In the era of accessible multimodal imaging, recently the MOLES acronym has been introduced to assist a wider range of eye practitioners in optimizing referral of melanocytic choroidal tumors to eye specialists. Thus, it is not focused on predicting growth, but rather assisting optometrists/ophthalmologist that recognizing certain features requires referral to an eye specialist. MOLES stands for the following: M for mushroom shape, O for orange pigment, L for large size, E for enlarging tumor, and S for SRF.

- There is always a difficult question as to whether to treat these lesions to permanently terminate the risk of future growth. The situation becomes more challenging if the lesion is near sensitive structures such as the macula or the optic disc, where treatment can lead to severe vision loss. Close monitoring at relatively

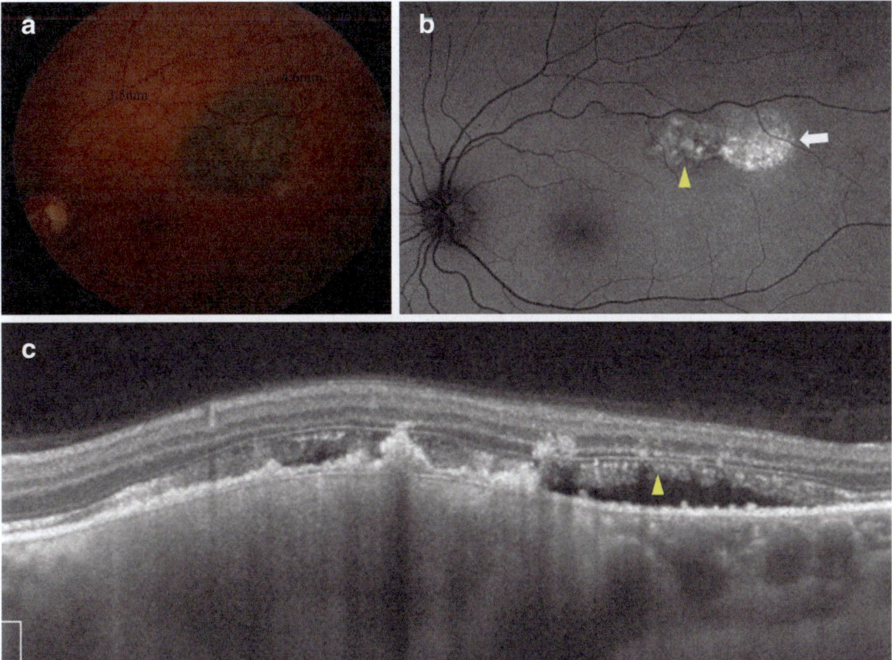

Fig. 3 (**a**) Indeterminate choroidal melanocytic lesion in the macula with orange pigment. (**b**) Hyperautofluorescence of orange pigment on FAF (arrow head) and adjacent subretinal fluid (SRF) (arrow). (**c**) Optical coherence tomography (OCT) detects SRF and shows "shaggy" photoreceptors (arrowhead)

shorter intervals is usually followed and treatment can be offered in some cases if the lesion is peripherally located away from sensitive structures or if there is evidence of growth.

- **Differential diagnosis:** several pigmented lesions, besides choroidal nevus, commonly confused with choroidal melanoma and referred to ocular oncology service for assessment. Below, we will elaborate briefly on most common such lesions. Figure 4 shows ophthalmoscopic appearance of some pigmented lesions that mimic choroidal melanoma.

1.4   Melanocytoma of the Optic Disc

- Congenital magnocellular peripapillary choroidal nevus that extends beyond the end of Bruch's membrane into epipapillary tissue and juxtapapillary retina. This explains why it appears to be encroaching over the optic disc (Fig. 4a). There is no racial predilection to melanocytoma which can affect any race equally.
- Melanocytoma of the optic disc tends to remain benign. It may cause enlargement of the blind spot; but malignant transformation is rare.
- The key differentiating features from choroidal melanoma include its darker color, characteristic fibrillar or feathery appearance due to extension into the nerve fiber layer, and absence of orange pigment and SRF.
- Periodic observation annually with lesion documentation using color photos and ultrasonography is required.

1.5   Vortex Vein Varix

- Occasionally confused for a melanocytic lesion (Fig. 4b). Can easily be identified by its anatomical location at the ampulla of vortex vein and by blanching on digital pressure or scleral depression (Fig. 4c). This sign can also be demonstrated by ultrasound and by OCT [4].
- No observation required being a normal anatomical variation.

1.6   Congenital Hypertrophy of the Retinal Pigment Epithelium (CHRPE)

- Congenital, asymptomatic, flat, very dark or black, sharply demarcated lesion usually located in the retinal periphery or mid-periphery (Fig. 4e). When long-standing it tends to develop spots of depigmentation, called lacunae. Although it

is believed to be congenital it is usually discovered accidentally later in life due to asymptomatic nature and peripheral location. Has no racial predilection and may grow in diameter slowly over many years.
- Periodic observation annually and documentation with color photos is adequate.

1.7   *Ocular and Oculodermal Melanocytosis (Nevus of Ota)*

- Congenital condition in which there is diffuse hyperpigmentation of the sclera and uveal tract. In the oculodermal version, cutaneous pigmentation is also seen. The condition is generally unilateral, but can occasionally be bilateral. The lifetime risk of developing uveal melanoma is 1/400, and 3% of all uveal melanoma cases are thought to be associated with ocular melanocytosis.
- Periodic examination with multimodal imaging for screening for uveal melanoma is required at 6-month interval for life.

1.8   *Peripheral Exudative Hemorrhagic Chorioretinopathy (PEHCR)*

- Peripheral age-related retinal degeneration resulting in the formation of peripheral choroidal neovascular membrane (CNVM) with consequent subretinal hemorrhage (Fig. 4f). Its location in the periphery and deep brown color can mimic uveal melanoma. Patients are typically elderly, and signs of age-related macular degeneration may be seen in the same eye and fellow eye. The color of the blood can also be more heterogeneous than the more brown uveal melanoma, and over time, blood at least partially absorbs while a choroidal melanoma would persist and grow [5].
- As compared to melanoma, The presence of hemorrhagic PED strongly supports a diagnosis of PEHCR [6]. IVFA shows blocked fluorescence due to bleeding followed by late hyperfluorescence from leakage. Ultrasonography shows heterogenous high reflectivity. In the context of marked subretinal hemorrhage, MRI with contrast can be very helpful in differentiating blood from melanoma [7].
- AMD-related submacular hemorrhage can also be occasionally confused for melanoma and is differentiated similarly.

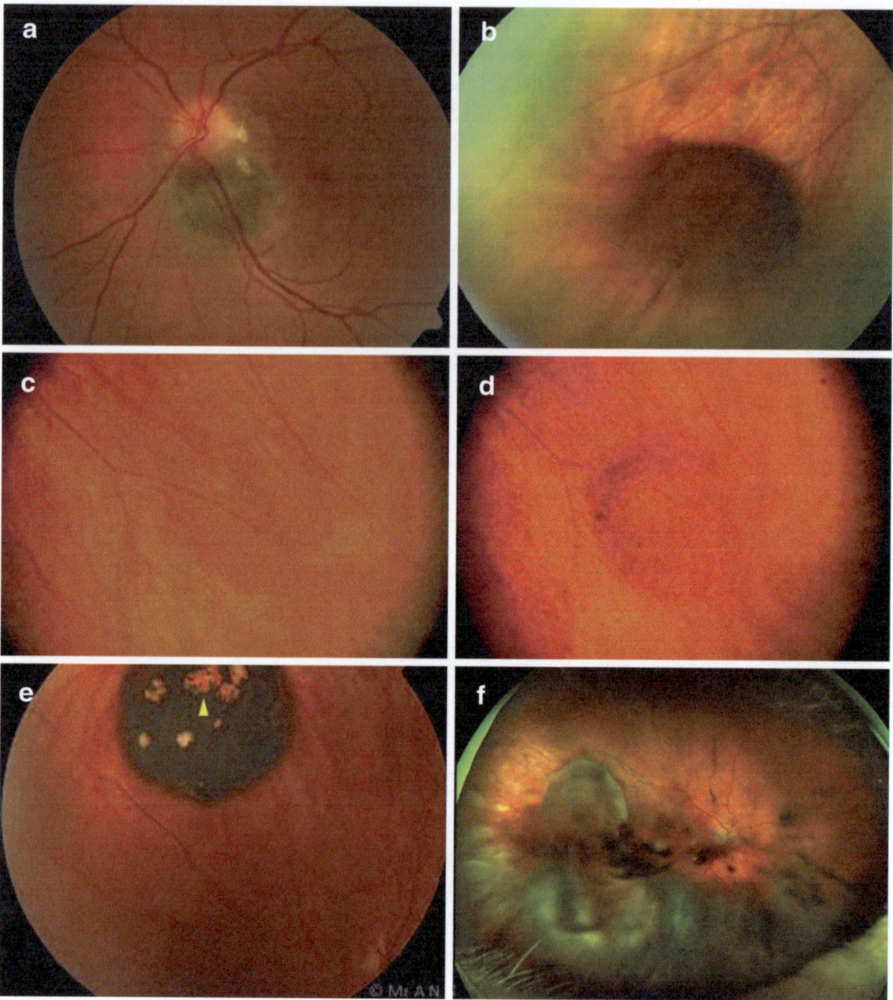

Fig. 4 (**a**) Optic disc melanocytoma. (**b**) Vortex vein varix. (**c**) Blanched ampulla of the vortex vein on scleral depression. (**d**) Prominent ampulla of the vortex vein on Valsalva maneuver. (**e**) Very dark sharply demarcated congenital hypertrophy of the retinal pigment epithelium (CHRPE). Note the hypopigmented spots, lacunae (arrowhead), indicating chronicity. (**f**) Peripheral exudative hemorrhagic chorioretinopathy (PEHCR) can also mimic peripherally located choroidal melanoma

2 Non-pigmented Uveal Tumors

2.1 Amelanotic Choroidal Nevus

- Previously discussed under choroidal nevus.

2.2 Amelanotic Choroidal Melanoma

- Previously discussed under choroidal melanoma.

2.3 Choroidal Metastasis

- Is the most common intraocular malignancy. Uveal metastases are most commonly carcinomas that spread to the uvea through a hematogenous route. Most common primary is breast cancer in women and lung cancer in men. Less commonly, the primary can be carcinoma of the alimentary tract, kidney, thyroid, pancreas, prostate, and other organs.
- Most patients have known history of primary malignancy; however, approximately 25% of patients have no known history of primary malignancy and the uveal metastasis is the initial presentation.
- **Clinical picture:** sessile or dome-shaped soft yellow mass, usually unilateral and unifocal but may be multifocal and bilateral. Secondary serous retinal detachment is common. Overlying retinal pigment epithelial changes give the characteristic "leopard spots." Untreated, the rate of growth is much faster than choroidal melanoma.
- **Imaging:** color fundus photographs are important for baseline and subsequent documentation. OCT shows characteristic "lumpy bumpy" configuration (Fig. 5c) and detects SRF. B-scan ultrasonography shows acoustic solidity and A-scan shows medium-high internal reflectivity (Fig. 5e, f).
- **Diagnosis:** complete medical history is key. Systemic evaluation and whole-body scan is necessary to identify the primary site.
- **Management:** small asymptomatic lesions can be observed. Some symptomatic lesions respond well to systemic chemotherapy administered for the primary cancer and show regression of choroidal lesion. Larger tumors with large exudative RD and vision loss despite chemotherapy may benefit from external beam radiotherapy (EBRT).

2.4 Choroidal Hemangioma

- Benign vascular hamartoma of the choroid that can present in diffuse and circumscribed variants. The former is associated with nevus flammeus or Sturge-Weber syndrome, where the latter is seen in patients with no systemic disorders.
- **Clinical picture:** circumscribed choroidal hemangioma is a well-defined elevated red/orange subretinal tumor (Fig. 6a), usually located postequatorially, commonly at the macula. Small lesions can be subtle and difficult to discern from surrounding retina. With time these lesions can cause alterations of overlying RPE, macular edema, central SRF, and decreased vision.

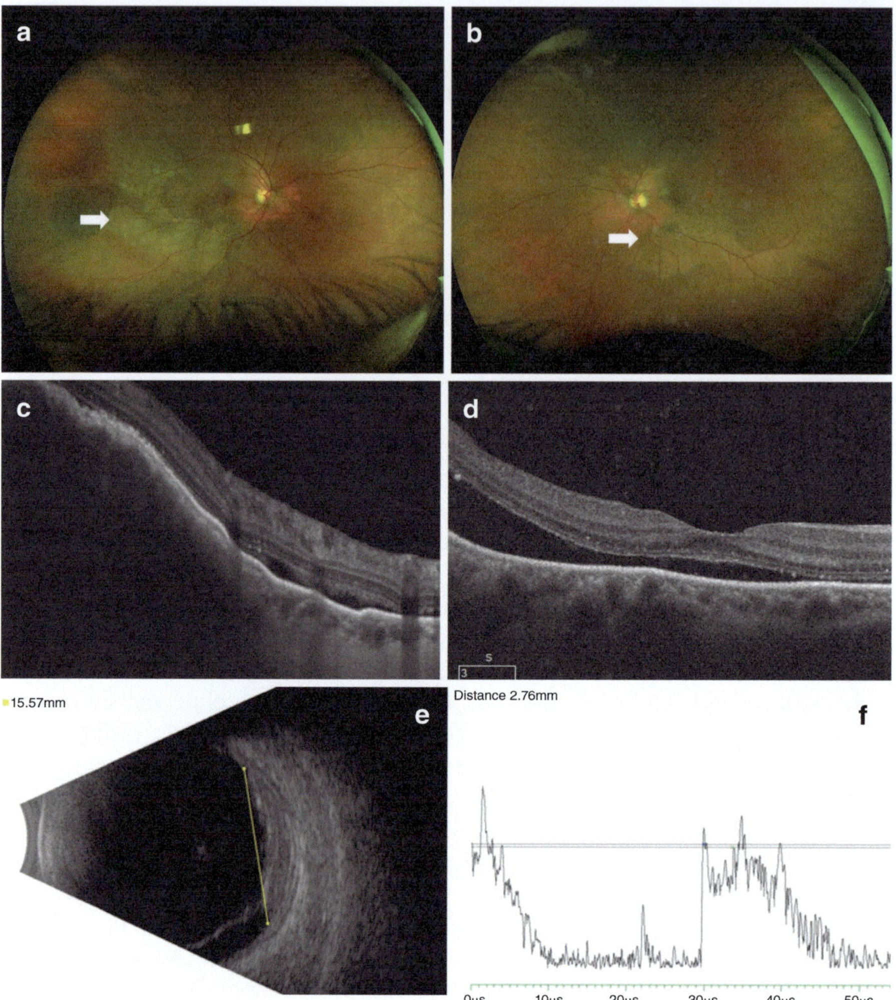

Fig. 5 (**a**, **b**) Ophthalmoscopic appearance of bilateral, asymmetric choroidal metastasis of breast carcinoma, more severe in the right eye. (**c**) Characteristic "lumpy pumpy" configuration on optical coherence tomography. (**d**) Subretinal fluid in active lesion. (**e**) Acoustic solidity on B-scan. (**f**) High internal reflectivity

- **Imaging:** OCT can detect the dome-shaped subretinal mass (Fig. 6b) and shows enlarged sub-RPE vessels. B-scan ultrasonography shows acoustic solidity and A-scan shows high internal reflectivity. IVFA may show early hyperfluorescence that gets more progressive in late phase and therefore has limited ability to identify tumor margin accurately for treatment purposes. Indocyanine green (ICG) angiography shows a characteristic early hyperfluorescence followed by late

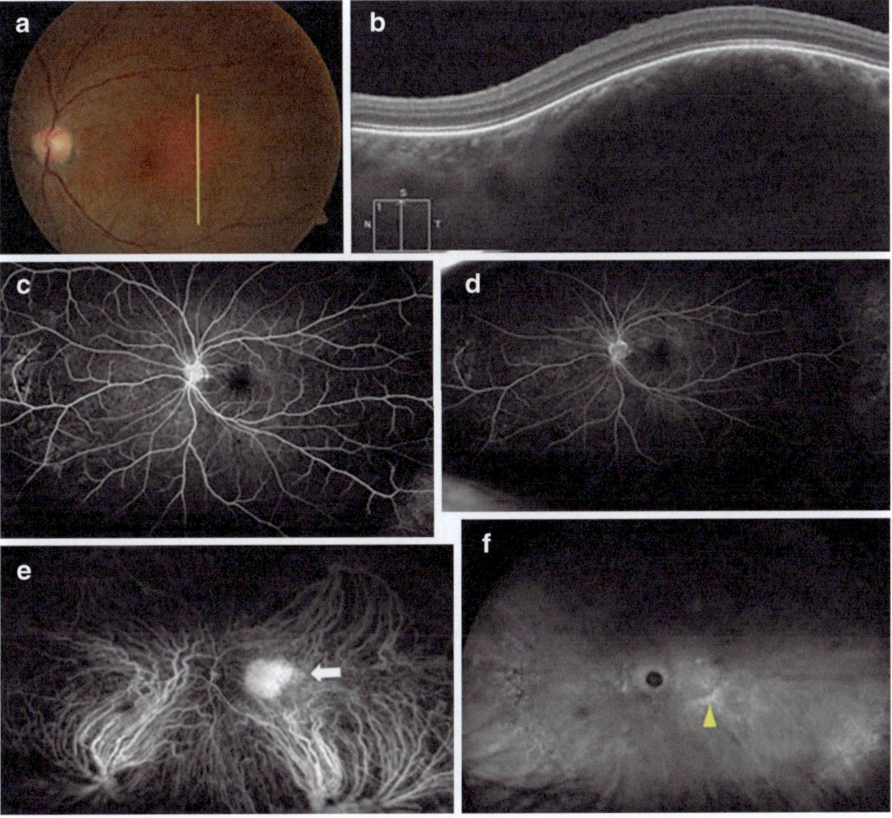

Fig. 6 (**a**) Well-defined orange/red choroidal hemangioma in the macula. (**b**) Optical coherence tomography appearance. (**c**, **d**) Unremarkable fluorescein angiography of the same lesion. (**e**) Indocyanin green angiography shows hyperfluorescence at 1 min (arrow). (**f**) Late "washout" gives more precise demarcation of the tumor margin

"washout" of hyperfluorescence (Fig. 6e, f); thus it is more helpful in identifying the tumor margin precisely for treatment planning. The combination of ICG + A-scan is usually successful in differentiating choroidal hemangioma from amelanotic melanoma.

- **Management:** observation is adequate for small asymptomatic tumors. Active tumors with SRF require treatment. Photodynamic therapy (PDT) is useful in lesions with thickness of 2 mm or less and usually shows resolution of leakage. Sometimes treatment may need to be repeated. Clinician should allow 3–4 months at least before considering further treatment. Larger lesions usually require low-dose plaque brachytherapy.
- **Pearl:** a limitation of Optos (Optos PLC, Dunfermline, UK) is color distortion due to the green filter used in the imaging. This may affect the ability to differentiate some lesions such as choroidal hemangioma vs. amelanotic melanoma based on their color.

2.5   *Intraocular Lymphoma*

- Intraocular lymphoma may affect different parts of the eye including the retina, vitreous, optic disc, and choroid.
- **Subtypes:** primary intraocular lymphoma (also known as vitreoretinal or large cell lymphoma) is the most common variant and is associated with primary central nervous system lymphoma (PCNSL), although it may present prior to any CNS involvement. It is more aggressive and usually masquerades as bilateral onset of uveitis in patients older than 50 years old, whereas choroidal lymphoma (visceral or systemic lymphoma) usually masquerades as chronic bilateral uveitis in patients in their fifth to seventh decade.
- **Clinical picture:** vitreoretinal lymphoma usually shows diffuse vitreous cells and subretinal yellow/white infiltrates. Decreased clarity of retinal details, due to dense vitreous cells, gives the characteristic sign of "headlight in the fog." RPE clumping is also common.
- Choroidal lymphoma presents as yellow subretinal infiltrate usually with no involvement of the retina or vitreous. In advanced disease both variants overlap clinically.
- **Diagnosis:** when intraocular lymphoma is suspected clinically the patient should undergo thorough systemic and neurological examination, lumbar puncture, and MRI of the brain. Vitreous sample with cytology by experienced pathologist who is familiar with the condition is key. Coordination with the pathologist prior to diagnostic vitrectomy is crucial. This can often be negative due to scanty sample and may need to be repeated. Tissue biopsy of the subretinal infiltrate may be needed. Refer to Chap. 26 'Vitreortinal Surgery in Uveitis'. In choroidal lymphoma the conjunctival fornices should be examined thoroughly for lymphoma involvement.
- Color fundus photos and IVFA helps with documentation of the lesion, but are less helpful in establishing the diagnosis.
- **Management:** in patients with choroidal lymphoma systemic involvement requires systemic evaluation by an experienced medical oncologist and is usually treated with systemic chemotherapy such as high-dose methotrexate or rituximab.
- Ocular involvement could be observed in asymptomatic cases or can be treated with fractionated radiotherapy for symptomatic lesions.
- In vitreoretinal lymphoma patients, systemic and intrathecal chemotherapy is generally considered along with intraocular methotrexate or rituximab. The intraocular route for methotrexate/rituximab becomes more crucial if systemic therapy is poorly tolerate or if the patient is maxed out on CNS radiotherapy. Fractionated radiotherapy is also effective but is usually reserved for cases that did not respond adequately to intraocular chemotherapy due to potential risk of visual loss post-irradiation especially if there is recurrence and treatment needs to be repeated.

2.6   Choroidal Osteoma

- Characteristic yellow-orange, sharply defined mass in the posterior pole with geographic margin with pseudopodia-like projections. Can be unilateral or bilateral.
- Ultrasonography shows calcified bone within choroid.
- Old-standing subfoveal lesions can cause decreased vision due to photoreceptor degeneration or secondary CNVM. These lesions should not be treated with PDT as treatment may promote photoreceptor atrophy. Associated CNVM may still be treated with anti-VEGF at the discretion of the clinician.
- Extrafoveal lesions can be treated by PDT which leads to decalcification and eradication of the tumor.

2.7   Ciliary Body Leiomyoma

- Rare smooth muscle tumor that arises from the ciliary body smooth muscles. Usually grow in the space between the uvea and sclera and grow as dome-shaped yellow mass in the fundus periphery that can simulate amelanotic melanoma.
- Diagnosis requires the clinician to be experienced and familiar with clinical features and variations of the condition. Ultrasonography may show intact choroid underneath the mass, but this is a subtle sign to elicit.
- Tumor growth can lead to multiple complications including secondary cataract, subluxation of the crystalline lens, retinal detachment, and scleral perforation. Therefore, surgical excision of the tumor is advisable and usually has favorable outcome.

3   Retinal Tumors

Retinal tumors can originate from the neural, vascular, or glial elements of the retina or from the retinal pigment epithelium or a mix of all these elements such as combined hamartoma of the retina and RPE. Retinoblastoma originates from the neural element of the retina. Vascular element of the retina can give rise to retinal capillary hemangioma, retinal hemangioblastoma, racemose hemangioma, or vasoproliferative tumors. Benign astrocytic hamartoma or astrocytoma arises from the glial element, whereas the RPE can give rise to RPE adenoma or RPE adenocarcinoma.

3.1 Retinoblastoma

- Is the most common intraocular malignancy in childhood and the second most common primary intraocular malignancy after uveal melanoma. It affects 1 live birth in every 14,000–20,000.
- **Genetics:** mutation of the retinoblastoma tumor suppressor gene RB1 located on the long arm of chromosome 13 at locus 14 (13q14) is universal in almost all cases. Positive family history of retinoblastoma is present in 10% of patients, whereas 90% of cases are sporadic. Bilateral disease indicates 98% chance of germline mutation; however, the percentage of germline mutation in sporadic unilateral cases is approximately 15%.
- **Clinical picture:** the most common presenting signs vary in different regions, and the mean age at presentation depends on disease laterality and family history. In the USA, the most common presenting signs are leukocoria, strabismus, and ocular inflammation and more than 90% of cases are diagnosed before the age of 3 years. The tumor starts as a gray white retinal lesion with a feeding artery and draining vein. With time, foci of calcification start to form. **Exophytic tumors:** grow underneath the retina and are usually associated with serous retinal detachment. **Endophytic tumors:** grow on the surface of the retina into the vitreous cavity and may shed vitreous seeds that are typically visible in the vitreous cavity on examination. Vitreous seeds may lead to tumor dissemination in the whole eye and may also migrate to the anterior chamber and settle on the iris forming iris nodules or settle inferiorly causing pseudohypopyon. There is risk also risk of neovascular glaucoma, rubeosis, and spontaneous hyphema. **Diffuse infiltrative retinoblastoma:** is a rare variant that represents a diagnostic dilemma due to often obscured view of the retina.
- **Diagnosis:** diagnosis is made clinically in the office. Examination under anesthesia (EUA) is mandatory for every case for full and precise assessment and documentation of all lesions. Complete medical history and physical examination must be carried out by a pediatric oncologist. Ultrasonography can detect tumor calcification and provide a clue to diagnosis. MRI is the key imaging modality to assess the optic nerve and orbit. Lumbar puncture may also be performed if optic nerve spread is suspected.
- **Differential diagnosis:** includes persistent fetal vasculature (also known as persistent hyperplastic primary vitreous PHPV), Coats disease, retinopathy of prematurity, toxocariasis, astrocytic hamartoma, uveitis, and choroidal coloboma.
- **Retinocytoma:** is considered by some as a benign variant of retinoblastoma that is clinically indistinguishable. However, it may show spontaneous calcification.
- **Primitive neuroectodermal tumor (PNET):** also known as trilateral retinoblastoma, which is coined to describe cases of bilateral retinoblastoma associated with pineoblastoma. This condition affects approximately 5% of children with RB1 germline mutation.
- **Management:** the collaboration of an experienced team that consists of ocular oncologist, pediatric ophthalmologist, pediatric oncologist, and radiation oncol-

ogist is necessary. The primary goals of treatment, in order, are to preserve life, then to preserve the eye as an organ, then to preserve vision as a function. Failure to treat retinoblastoma adequately leads to risk of metastasis and compromises survival. Treatment options include:

- **Enucleation:** remains a valid treatment that achieves complete removal of the tumor. It is usually considered when the tumor involves >50% of the globe, when optic nerve involvement is suspected, when neovascular glaucoma is present, or for an eye with guarded visual prognosis. Great care must be exercised to avoid globe penetration and resection of at least 10 mm of the optic nerve or more is important.
- **Chemotherapy (chemoreduction):** systemic chemotherapy using variable combinations of carboplatin, vincristine, and etoposide has been successful in achieving initial regression of the tumor, which can then be followed by laser therapy, cryotherapy, or brachytherapy. Intraarterial chemotherapy (IAC) by direct injection of chemotherapy through selective cannulation of the ophthalmic artery has gained more popularity recently to minimize systemic complications of chemotherapy such as second tumor or ototoxicity.
- **Laser therapy:** usually 810 nm infrared diode laser can be used as primary therapy or following chemotherapy.
- **Cryotherapy:** triple freeze-thaw technique under direct visualization through indirect ophthalmoscopy can be used for anteriorly located tumors <3 mm in maximum thickness.
- **Plaque brachytherapy:** may be used as primary or secondary therapy for localized small or medium tumors <16 mm in basal diameter and < 8 mm in maximum thickness.
- External beam radiotherapy: reserved for cases that failed to respond to other modalities. There is a concern of exacerbation of the already existent risk of developing second independent malignancies (such as osteosarcoma) in cases with RB1 germline mutation.

3.2 *Retinal Astrocytoma (Astrocytic Hamartoma)*

- Benign retinal glial tumor that arises from the retinal nerve fiber layer as a small white glistening tumor overlying the retinal vessels. They are commonly associated with tuberous sclerosis and occasionally neurofibromatosis. It may present with single or multiple lesions and can be unilateral or bilateral and may grow and calcify.
- Occasionally, the lesion may arise from the optic nerve head and is called "giant drusen."
- **Diagnosis:** typically through dilated ophthalmoscopy. B-scan ultrasonography can detect calcification which may cause acoustic shadowing.
- **Management:** most cases do not progress and therefore do not require treatment. However, evaluation for tuberous sclerosis is necessary for all patients.

3.3 Acquired Retinal Astrocytoma

- Unlike congenital astrocytoma, the acquired variant is not associated with tuberous sclerosis and is more aggressive. It appears as pink/yellow mass near the optic disc which tends to grow and assume a pedunculated configuration and can have numerous blood vessels on the surface. It may cause secondary serous retinal detachment and VH.
- **Management:** laser photocoagulation and PDT are useful to control the lesion and reduce the risk of subretinal exudation or VH.

4 Retinal Reactive Astrocytic Tumors (Formerly Retinal Vasoproliferative Tumors)

4.1 Retinal Capillary Hemangioblastoma

- Rare retinal vascular hamartoma with an incidence of 1/40,000 that can occur as a unilateral solitary lesion due to sporadic mutation or as bilateral or multiple lesions that are associated with chromosome 3 mutation and Von Hippel-Lindau (VHL) disease. Lesions are usually diagnosed in the second or third decade of life [8].
- **Clinical picture:** red/orange retinal mass with dilated tortuous feeding artery and draining vein. Subretinal exudation is common and has a predilection to involve the macula. If the macula is involved this leads to significant vision loss regardless of tumor size or location. Some lesions may arise from the optic nerve head.
- **Diagnosis:** is based on clinical examination. Ancillary tests such as IVFA are not necessary to establish diagnosis, but can show rapid filling of feeder vessels and late leakage. OCT can show the extent of macular exudation and detect an epiretinal membrane.
- If VHL disease is suspected, screening for systemic vascular anomalies such as cerebellar hemangioblastoma and malignancies such as renal carcinoma and pheochromocytoma is necessary to reduce mortality. Further, genetic consultation is offered to the patient and family members.
- **Management:** early detection of retinal lesions is key to good outcome. Small lesions can be treated with laser photoablation. Larger and more peripheral lesions may benefit from cryotherapy. Larger non-responsive lesions with large exudative RD may require plaque brachytherapy or proton beam radiotherapy. Anti-VEGF injection may be employed to help with macular edema. Lesions overlying the optic nerve head are the most challenging to treat. Recently, intravitreal propranolol has been reported to show favorable response for such lesions. Surgical excision through vitrectomy is useful in selected cases that are centrally located within the macular area.

4.2 Retinal Cavernous Hemangioma

- **Clinical picture:** a cluster of dark intraretinal venous aneurysms usually referred to as "bunch of concord grapes." The lesion does not have any associated feeding vessels and is usually located along the course of a retinal vein. Presentation can range from asymptomatic to variable degree of visual loss most commonly due to vitreous hemorrhage (VH).
- **Diagnosis:** usually based on characteristic findings on clinical examination. IVFA shows a unique sign of "fluorescein-erythrocyte interface" where the fluorescein dye pools in the superior portion of the cavernous space and the erythrocytes collect in the inferior portion.
- **Management:** usually no treatment is required. In the rare incident of VH it may be observed or treated with vitrectomy as needed. If VH is recurrent cryotherapy, PDT or plaque brachytherapy may be used to sclerose the cavernous spaces.

4.3 Racemose Hemangioma (Arteriovenous Communication)

- This is a simple or complex arteriovenous communication that occurs either as solitary lesion or as part of Wyburn-Mason syndrome.
- **Clinical picture:** characteristic large dilated tortuous retinal artery that travels for a variable distance into the fundus until it communicates directly with a similarly dilated tortuous vein.
- **Management:** systemic evaluation for Wyburn-Mason syndrome and imaging studies to detect vascular abnormalities in the brain are required. Observation of retinal lesion is usually adequate.

4.4 Retinal Vasoproliferative Tumor

- Acquired vasoproliferative tumor is a vascular mass that may occur as a primary lesion or secondary to intermediate uveitis, retinitis pigmentosa, or Coats disease. There is no known systemic association.
- **Clinical picture:** sessile or dome-shaped gray/pink mass usually located inferotemporally anterior to the equator. The mass can be well-circumscribed or can be ill-defined if the margin is masked by exudation. The feeding vessels are not prominent, unlike hemangioblastoma.
- Retinal vasoproliferative tumor can cause several complications that lead to decreased vision including intraretinal and subretinal exudation that usually tend to be present around the tumor base, SRF, remote cystoid macular edema (CME), epiretinal membrane and tractional retinal detachment.

Table 1 Key differentiating features of retinal vascular tumors

Name of the lesion	Clinical features on fundoscopy	Location	Exudation	Association with systemic diseases
Retinal capillary hemangioblastoma	Reddish pink lesion(s) with tortuous feeding and draining vessel. Exudation +/− vitreoretinal traction	Peripheral, mid-peripheral, or optic disc	In the posterior pole, commonly macular	Von Hippel-Lindau
Retinal cavernous hemangioma	Small cavernous spaces along the course of retinal vein Bunch of concord grape appearance	No specific location	No	CNS hemangioma
Racemose hemangioma (arteriovenous communication)	An arteriovenous communication rather than an actual tumor Characteristic large dilated tortuous vessels	Diffuse	No	Wyburn-Mason syndrome
Retinal vasoproliferative tumor	Sessile or dome-shaped lesion, typically present inferotemporally at equatorial level	Peripheral, most commonly inferotemporal	Surrounding the base of the lesion	No

- **Diagnosis:** Ophthalmoscopic findings are usually diagnostic. IVFA may show the high internal vascularity of the lesion. OCT can show CME and ERM.
- **Management:** small asymptomatic lesions may be observed closely if no leakage. Small lesions with active leakage can be treated with laser photocoagulation, PDT, and cryotherapy with some response. Plaque brachytherapy is an effective treatment in case of inadequate response to previous treatment modalities.
- Persistent CME after control of the tumor may be treated with anti-VEGF therapy. Sub-tenon's steroid can be helpful to control inflammatory reaction caused by treatment if necessary see Table 1. Tractional retinal detachment in the context of retinal vasoproliferative tumour can be very challenging and is best to be conservative during membrane dissection and avoid iatrogenic retinal tears [9].

5 Tumors of the Retinal Pigment Epithelium

5.1 CHRPE

- Previously discussed in the differential diagnosis of posterior uveal melanoma.

5.2 Combined Hamartoma of the Retina and RPE

- **Clinical picture:** usually solitary juxtapapillary lesion adjacent or encroaching over the optic disc with variable pigmentation and tractional stretching and tortuosity of the overlying retinal vessels. It may be a manifestation of neurofibromatosis II. The fovea may exhibit distorted macular striae. With time, vitreoretinal traction may result in subfoveal exudation, retinoschisis, or retinal hole.
- The lesion can also be present in the peripheral fundus causing significant dragging of retinal vessels toward the lesion.
- **Diagnosis:** usually based on clinical examination findings. Color photos may be used for documentation of the lesion. intravenous florescein angiograpghy (IVFA) shows late staining of the lesion and OCT demonstrates vitreoretinal traction.
- **Management:** most cases are observed. Visually symptomatic vitreoretinal traction may require vitrectomy with membrane peeling.

5.3 RPE Adenoma and Adenocarcinoma

- Benign RPE adenoma and malignant RPE adenocarcinoma are rare neoplasia of the RPE that show local growth with no tendency to metastasize.
- **Clinical picture:** oval black or very dark lesion in the retinal periphery with abrupt elevation of its margin. Occasionally, a dilated tortuous feeding artery and draining vein can be present.
- **Diagnosis:** B-scan ultrasonography shows acoustically solid mass with abrupt elevation. A-scan shows high internal reflectivity. Fine needle biopsy can be considered if diagnosis is uncertain.
- **Management:** small asymptomatic lesions can be observed. Large tumors may require surgical resection with lamellar iridocyclectomy. Response to plaque brachytherapy has been variable and unpredictable (Table 2).

Key Points
- Choroidal nevus is the most commonly encountered pigmented fundus tumor. It is important to be familiar with its clinical appearance and the clinical features that predict high risk of growth.
- Choroidal melanoma is the most common primary intraocular tumor, which can lead to loss of vision, loss of the eye, liver metastasis, and death if untreated. It is essential for clinicians to able to identify lesions suspicious for uveal melanoma and refer timely to specialized service.
- Several benign pigmented lesions can mimic uveal melanoma such as CHRPE, subretinal hemorrhage, and vortex vein varix. These can easily be differentiated from melanoma using findings from clinical examination and multimodal imaging.

Table 2 Provides a summary of common fundus lesions encountered during ophthalmoscopy and a color-coded guide to differential diagnosis

Pigmented (brown/dark)	Non-pigmented (yellowish/white)	Red/orange
Choroidal melanoma • Orange pigment, SRF, evidence of growth over short span of time • Acoustic hollowness on B-scan	Amelanotic choroidal melanoma • Clinical features are identical to those of melanoma with nonpigmented appearance	Choroidal hemangioma • Usually postequatorial, commonly in the macula • Enlarged choroidal vessels on OCT • Acoustically solid and high internal reflectivity on ultrasonography
Choroidal nevus • Overlying drusen, RPE degenerative changes, or hyperplasia • Preserved choriocapillaris layer on OCT	Amelanotic choroidal nevus • Clinical features are identical to those of choroidal nevus with nonpigmented appearance	Metastatic carcinoid tumor • Complete medical history and systemic evaluation is key
Indeterminate melanocytic lesion • Presence of risk features, e.g., orange pigments and SRF without definitive diagnosis of melanoma	Choroidal metastasis • History of lung or breast cancer • Lumpy pumpy appearance on OCT • Commonly bilateral and multifocal	Metastatic thyroid carcinoma • Complete medical history and systemic evaluation is key
CHRPE • Flat, sharply demarcated, black or very dark, mid-peripheral or peripheral	Choroidal detachment • "Double spike" on A-scan and clinical context such as postoperative, etc.	Metastatic renal cell carcinoma • Complete medical history and systemic evaluation is key
Melanocytoma of the optic nerve • Overlying the optic disc with fibrillar or feathered appearance • The lesion is very pigmented/black	Chorioretinal inflammatory granuloma • Coexisting uveitis such as TB or sarcoidosis	
Vortex vein varix • Follows anatomical location of vortex vein varix • Enlarges on Valsalva and blanches on scleral indentation	Choroidal osteoma • Yellow-orange with sharply defined geographic margin with pseudopodia-like projections	
Ocular melanocytosis • Flat diffuse pigmentation • Anterior segment pigmentation: Iris and sclera.	Uveal lymphoma • Yellow/white subretinal infiltration with greasy appearance	
PEHCR • Elderly patient with signs of AMD such as drusen • Subretinal, and often vitreous, hemorrhage of various age	Ciliary body leiomyoma • Diagnosis by exclusion. Very similar to amelanotic melanoma	

Table 2 (continued)

Pigmented (brown/dark)	Non-pigmented (yellowish/white)	Red/orange
AMD-related subretinal hemorrhage • History of AMD	Neurilemmoma • Exceedingly rare tumor that arises from Schwann's cells. Very similar to amelanotic melanoma	
Combined hamartoma of the retina and RPE • Usually located juxtapapillary • Associated vitreoretinal traction with macular striae and distorted retinal vessels	Posterior scleritis • Pain • Characteristic T-sign on B-scan	
RPE adenoma • Very dark or black lesion in the retinal periphery with abrupt elevation of the margin, feeding artery, and draining vein • Acoustically solid on B-scan	Sclerochoroidal calcification • Multiple discrete yellow placoid lesions usually along superotemporal arcade	
RPE adenocarcinoma • As adenoma with evidence of rapid local growth	Retinal astrocytoma • Small whitish lesion at the retinal nerve fiber layer typically near the optic disc • Commonly associated with tuberous sclerosis	

CHRPE congenital hypertrophy of the retinal pigment epithelium, *PEHCR* peripheral exudative hemorrhagic chorioretinopathy, *RPE* retinal pigment epithelium

- Choroidal metastases are the most common intraocular malignancy. They are seen much less frequently in clinical practice compared with uveal melanoma because patients can be severely unwell which reduces rate of seeking ophthalmological assessment. Another reason is that these lesions commonly respond to systemic chemotherapy and be present but asymptomatic.
- Retinoblastoma is the most common intraocular tumor in childhood. Diagnosis is usually established clinically, and it is important to be familiar with the common differential diagnosis of leukocoria.

References

1. Shields CL, et al. Choroidal NEVUS transformation into melanoma per millimeter increment in thickness using multimodal imaging in 2355 cases: the 2019 Wendell L. Hughes lecture. Retina. 2019;39(10):1852–60.
2. Hawkins BS. Collaborative ocular melanoma study group. The collaborative ocular melanoma study (COMS) randomized trial of pre-enucleation radiation of large choroidal melanoma: IV. Ten-year mortality findings and prognostic factors. COMS report no. 24. Am J Ophthalmol. 2004;138(6):936–51.

3. Kivelä T, Simpson SR, Grossniklaus HE, et al. Uveal melanoma. In: Amin MB (ed.) AJCC cancer staging mannual. 8th ed. New York: Springer, 2016, pp. 805–17.
4. Ismail RA, Sallam A, Zambarakji HJ. Optical coherence tomographical findings in a case of varix of the vortex vein ampulla. Br J Ophthalmol. 2011;95(8):1169–70, 1182.
5. Safir M, Zloto O, Fabian ID, Moroz I, Gaton DD, Vishnevskia-Dai V. Peripheral Exudative Hemorrhagic Chorioretinopathy with and without treatment-Clinical and multimodal imaging characteristics and prognosis. PLoS One. 2022;17(9):e0275163.
6. Sodhi GS, Singh N, Wrenn J, Singh AD. Peripheral Hemorrhagic Chorioretinopathy: Differentiating Features from Choroidal Melanoma. Ocul Oncol Pathol. 2023;9(1–2):1–8.
7. Safir M, Zloto O, Fabian ID, Moroz I, Gaton DD, Vishnevskia-Dai V. Peripheral Exudative Hemorrhagic Chorioretinopathy with and without treatment-Clinical and multimodal imaging characteristics and prognosis. PLoS One. 2022;17(9):e0275163. PMID: 36166419; PMCID: PMC9514609.
8. Shields JA, Shields CL. Intraocular tumors: an atlas and textbook. Philadelphia: Lippincott Williams & Wilkins; 2016.
9. Jennifer OA, Samantha RG, Brian M, Alan S, Jules W, Talia RK. Repair of a Tractional Retinal Detachment in the Setting of an Idiopathic Vasoproliferative Tumor. Ophthalmic Surgery Lasers and Imaging Retina. 2023;54(8):485–88.

Vitreoretinal Endoscopy

Christopher D. Riemann

1 Background

The Greek etiology of the word "endoscopy" stems from the words "scopy"—to look—and "endo" within. Endoscopy is in wide use today with a multitude of medical and industrial applications. Technologies including optical, fiber optic, and Grindrod designs were used for different applications.

Ocular endoscopy in cadaver eyes was first described in 1952 [1] and clinical in vivo ocular endoscopy was first performed in 1986 [2].

One mm (19-g) fiber optic ophthalmic endoscopes typically are deployed into the eye through a limbal paracentesis or through a pars plana sclerotomy. 0.7 mm (23-g) endoscopes can be used through a paracentesis or a standard 23-gauge vitrectomy trocar system. The endoscope units are connected to a central unit that houses a camera module, a 810 nm laser module, and an illumination source, each of which is connected to the respective fibers in the endoscope (Fig. 1). The 19-gauge imaging fiber bundle consists of 17,000 ultrathin fibers. The 23-g imaging fiber bundle has 10,000 fibers creating very low resolution but functional views of target structures especially when the endoscope is moved close to structures of interest to maximize magnification (Fig. 2a, b).

Endoscopic surgery can be utilized in a broad spectrum of ophthalmic surgery. Some representative examples include:

- Glaucoma. Endocyclophotocoagulation ablates the ciliary under direct visualization to lower the intraocular pressure (IOP) [3]. Endoscopic visualization of angle structures may aid in diagnosing and repairing angle defects such as cyclodialysis clefts and can aid in placing angle-based glaucoma drainage devices when gonioscopy is not possible.

C. D. Riemann (✉)
Cincinnati Eye Institute and University of Cincinnati, Cincinnati, OH, USA

© The Author(s), under exclusive license to Springer Nature Switzerland AG 2024

A. B. Sallam et al. (eds.), *Practical Manual of Vitreoretinal Surgery*,
https://doi.org/10.1007/978-3-031-47827-7_31

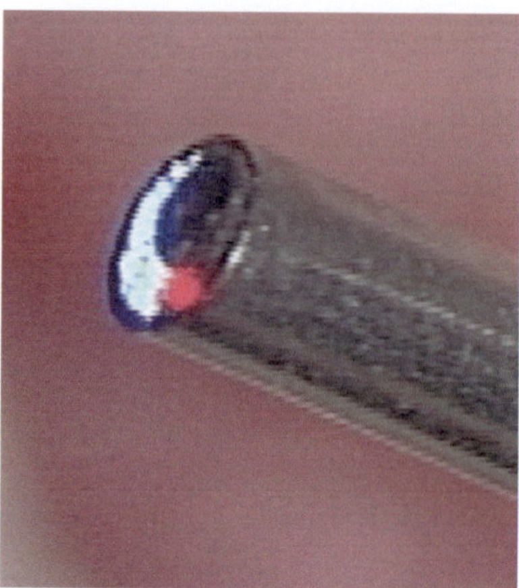

Fig. 1 High magnification view of a 19-g ophthalmic endoscope with a single 200-micron laser delivery fiber, approximately 75–100 illuminating fibers, and a 600-micron-diameter imaging fiber bundle with 17,000 fibers. (Courtesy of Christopher Riemann, MD, USA)

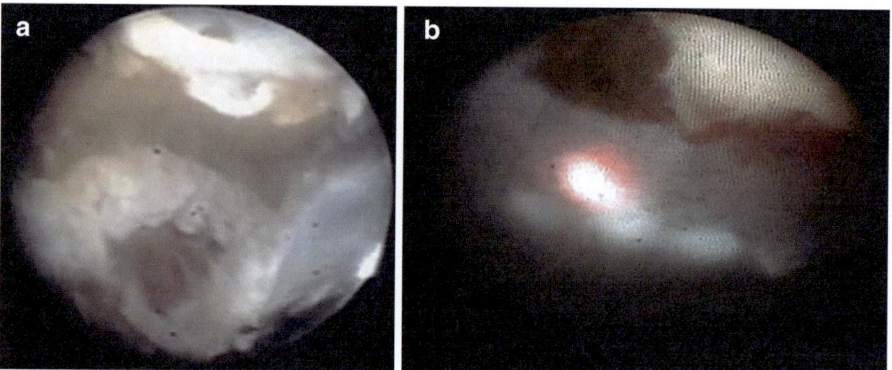

Fig. 2 (**a**) 19-gauge endoscopy of a 20 g forceps removing massive tractional epiciliary membrane causing profound hypotony and globe collapse. Photo credit – Christopher Riemann MD. (**b**) 23-g endoscopy of the pars plana with pars plana scarring, the ora serrata, fresh laser burns, and an endoscope laser aiming beam. (Courtesy of Christopher Riemann, MD, USA)

- Anterior segment. Sutured posterior chamber intraocular lens (PCIOL) and iris prosthesis cases can be performed with precise confirmation of ciliary sulcus placement of sutures, endo-rotation of knots, and IOL position. [4] UGH syndrome etiology can be visualized directly. Anterior segment maneuvers can be performed in the setting of corneal media opacity.
- Oculoplastics. Endoscopic approaches for brow and facelifts are common as are corrugator muscle lyses. Endoscopic visualization can also aid in dacryocystorhinostomy, orbital decompression for thyroid eye disease, and orbital fracture repair [5].
- Retina. See below.

2 Endoscopic Vitrectomy Case Selection

There are three types of scenarios where endoscopic PPV may be useful [6].

– Eyes with media opacity and limited visualization precluding repair of posterior segment pathology:

> Cornea/anterior chamber media opacity.
> Permenant keratoprosthesis.
> Previous iris repair or iris prosthesis [7]
> Endophthalmitis [8]
> Trauma.

– Eyes with retro-iris very anterior pathology:

> Hypotony with or without epiciliary membrane.
> Anterior loop proliferative vitreoretinopathy (PVR), anterior-posterior PVR, anterior circumferential PVR.
> Anterior intraocular foreign body.
> Anterior tumor.
> Trauma.
> Primary sutured PCIOL [9]
> Sutured PCIOL revision.
> Aniridia fibrosis syndrome.
> Sutured fluocinolone or ganciclovir implant placement [10]
> Need for pars plana tube shunt placement in the setting of limited visualization [11].
> Endoscopic facilitation of suprachoroidal approach to subretinal surgery [12, 13].

– Eyes where "less is more" are particularly amenable to the lighter touch and more gentle surgical approach afforded by endoscopic vitrectomy with less aggressive scleral depression and globe manipulation:

> Uveitis.
> Corneal disease with stem cell deficiency and/or low endothelial cell count.
> Ischemic eyes (diabetics, ocular ischemic syndrome).
> Multiply operated eyes.

3 Limitations of Ocular Endoscopy

– One endoscopic optical pathway precludes any stereopsis or depth perception. Surgeon must rely on monocular cues which are subtle to appreciate and difficult to master.
– Very low image resolution. To put this into meaningful perspective, consider:

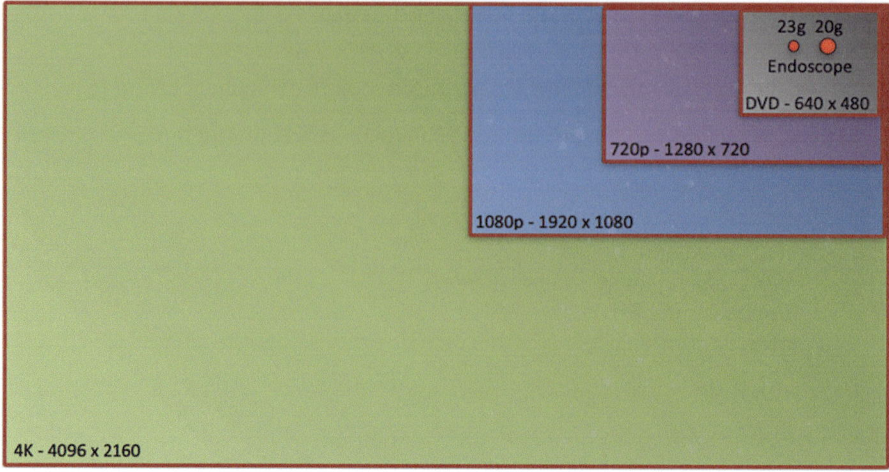

Fig. 3 Graphic visually representing relative amounts of visual information of 4 K (green) (see Chap. 32), 1080p (blue), 720p (violet), and 480p (gray) video formats and currently approved fiberoptic ophthalmic endoscopes (red)

> 4 K television at a resolution of 4096 x 2160 = 8,847,360 pixels (8.8 megapixels)
> 1080p HD television at 1920 x 1080 = 2,073,600 pixels (2.1 megapixels)
> Standard definition video at 640 x 480 = 307,200 pixels (0.3 megapixels).
> 19-g endoscope with 17,000 fibers = 17,000 "pixels" (0.017 megapixels)
> 23-g endoscope with 10,000 fibers = 10,000 "pixels" (0.01 megapixels) (Fig. 3).

- Rigid scopes make anterior imaging structures in phakic patients challenging.
- Poor illumination especially as semi-disposable endoscopes approach the end of their life cycle.
- Head turn away from microscope to operate off endoscope screen.
- Rotational orientation is sometimes counterintuitive—especially when operating on the superior hemiglobe.
- Limited oppurtunity for bimanual dissection.
- Substantial capital investment plus the ongoing expense of semi-disposable probes. Very poor reimbursement in the US medical system.
- Steep learning curve—technically difficult.
- No possibility for bimanual surgery.

4 Alternatives to Endoscopic Vitrectomy

- Don't operate.

> Repeated tap and inject procedures for endophthalmitis.
> Observe luxed PCIOL and treat functional aphakia with contact lens.

Wait for media opacity to clear.
If prognosis is very guarded, rely on the healthy contralateral eye.
Heroic surgery is not always the best choice for every patient:

> Disease state and prognosis for operative eye.
> Realistic goals—recovery of vision versus globe retention.
> Age.
> Medical comorbidity.
> Condition and health of contralateral eye.

– Altered surgical approach with a compromise—do what is feasible:

> Silicone oil fill without epiciliary peeling for hypotony.
> Large retinectomy for anterior PVR.

– "May the force be with you" vitrectomy:

> Core and very limited vitrectomy is possible without internal view.
>
> > Clinical preoperative B scan must rule out large choroidals or RD.
> > Careful attention to extraocular hand and instrument position.
>
> Surgical fact pattern must be straightforward.
> No precise dissection or manipulation is possible.

– Advanced conventional viewing techniques:

> Aggressive scleral depression:
>
> > May sometimes offer adequate visualization.
> > Significant inflammation can complicate the postoperative course.
>
> Conventional eccentric viewing through windows of lesser media opacity.
> Digital screen-based viewing techniques—see screen-based surgery Chap. 32:
>
> > Low illumination and maximum camera aperture reduce light scatter and improve visualization through the corneal haze and other light-diffusing media opacity.
> > High illumination level and small camera aperture create a pinhole-type viewing scenario which reduces the effect of refractive-type media opacity from extreme irregular astigmatism and other higher-order optical aberrations.
>
> Temporary keratoprosthesis:
>
> > Longer and more complex surgery. Please refer to Chap. 33 "Vitrectomy in the Presence of Opaque Cornea".
> > Associated with more inflammation.
> > Requires corneal surgery techniques and possibly a corneal surgeon.
> > Requires full-thickness corneal transplant to follow.
> > Corneal transplant may not be needed and may complicate postoperative course.

5 Clinical Pearls: Getting Started

Despite very real challenges and drawbacks, endoscopic vitrectomy techniques are highly relevant and useful to mainstream vitreoretinal surgery practice. A graduated approach with careful attention to detail is essential to avoid frustration and ensure successful skill set acquisition.

- Start by using the endoscope as light pipe for conventional 23-g cases and compare the endoscopic view to conventional visualization frequently to orient yourself.
- Always start with maximum illumination on the endoscope.
- Maximize magnification by filling the endoscopic image with the area of surgical interest. Use all the available resolution by moving close to the target area with the endoscope.
- Reduce illumination when video whites out as you move closer to increase magnification.
- Consider a chandelier to improve the brightness of dim endoscopes and to create better shadows for monocular depth clues.
- Frequently wipe the endoscope tip with a moist instrument wipe.
- Endoscopically visualizing and operating the inferior hemiglobe is much more intuitive than the superior hemiglobe where point-of-view realities can make everything appear inverted and unintuitively rotated. Operating superiorly requires repeat practice with cadaver, animal, or model eyes.
- Endoscope trocar entry points are best placed nearly 180 degrees apart for the greatest disparity between right- and left-handed entry sites.
- Low threshold for third (often superior) entry port to be able to both visualize and surgically access the subtrocar anterior ocular structures.
- Limbal entry with a larger higher-resolution (17,000 or higher) endoscope whenever possible.
- Suggest integrating endoscopic viewing into digital screen-based surgery with same screen/split screen viewing for improved ergonomics and faster switching between conventional surgical and endoscopic viewing. [14]
- Store the endoscope in a cup of BSS when not in use to avoid heat from illumination fibers baking debris onto the end of the endoscope.

6 Conclusion

Vitreoretinal endoscopy is a skill set that has a steep learning curve and is difficult to master. Notwithstanding, an expanded vitreoretinal surgical repertoire including endoscopic techniques is incredibly rewarding. Endoscopy opens an entire world of surgical possibilities previously not feasible and changes the definition of impossible or inoperable. Globes previously destined for removal can be saved and unsalvageable vision can be restored. Endoscopic vitrectomy is a "labor of love" that is rewarded with frequent complex surgical referrals, plenty of respect from colleagues, and more time in the operating room.

7   Case Scenario

A 45-year-old monocular female patient with congenital aniridia presents with 24 hours duration of painful visual loss. Best corrected visual acuity was 20/125 two months ago. Exam reveals light perception visual acuity and an IOP of 56 on maximum medical therapy. There is a decompensated previous penetrating keratoplasty with 4+ epithelial and stromal edema. B scan ultrasonography was normal. This surgical dilemma is optimally addressed with endoscopic vitrectomy and pars plana tube shunt placement (Fig. 4).

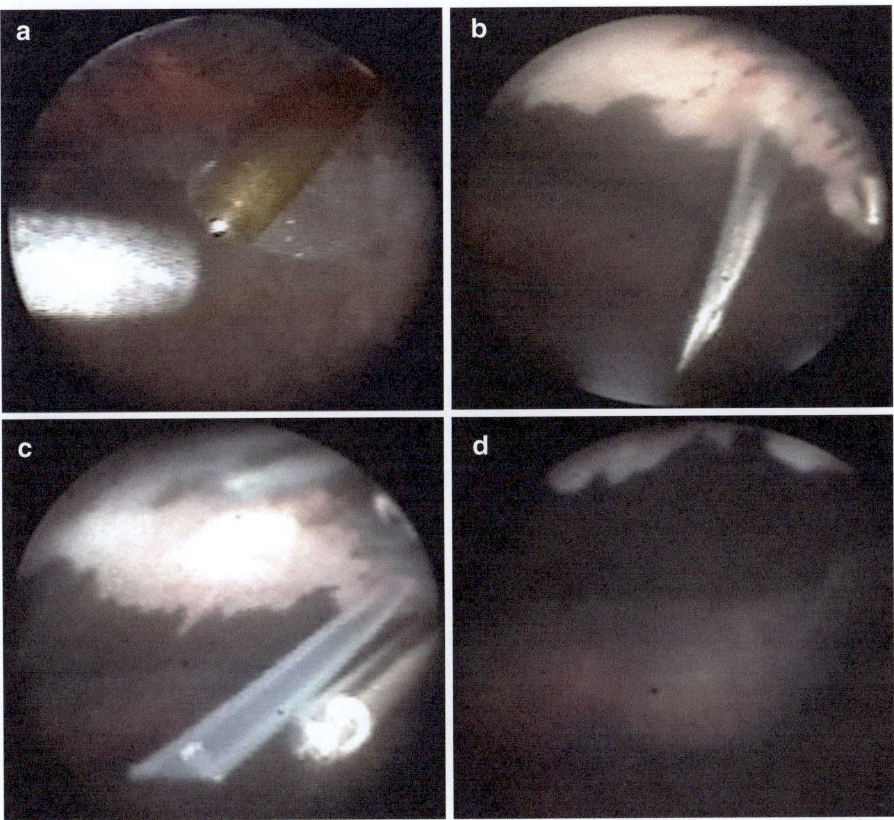

Fig. 4 Endoscopic core and peripheral vitrectomy are performed (**a**). A 23-g needle is used to create the tube shunt tract and is confirmed to be within the pars plana – note the extensive scarring from previous trans-scleral cyclophotocoagulation (**b**). The tube shunt tube is placed and confirmed to be in the vitreous cavity and free of any vitreous material. (**c**) Scleral depression is performed and does not reveal any iatrogenic breaks. (**d**). The patient achieves immediate IOP control and undergoes successful limbal stem cell transplantations and penetrating keratoplasty 3 months later with recovery to baseline 20/125 visual acuity. (Courtesy of Christopher Riemann, MD, USA)

Key Points

- Endoscopic posterior segment surgery is particularly valuable in eyes with optical media opacity hindering traditional repair, those with very anterior pathologies, involving the ciliary body and the peripheral retina.
- Mastering endoscopic techniques demands persistence and practice starting with simple cases.
- Surgeons must navigate the lack of stereopsis, low image resolution, and orientation challenges posed by endoscopy.
- Compared to 23-g endoscopes, 19-g probes have acceptable resolution enabling surgeons to perform intricate maneuvers even in challenging scenarios.
- Surgeons must navigate the lack of stereopsis, low image resolution, and orientation challenges posed by endoscopy.

References

1. Butterworth RF, Bignell JL. A new type of eye endoscope. Brit J Ophthalmol. 1952;36:217–20.
2. Lecoq PJ, Billotte C, Combe JC. Value of vitreoretinal video-endoscopy. J Fr Ophtalmol. 1986;9(6–7):427–9.
3. Uram M. Endoscopic cyclophotocoagulation in glaucoma management. Curr Opin Ophthalmol. 1995;6(2):19–29.
4. Sasahara M, Kiryu J, Yoshimura N. Endoscope-assisted transscleral suture fixation to reduce the incidence of intraocular lens dislocation. J Cataract Refract Surg. 2005;31(9):1777–80.
5. Zhou G, Tu Y, Yu B, Wu W. Endoscopic repair of combined orbital floor and medial wall fractures involving the inferomedial strut. Eye (Lond). 2020;35:2763.
6. Riemann CD. Vitreoretinal surgeons pick up endoscopes. Retina Today. 2007.
7. Toygar O, Snyder ME, Riemann CD. Pars Plana vitrectomy through a custom flexible iris prosthesis. Retina. 2016 Aug;36(8):1474–9.
8. De Smet MD, Carlborg EA. Managing severe endophthalmitis with the use of an endoscope. Retina. 2005;25(8):976–80.
9. Boscher C, Lebuisson DA, Lean JS, Nguyen-Khoa JL. Vitrectomy with endoscopy for management of retained lens fragments and/or posteriorly dislocated intraocular lens. Graefes Arch Clin Exp Ophthalmol. 1998;236(2):115–21.
10. KochFH GHOC, Hattenbach LO, Ohrloff C. Endoskopische Kontrolle von pars plana implantierten ganciclovir-Medikamenten zur Verbesserung der Langzeitprognose bei der Behandlung der Cytomegalievirusretinitis = intravitreal endoscopic visualization of intraocula ganciclovir devices : improved long-term treatment of CMV retinitis. Klinische Monatsblaetter fuer Augenheilkunde. 1999;214(2):107–11.
11. Shaikh AH, Khatana AK, Zink JM, Miller DM, Petersen MR, Correa ZM, Riemann CD. Combined endoscopic vitrectomy with pars plana tube shunt procedure. Br J Ophthalmol. 2014;98(11):1547–50.
12. Koch FH, Luloh KP, Augustin AJ, el Agha MS, Guembel H, Ohrloff C, Grizzard WS, Hammer ME, Sinclair S. Subretinal microsurgery with gradient index endoscopes. Ophthalmologica. 1997;211(5):283–7.

13. Ho AC, Chang TS, Samuel M, Williamson P, Willenbucher RF, Malone T. Experience with a subretinal cell-based therapy in patients with geographic atrophy secondary to age-related macular degeneration. Am J Ophthalmol. 2017;179:67–80.
14. Brooks CC, Kitchens J, Stone TW, Riemann CD. Consolidation of imaging modalities utilizing digitally assisted visualization systems: the development of a surgical information handling cockpit. Clin Ophthalmol. 2020;14:557–69.

Digitally Assisted, Screen-Based Vitreoretinal Surgery

Christopher D. Riemann

1 Background

The operating room microscope (TOM) has been a fixture in the vitreoretinal operating room since the very first vitrectomies over half a century ago. Stunning innovation in vitreoretinal surgery technologies has been less notable for the retinal operating room microscope and primary surgical visualization which have remained remarkably unchanged—especially over the past 25 years. With the evolution of micro-processing capabilities for digital image acquisition, processing, and display over the past decade, primary digital visualization with 3D high definition (HD) screen-based surgery is now feasible [1] and commercially available systems are available [2]. Digitally assisted screen-based vitreoretinal surgery (DSVS) has arrived.

2 Basics

Digital video consists of serially projected digital images. Primary digital surgical visualization requires:

- Spatial pixel resolution digitally approximating 1 min of arc—20/20 visual acuity.
- Viewing geometry analogous to the 60-degree field of view of the analog microscope.
- Temporal resolution of at least 30 frames per second (fps)—preferably 50–60 fps.
- Dynamic range image acquisition and display equivalent to human photopic function.

C. D. Riemann (✉)
Cincinnati Eye Institute and University of Cincinnati, Cincinnati, OH, USA

© The Author(s), under exclusive license to Springer Nature Switzerland AG 2024

A. B. Sallam et al. (eds.), *Practical Manual of Vitreoretinal Surgery*,
https://doi.org/10.1007/978-3-031-47827-7_32

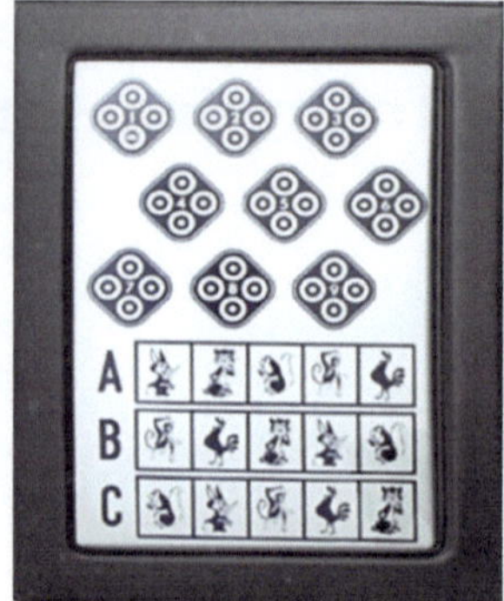

2D Visual Acuity	Digital Microscopy Video Format Equivalent	Titmus Circles	Stereopsis (sec of arc)
20/200	480i SD (Moving Image)	1	800
20/100	480i SD (Still Image)	2	400
20/80		3	200
20/70		4	140
20/60		5	100
20/50		6	80
20/40	1080p HD	7	60
20/30		8	50
20/25		9	40
≥ 20/20	Optimized 1080p or 4K	≥ 9	Hyperstereo

Fig. 1 Excellent two-dimensional visual acuity is required for high-grade stereopsis. The table (left) shows stereopsis in Titmus™ circles (pictured to the right) and seconds of stereo arc as a function of 2D visual acuity. The approximate equivalent visual acuity of different digital microscopy video formats is also tabulated. (Courtesy of Christopher Riemann, MD, USA)

– Digital delay or latency of <100 ms—preferably <75 ms.
– Synchronized left and right video independently delivered to each eye of the observer.

Stereopsis is directly impacted by 2D spatial resolution [3, 4] (Fig. 1), and the advent of 3D high-definition video standards (1080p or greater) meeting the above criteria has created the opportunity for digital visualization systems that afford visualization and other benefits superior to analogue optical viewing.

3 Advantages of Digital Visualization

– **Better Ergonomics:** 50–80% of ophthalmologists develop symptomatic c-spine disease. Estimates are that 10% end their careers prematurely due to back and neck problems, and up to 3% require surgery. Suboptimal physician positioning is a problem in clinic at the slit lamp as well as in surgery at TOM. While slit lamp examinations occur over a span of a few seconds to a few minutes, the longer duration of unergonomic positioning in the operating room routinely lasts from many minutes to several hours. The surgeon is functionally tethered—motionless and with neck unphysiologically craned forward to reach the microscope oculars—for the duration of the surgical case [5–14]. DSVS mechanically uncouples the surgeon from the microscope allowing a proper physiologic seated position (Fig. 2).
– **High Dynamic Range/Low Light Surgery:** Combining digital cameras with high dynamic range (HDR) algorithms results in superior low light performance compared to the human eye. DSVS allows for surgery to be performed with excellent visualization at much lower illumination levels [15]. The author rou-

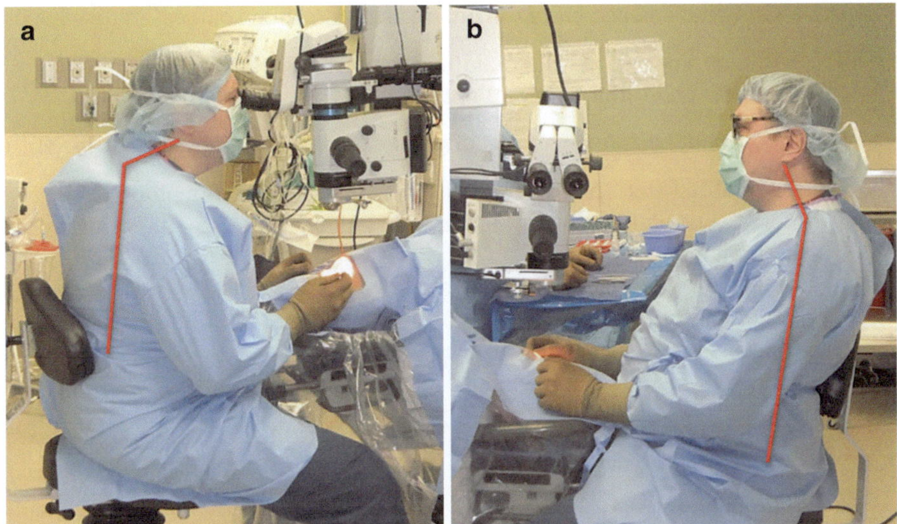

Fig. 2 (**a**) Photo of the author operating with the analogue microscope. Note abdomen against the wrist rest and significant c-spine flexion to reach the microscope oculars. (**b**) Photo of the author operating with a digital visualization system. The screen (not pictured) is to the left. The surgeon oculars have been replaced with a digitally assisted screen-based vitreoretinal surgery (DSVS) camera (black) and only the assistant oculars are visible. Note much less c-spine flexion, lumbar spine against the operating room stool backrest. (Courtesy of Christopher Riemann, MD, USA)

tinely uses a light pipe setting of 35% on the Alcon Constellation™ and 80–100% on the DORC EVA™ machines when operating with TOM. Light pipe settings are reduced to 5–15% and 20–50% respectively when operating with DSVS. Phototoxicity has become happily uncommon with modern illumination systems, but remains a concern in certain situations where lower light levels of DSVS may be beneficial:

> Longer complex cases with long macular instrumentation times.
> Multiple light sources in use.
> More light needed to compensate for media opacity.
> Less experienced surgeons.
> Trainees and teaching institutions.
> Diseased, at-risk maculas.
>
>> Age related macular degeneration.
>> Retinovascular disease.
>> Inherited retinal diseases.

– **Digital Signal Processing (DSP):** DSVS allows for never-before-possible active real-time manipulation of the video feed from the primary surgical field. While the possibilities are many and remain to be fully elucidated, several beneficial DSP algorithms have been implemented into commercially available DSVS systems.

Camera white balance tuning to different illumination sources.

Different microscope external illumination sources.
Different endo-illumination light sources.

Color channel adjustments to modify displayed color information (Fig. 3).

"Digital red-free" helps to improve visualization through blood [16].
"Green boost" for use with indocyanin green (ICG) dye—the author used ¼ strength ICG.
"Blue boost" for use with blue colored vital dyes.
Yellow boost.
Contrast boost.
Monochrome black and white.

Digital overlays (Fig. 4).

Real-time machine fluidics.
Illumination levels.
Laser settings.
Video recording functions.
Elapsed case time.
Elapsed elevated intraocular pressure tamponade time.
Capsulorrhexis and intraocular lens (IOL) incision templates.
Toric IOL alignment templates.

Auxiliary video handling. Same-screen simultaneous viewing of the surgical field and other ancillary video feeds promotes efficient, ergonomic acquisition, display, and interpretation of ancillary video information facilitating surgical decision making [17, 18, 19, 20].

Ocular endoscopy (Fig. 5).
Intraoperative optical coherence tomography (iOCT) (Fig. 6).

– Better teaching and observation:

Scrub tech and circulating nurse are more informed and remain engaged.
Better surgical teaching for surgical trainees.

Less attending anxiety.

Attending and trainee see the exact same image eliminating differences form disparate optical paths of the primary and teaching scope oculars.
Trainee/attending accommodation and focus disparities are eliminated.
Faster surgical "switch" without need to adjust pupillary diameter and instrument myopia settings.
Better ergonomics—contortionist maneuvers at the teaching scope are eliminated.

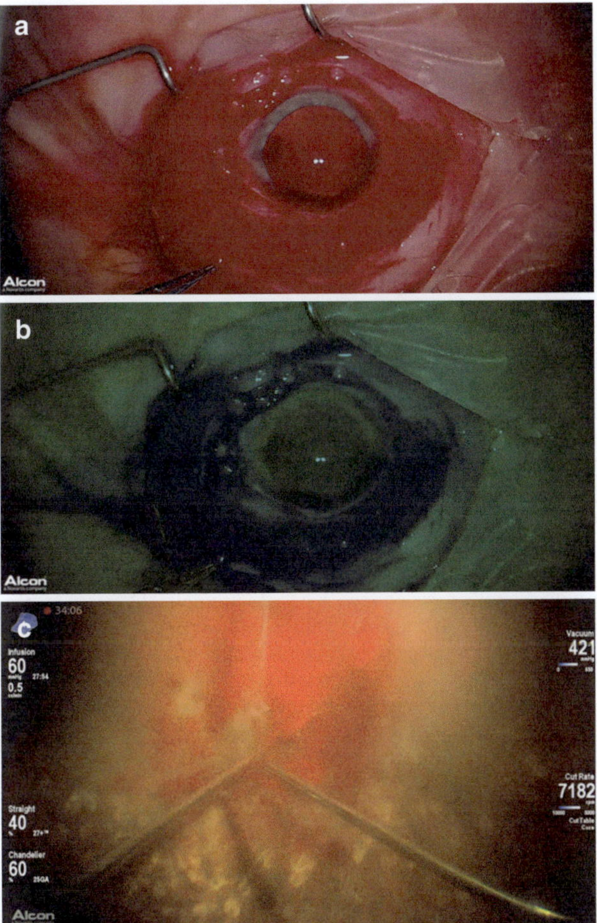

Fig. 3 Examples of digital signal processing (DSP) during digitally assisted screen-based vitreo-retinal surgery (DSVS). (**a**) Video frame grab after opening conjunctiva and Tenon's capsule for scleral buckling on a patient anticoagulated with coumadin. Hemorrhage is everywhere and compromises visualization. Surgery cannot proceed without addressing the bleeding. (**b**) The same surgical view 20 ms after employing "digital red-free" DSVS settings. Note markedly improved visualized detail. Tenon's capsule and conjunctival edges are visible which is enough for surgery to continue. (**c**) Video frame grab during vitrectomy for advanced proliferative diabetic retinopathy with machine overlays activated. Information displayed is comprehensive. Note clockwise from top right corner. Actual vacuum is 421 mmHg. Machine settings are 0–650 mmHg. Actual cut rate is 7182 cpm. Machine settings are dual liner 10,000 to 5000 cpm. Port bias is set to open or "core." A 25-g chandelier is in use and illumination is 60%. A 27-gauge (**g**) light pipe is plugged into the machine and is set to 40% illumination but is not visible in the surgical field so bimanual dissection is in progress. The infusion is set to 60 mmHg and has been for the past 27 min and 54 s. Actual infusion flow is 0.5 cc/min. The machine foot pedal is currently in position 1. Total elapsed case time from camera activation is 34 min and 6 s and video recording is active (red dot). (Courtesy of Alan J Franklin, MD, USA)

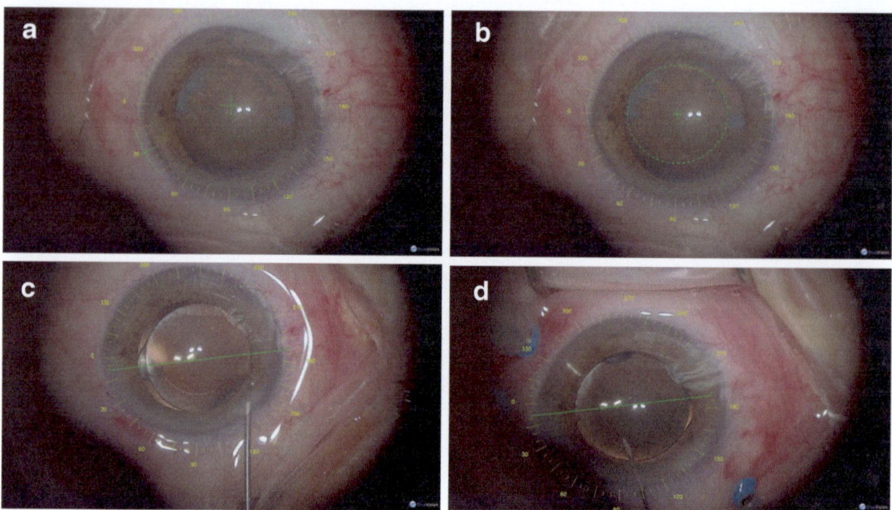

Fig. 4 Surgical alignment templates during a combined phaco-vitrectomy-membrane peeling procedure with toric intraocular lens (IOL) implantation performed by the author in August of 2014 with a first-generation digitally assisted screen-based vitreoretinal surgery system. (**a**) Phaco incision template. Note incision at 30 degrees. (**b**) Five-millimeter-diameter capsulorrhexis template. (**c**) The toric alignment template is guiding rough IOL alignment prior to the vitrectomy. (**d**) The toric alignment template guides IOL alignment fine-tuning to an axis of 8 degrees with a 30-g needle after completion of the vitrectomy, membrane peeling, and scleral depressed examination of the retinal periphery. (Courtesy of Christopher Riemann, MD, USA)

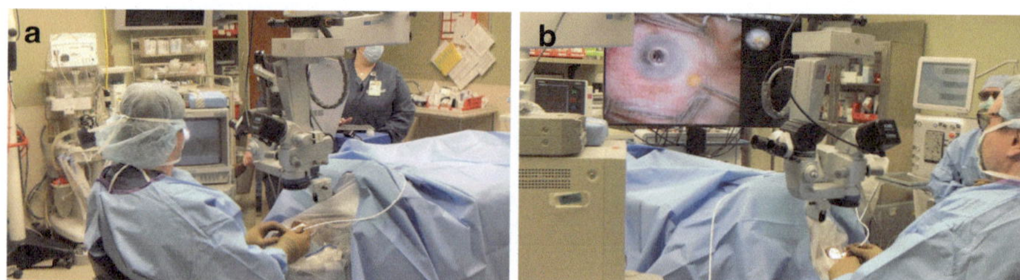

Fig. 5 (**a**) Operating with the ophthalmic endoscope typically involves an awkward face turn away from the operating room microscope (TOM) oculars or primary digitally assisted screen-based vitreoretinal surgery (DSVS) screen. Note DSVS camera in place of TOM oculars. (**b**) Same-screen simultaneous viewing of the ophthalmic endoscope and primary 3D surgical video eliminates the awkward face turn and facilitates rapid alternating viewing of both video feeds. Note pars plana vitrectomy is being performed on an eye with a Dohlman type 2 keratoprosthesis. The 3D primary surgical field video is displayed on the left side of the screen and the endoscope is about to be inserted into the supero-nasal trocar. The endoscope video feed showing an *en-face* view of the trocar is visible on the right side of the screen. Surgeon positioning is comfortable and ergonomic. (Courtesy of Christopher Riemann, MD, USA)

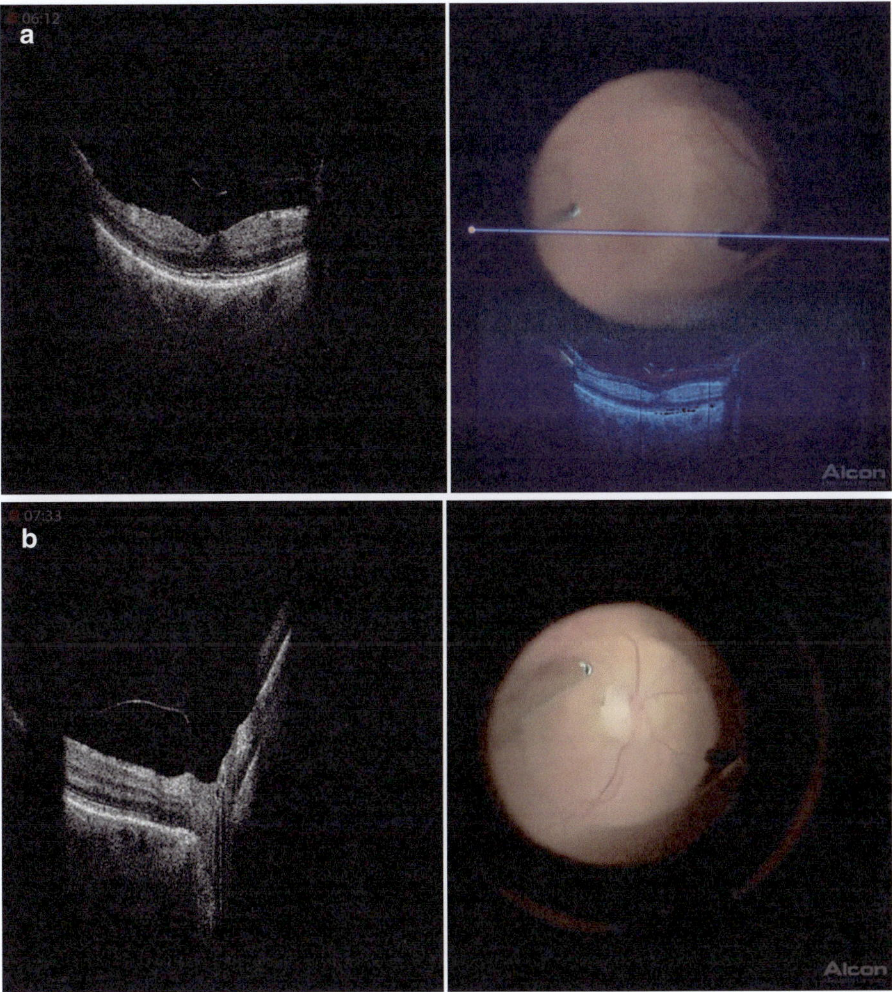

Fig. 6 Video frames of same-screen simultaneous viewing of the intraoperative optical coherence tomography (iOCT) (left) and primary 3D surgical videos (right) in a patient operated for macular pucker and vitreomacular traction (VMT). (**a**) Macular pucker and vitreomacular traction are evident at the beginning of the case. Full-resolution iOCT image resolution is much better than optical image injected iOCT video overlayed on the surgical video. (**b**) Induced vitreo-papillary traction is seen on iOCT as the posterior hyaloid is elevated with suction from the vitreous cutter. (**c**) The hyaloid has been removed, the vitrectomy is finished, and indocyanin green staining is complete. (**d**) iOCT during the membrane peel clearly shows areas where epiretinal membrane (ERM) and internal limiting membrane (ILM) have been removed. (**e**) iOCT confirms complete removal of VMT, ERM, and ILM. Note elapsed case time of 18 min and 41 s (top left corner)

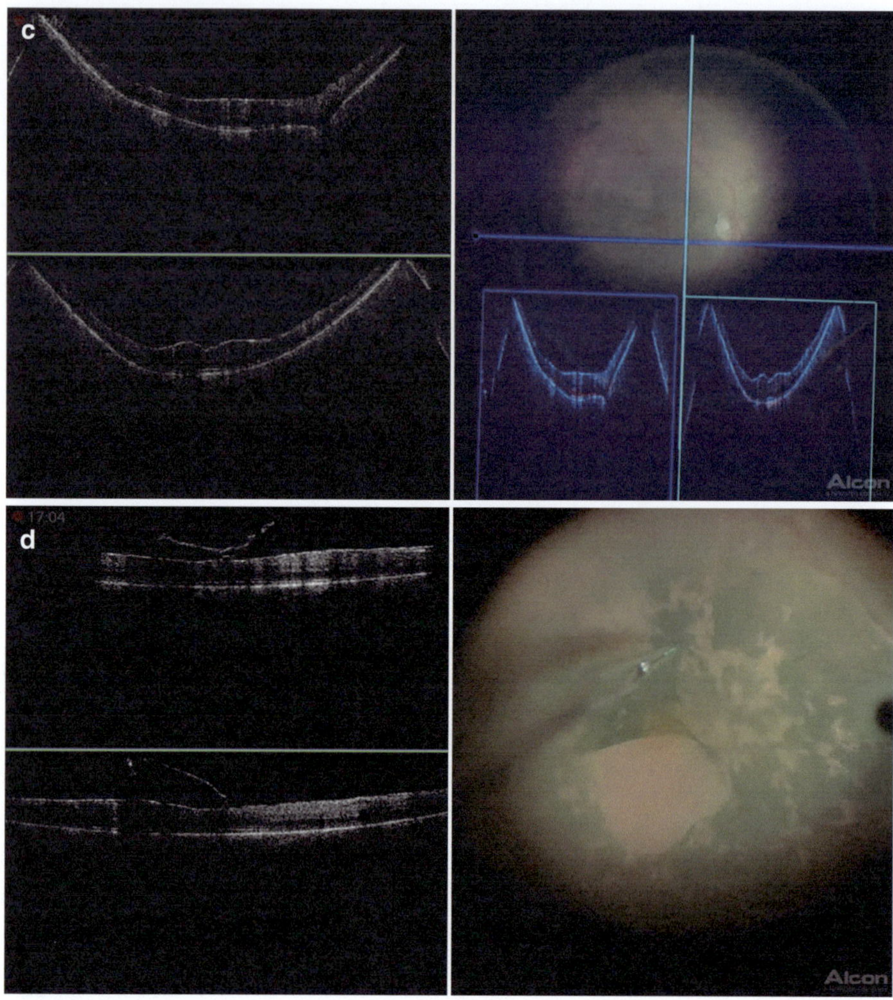

Fig. 32.6 (continued)

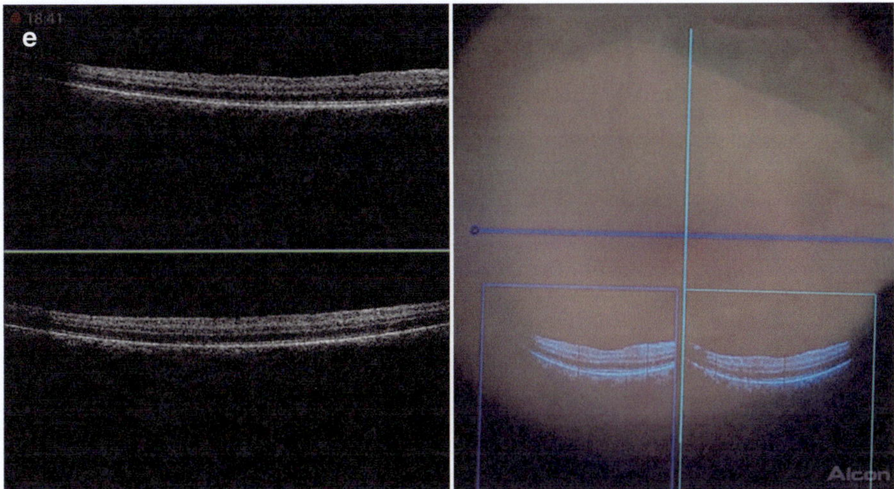

Fig. 32.6 (continued)

Less trainee anxiety.

Illusion of independence with attending sitting behind trainee.
No convergence/accommodation disparity.
Screen is a familiar viewing interface for younger doctors.

Multiple medical students and other observers can have simultaneous immersive experiences by looking over the surgeon's shoulder.
3D live surgical streaming for conferences.
Cloud educational sites.

Eyetube
RetinaLink

- Higher total maximal magnification.
- Better 3D resolution (stereopsis):

Hyper-stereo better than TOM possible under high magnification.
Need screen viewing distance of <1.8 m.
Beneficial for macular peeling.

- Better depth of field:

Up to 590% better instantaneous depth of field without accommodation
Up to 250% better depth of field with moderate accommodation

- Active aperture management—allows better viewing through media opacity:

Low illumination and large aperture size.

Capitalizes on superb low light functionality of camera sensors.
Reduces light scatter and glare.

Improved visualization through cataract, corneal haze, and fibrosis.
"Let the camera gain do the work".

Max light and small aperture size.

Significantly increases depth of focus/depth of field.
Improved visualization through refractive media opacity
Multifocal IOL.
Air or gas fill.
Silicone oil marring of posterior chamber IOL.
Higher-order aberrations and irregular astigmatism.

Corneal sutures.
Cataract.

"Let enhanced depth of field do the work"

– Platform for unlimited future advances. Possibilities include (very partial list):

Improved latency
Better 2D and 3D resolution
Improved dynamic range and low light capability
Auto-focus and auto-centration
Automatic instrument tip tracking
Better DSP.

Contrast
Edge enhancement
Color space transformation
False color imaging
Virtual staining of vitreous and retinal membranes

Integration and synergy with vitrectomy machine platforms and electronic medical records.
Expanded electromagnetic bandwidth visualization.

Near ultraviolet.
Near infrared.

Hyperspectral imaging.
Eulerian motion and color magnification.
Real-time remote mentoring.
Headset-based virtual reality and augmented reality visualization.
Registered overlays.

Preoperative diagnostic testing.
Autorotated ocular endoscopy.
Intraoperative OCT.
Premium IOL placement tools and intraoperative aberrometry.

Artificial intelligence and deep learning algorithms that look for and alert surgeon to occurrences on the surgical field they may not have noticed.
All digital microscope without oculars and with camera on a robotic arm.

4 Disadvantages of Digital Visualization

- Cost of an expensive capital equipment acquisition.
- Field of View: DSVS has less vertical field of view:

    60 × 32 degrees (rectangular width x height) for DSVS.
    60 × 60 degrees (round) for TOM.
    Difference not clinically relevant.
    Horizontal field of view is more important.

- Increased latency: [21, 22]

    Digital delay <100 ms is required for primary digital surgical visualization.
    Digital delay >50 ms is noticeable.

      More so in faster-moving cataract procedures
      Less so in slower-moving vitreoretinal surgery

    Current range is 30–70 ms.

      Trade-off.
      Faster systems have less DSP features.
      "faster-moving" and "slower-moving"
      Slower systems have more DSP features (HDR, color channels, etc.).

    Average motor feedback reaction time.

      To simple stimulus is 270 ms.
      To complex stimulus is 1000–2000 ms.

    Digital latency of 30–75 ms increases.

      Photon flight time from surgical field to surgeon 10,000–25,000x.
      Motor response to simple stimulus 1.1–1.3x.
      Motor response to complex stimulus 1.01–1.08x.

    For perspective, difference in reaction time 50- vs. 25-year-old = 8%.
    Digital delay in all systems currently for sale is not clinically important and should not represent a barrier to adoption of DSVS.

5 Clinical Pearls: Getting Started

Transitioning to digital viewing and DSVS involves a brief and easy to master learning curve. Younger surgeons—raised in front of screens—easily and readily transition from TOM to DSVS without any significant learning curve. The learning curve for older surgeons is short and manageable. Some clinical pearls :

- Attention to surgeon ergonomic positioning:

    Sit upright and let your torso move away from the surgical field.
    Slight extension of elbows.

Use OR chair lumbar spine support.
Slight lateral face turn toward screen without unbalanced lateral movement.
Make physiologic small head and neck movements during surgery.

> To maintain blood flow and prevent c-spine stiffness.
> Not possible when tethered to oculars of TOM.
> OK to crack neck while operating.

Wrist rest as needed.
Patient height to eliminate excessive leg flexion and extension when seated.

– Install the correct camera footplate for microscope model.
– White balance to your illumination sources monthly:

> Color temperature can vary from machine to machine.
> Color temperature varies during lifecycle of each bulb/LED.

– Careful attention to screen position:

> Facing surgeon's head precisely
>
>> Left-right rotation
>> Up-down tilt
>> Height
>
> 1.4 to 1.8 meters distance to surgeon

– Set aperture between 25–50%:

> More open for more light and brighter image
> More closed for greater depth of field

– Zero (XY and focus) the microscope at the beginning of the case.
– Max magnification and then focus to establish parfocality.
– Significantly decrease illumination levels compared to TOM.
– If image is grainy, reduce illumination to increase auto-exposure time and reduce noise.
– "Mag is your friend"—magnify appropriately to use all available screen pixels:

> "Fill the screen with the circle".
> Wide-angle lens image to vertically fill the screen during peripheral vitrectomy.
> Pupil to vertically fill the screen during core vitrectomy, lifting posterior hyaloid and membrane peeling.
> Even higher magnification during complex macular dissection maneuvers.

– Suturing is best with lowest possible magnification and maximum field of view.
– "Dance on the microscope foot pedal":

> Focus—don't let expanded depth of field make you complacent about meticulous focusing. Especially important when aperture is more open.
> Centration to maintain optical path through the optical axis of the globe.
>
>> Center of cornea.

    Center of pupil and IOL.
    Center of wide-angle viewing system.
    Wide-angle lens as close to eye as possible without corneal touch.

    Decentered view in conjunction with globe rotation in the opposite direction to use off-axis prismatic effect for extended view into periphery.

- If you are struggling with peripheral visualization:

    It's probably you and not the DSVS system!
    "Back to basics."
    Pay attention to media opacity.

        Dry cornea
        Corneal edema
        Anterior chamber heme and debris.
        Cataract.

    Pay attention to optical path centration.

        Easy to lose these without head and upper body tethered to TOM oculars—brief learning curve.
        Use wrist rest.
        Assure alignment of ocular axis with microscope mag-tube barrel.

            Patient face turn.
            Patient head/neck flexion and extension.
            Rotation of the globe.

- Color channels:

    Start with digital red-free for vitreous hemorrhage.
    Then green or blue boost for peeling after stain.
    Others per surgeon preference.
    Don't be afraid to experiment with surgeon-specific custom settings.

- If you typically eschew scleral buckling, consider a chandelier/DSVS approach.
- Integrating endoscopic and iOCT viewing into digital screen-based surgery with same-screen/split-screen viewing greatly improves ergonomics and the usability of endoscopy and iOCT with faster switching between viewing the surgical field and ancillary video feeds.

6 Conclusion

Digitally assisted screen-based vitreoretinal surgery is now over 10 years old and is steadily gaining adoption. The advantages of this form of surgical visualization are many and far outweigh the few relative disadvantages. Transitioning to DSVS is straightforward and well within the skill set of any competent vitreoretinal surgeon.

The learning curve is easy, simple to master, and well worth the effort. The future potential of this first-in-a-generation disruptive technological platform is astounding. It is a fantastic time to be a vitreoretinal surgeon.

Key Points
- DSVS addresses the ergonomic challenges faced by surgeons during traditional microscope-based surgery, reducing the risk of surgeons' musculoskeletal issues.
- DSVS allows the surgeon to operate at a high magnification without degrading the resolution which is of advantage in macular surgery.
- DSVS combines digital cameras with high dynamic range algorithms to enable superior surgical visualization under lower illumination levels.
- While DSVS involves initial costs and some limitations, its potential for continued technological advancements, such as digital optimization of retinal structures, AI integration and virtual reality, holds promise for further transforming vitreoretinal surgery.

References

1. Riemann CD. Machine vision and vitrectomy—three dimensional high definition (3DHD) video for surgical visualization in vitreoretinal surgery. Proceedings of SPIE Volume 7863. Stereoscopic displays and applications XII. 2011. Paper 7863–19.
2. Eckardt C, Paulo EB. HEADS-UP surgery for vitreoretinal procedures: an experimental and clinical study. Retina. 2016;36(1):137–47. PMID: 26200516.
3. Levy NS, Glick EB. Stereoscopic perception and Snellen visual acuity. Am J Ophthalmol. 1974;78(4):722–4.
4. Donzis PB, Rappazzo JA, Burde RM, Gordon M. Effect of binocular variations of Snellen's visual acuity on titmus stereoacuity. Arch Ophthalmol. 1983;101(6):930–2.
5. Al-Marwani Al-Juhani M, Khandekar R, Al-Harby M, Al-Hassan A, Edward DP. Neck and upper back pain among eye care professionals. Occup Med (Lond). 2015;65(9):753–7. Epub 2015 Sep 28. PMID: 26416844.
6. Chatterjee A, Ryan W, Rosen E. Back pain in ophthalmologists. Eye. 1994;8:473–4.
7. Dhimitri KC, McGwin G Jr, McNeal SF, Lee P, Morse PA, Patterson M, Wertz FD, Marx JL. Symptoms of musculoskeletal disorders in ophthalmologists. Am J Ophthalmol. 2005;139(1):179–81. PMID: 15652844.
8. Hyer JN, Lee RM, Chowdhury HR, Smith HB, Dhital A, Khandwala M. National survey of back & neck pain amongst consultant ophthalmologists in the United Kingdom. Int Ophthalmol. 2015;35(6):769–75. Epub 2015 Jan 22. PMID: 25609503.
9. Kaup S, Shivalli S, Kulkarni U, Arunachalam C. Ergonomic practices and musculoskeletal disorders among ophthalmologists in India: an online appraisal. Eur J Ophthalmol. 2020;30(1):196–200.
10. Shaw C, et al. Mechanical exposure of ophthalmic surgeons: a quantitative ergonomic evaluation of indirect ophthalmoscopy and slit-lamp biomicroscopy. Can J Ophthalmol. 2017;52(3):302–7.
11. Kitzmann AS, Fethke NB, Baratz KH, Zimmerman MB, Hackbarth DJ, Gehrs KM. A survey study of musculoskeletal disorders among eye care physicians compared with family medicine physicians. Ophthalmology. 2012;119(2):213–20. Epub 2011 Sep 16. PMID: 21925736.

12. Venkatesh R, Sumit K. Back pain in ophthalmology: National survey of Indian ophthalmologists. Indian J Ophthalmol. 2017;65(8):678–82.
13. Marx JL. Ergonomics: back to the future. Ophthalmology. 2012;119(2):211–2.
14. Sivak-Callcott JA, Diaz SR, Ducatman AM, Rosen CL, Nimbarte AD, Sedgeman JA. A survey study of occupational pain and injury in ophthalmic plastic surgeons. Ophthalmic. Plast Reconstr Surg. 2011;27(1):28–32. PMID: 20859236.
15. Kunikata H, Abe T, Nakazawa T. Heads-up macular surgery with a 27-gauge microincision vitrectomy system and minimal illumination. Case Rep Ophthalmol. 2016;7(3):265–9.
16. Franklin AJ, Lin Y, Sarangapani, R, Tripathi B, Reed D, Riemann CD. Digital filters enhance contrast and visualization during 3DHD retinal surgery. Poster Presentation at the Annual Meeting of The Association for Research in Vision and Ophthalmology (ARVO). (#AO250) Vancouver, Canada. 2019.
17. Ehlers JP, Uchida A, Srivastava SK. The integrative surgical theater: combining intraoperative optical coherence tomography and 3D digital visualization for vitreoretinal surgery in the discover study. Retina. 2018;38 Suppl 1(Suppl 1):S88–96.
18. Brooks CC, Kitchens J, Stone TW, Riemann CD. Consolidation of imaging modalities utilizing digitally assisted visualization systems: the development of a surgical information handling cockpit. Clin Ophthalmol. 2020;14:557–69.
19. Ehlers JP, Kaiser PK, Singh RP, et al. Application of intraoperative OCT to ophthalmic surgery: PIONEER 18-month iOCT vitreoretinal results. Toronto: American Society of Retina Specialists Annual Meeting; 2013.
20. Ehlers JP, Modi YS, Pecen PE, et al. The DISCOVER study 3-year results: feasibility and usefulness of microscope-integrated intraoperative OCT during ophthalmic surgery. Ophthalmology. 2018;125(7):1014–27.
21. Olson PL. Driver perception response time. Accident Reconstruction Journal. 1991;3(1):16–21, 29.
22. McGehee DV, Mazzae EN, Baldwin SGH. Driver reaction time in crash avoidance research: validation of a driving simulator study on a test track. In: Proceedings Of The IEA; 2000. p. 320–3. 2000/hfes 2000 Congress.

Vitrectomy in the Presence of Opaque Cornea

Michael Mikhail, Giampaolo Gini, and Faisal Fayyad

This chapter discusses the management of vitreoretinal pathology requiring vitrectomy surgery in the presence of opaque cornea limiting the ability to carry out the surgery. We also share our experience of operating such cases with temporary keratoprosthesis (TKP).

1 Important Causes/Risk Factors of the Opaque Cornea in the Vitreoretinal Setting

1. Corneal scarring.

    (a) Inherited corneal dystrophy.
    (b) Previous trauma/infection.
    (c) Corneal blood staining after hyphema.

Supplementary Information The online version contains supplementary material available at https://doi.org/10.1007/978-3-031-47827-7_33.

M. Mikhail
Vitreoretinal Department, Kabgayi Eye Unit, Gitarama, Rwanda

G. Gini
Department of Ophthalmology, University Hospitals Sussex NHS Foundation Trust, Worthing, West Sussex, UK

F. Fayyad (✉)
Ophthalmology Department, Jordan Hospital, Amman, Jordan

443

A. B. Sallam et al. (eds.), *Practical Manual of Vitreoretinal Surgery*, https://doi.org/10.1007/978-3-031-47827-7_33

2. Dysfunctional endothelium.

   (a) Fuchs' endothelial dystrophy.
   (b) Complicated anterior segment surgery.
   (c) Acute glaucoma.
   (d) Uveitis.
   (e) Prolonged surgery or vitrectomy combined with cataract surgery.

3. Epithelial instability and toxicity.

   (a) Diabetes.
   (b) Glaucoma drops.

2 Preoperative Assessment

Preoperative assessment should be thorough enough to identify potential issues with surgery and different options to mitigate vitreoretinal surgery in the presence of a diseased cornea.

- Assess the location, level, and density of the corneal scar.
- Review patients drug charts and try to avoid toxic eye drops containing preservatives.
- Check intraocular pressure (IOP) and uveitis – aim for optimum IOP and uveitis control to reduce further risk of endothelial dysfunction.
- For trauma cases with a sutured corneal wound, ensure it is done appropriately and not leaking to withstand pressure during vitrectomy surgery as this may need to be re-sutured prior to vitrectomy especially for sutures outside the area of planned trephination if planned TKP.

If a corneal procedure is contemplated, best to involve your cornea team as some of these cases require a multidisciplinary approach for onward graft management.

3 Intraoperatively

- Despite the hazy fundus view during the preoperative examination, it is quite often that the intraoperative view can be better than expected. It may be sufficient to do the surgery with contemporary endoillumination and widefield viewing systems. The reason is that when light hits the corneal surface from an indirect ophthalmoscope or operating microscope, it causes light to backscatter which is troublesome to the surgeon. However, having illumination from light pipe inside the eye eliminates the backscatter and reflection from the cornea and therefore enhances visualization up four times compared to external light from slit-lamp, indirect ophthalmoscope, or microscope [1].

- Avoid high/low IOP intraoperatively.
- Maintain corneal hydration and avoid corneal dryness with the use of viscous gel.If there is significant corneal edema, the corneal epithelium may have to be scraped to obtain optimum visualization of intraocular maneuvers. This is easily performed if the corneal epithelium is already edematous. The way to do this is by rubbing a cotton tip applicator firmly on the epithelium till it separates from Bowman's membrane. Alternatively, you could use a flat blade.
- In the presence of stromal edema or folds in Descemet's membrane, the anterior chamber can be filled with an ophthalmic viscoelastic device (e.g., Viscoat). This will be a physical barrier to fluid movement into the cornea "no water, no edema." Also, its increased viscosity compared to the corneal stroma may remove some of the accumulated fluid [2]. In the presence of a coexisting stromal scar. One way to deal with this is by doing deep anterior lamellar dissection and operating through Descemet's membrane. If you are not proficient in corneal surgery, a cornea colleague can be pretty handy at this stage. As the Descemet's membrane is resilient and provided it is left intact, it will be sufficient to perform vitrectomy surgery without TKP. After finishing vitrectomy surgery, either one's own cornea or a lamellar corneal button can be sowed in place [3]. For a full-thickness corneal scar, you have two options: either TKP or endoscopic vitrectomy. The TKP is our favored option as it allows bimanual surgery with excellent view and surgeons' usual technique and setup [4, 5]. Endoscopic vitrectomy will bypass anterior segment structures altogether, but its use requires special training and may not be readily available for most surgeons. Please refer to Chap. 31 "Vitreoretinal Endoscopy" on endoscopy use in retina surgery.
- Recently, Skevas et al. demonstrated that a soft contact lens sutured to the globe over the trephination site may function well as an alternative to TKP if it is unavailable or not possible to use because of a small trephination opening [6].
- As a last resort, the eye can be operated using an open-sky approach. Ideally, the time when the eye is open should be as short as possible because fluid outflow will be very high which can cause hypotony-related complications especially catastrophic suprachoroidal hemorrhage. Also, in the presence of hypotony, chorioretinal folds and collapse of the globe may occur which will make certain maneuvers difficult, e.g., membrane peeling. To partially overcome this, a scleral fixation ring can be secured to the sclera.

4 Temporary Keratoprosthesis (TKP)

- TKP has revolutionized the approach to retinal surgery in those eyes with concurrent corneal pathologies limiting the optimum view for carrying out the surgery.
- It has been used intraoperatively to replace pathologic cornea, allowing proper posterior segment visualization and surgical maneuvers.
- There are two main designs of TKPs: one made from polymethyl methacrylate (PMMA) (Landers) (Fig. 1) and the other made from silicone (Eckardt) (Fig. 2)

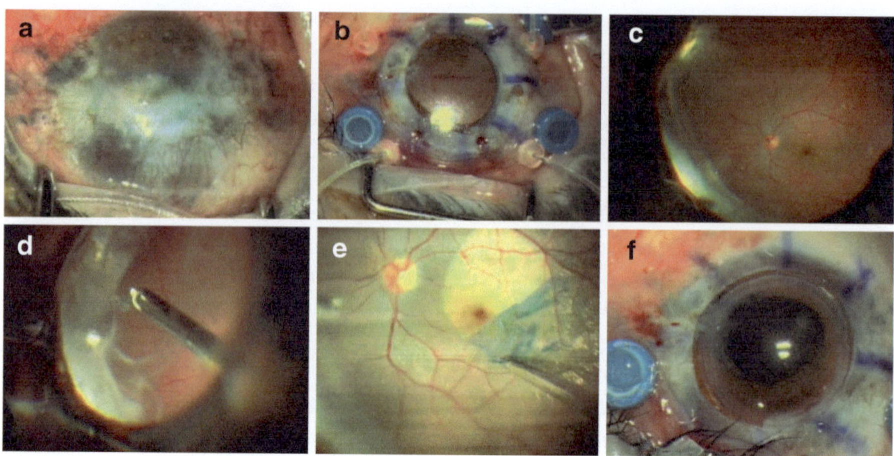

Fig. 1 Landers 8.2 mm temporary keratoprostheses (TKP) in a patient with corneal scarring and intraocular foreign body (IOFB) (**a**). TKP in place after corneal trephination (**b**). Wide-field fundus view with TKP (**c**, **d**). The central view was adequate for internal limiting membrane (ILM) peel (**e**). Corneal graft replacing the TKP (**f**)

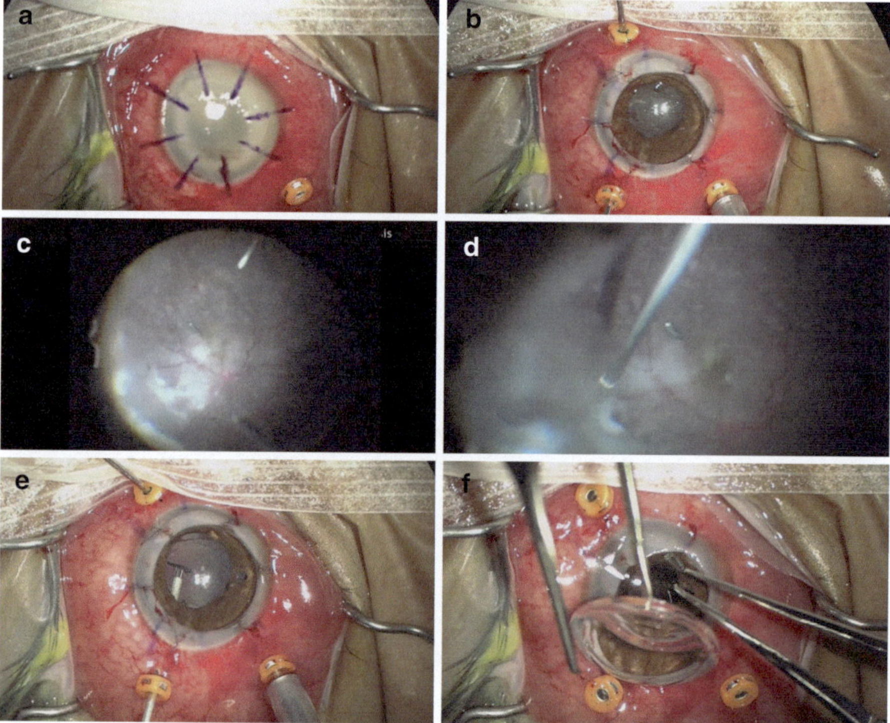

Fig. 2 Eckardt 8 mm temporary keratoprostheses (TKP) in corneal opacification (**a**) from traumatic endophthalmitis with intraocular foreign body (IOFB). TKP in place after corneal trephination (**b**). Widefield fundus view with TKP showing vitreous opacification and IOFB (**c**, **d**). IOFB was placed over the iris using a backflush needle (**e**) and then removed from the eye by cutting the sutures fixing the TKP (**f**)

Table 1 Commonly used temporary keratoprosthesis designs

Type/size	Material/design	Suitability by lens status
Landers wide field, 7.2 mm	Polymethyl methacrylate (PMMA) Trunkless	All
Landers wide field, 8.2 mm	PMMA Trunkless	All
Eckardt, 7 mm, 2.8 depth	Silicone; 2.8 mm central trunk	Aphakic/pseudophakic
Eckardt, 7 mm, 1.6 depth	Silicone; 1.6 mm central trunk	Phakic
Eckardt, 8 mm, 2.5 depth	Silicone; 2.5 mm central trunk	Aphakic/pseudophakic

(Video 1). Both designs have equal merits and provide a good macular and peripheral retinal view [4, 5]. The silicone made of the Eckardt TKP helps optimize peripheral molding and sealing of irregular corneal defects. However, it is more liable to damage with re-use than the Landers PMMA TKP.

- The combination of TKP and PPV has been widely published in the literature with successful outcomes [4, 5]. Table 1 summarizes the current most used TKP designs.
- We here provide a summary of the steps of combined TKP/pars plana vitrectomy (PPV) surgery:

  - Best to start by placing a scleral fixation ring (Flieringa) to decrease the risk of globe collapse in aphakic eyes or eyes that will be rendered aphakic. This is sutured with 7–0 Vicryl using a half-thickness scleral bite. The tension should be enough to fix the ring but not to compress the eye.
  - Place 23/25-g 3 port PPV while the globe is formed (do not open infusion). If the infusion cannula cannot be seen in the vitreous cavity, you can check that once you are open sky (i.e., before suturing TKP). Alternatively, the anterior chamber (AC) maintainer can be placed later.
  - Select the size and place of trephination. The actual size is determined by the size of the available TKP device. The trephine is ideally 0.25–0.5 mm smaller than the barrel of the TKP to achieve a good fit. The place of trephination is judged by the location of pathology and the visual axis. Generally, it is best to use a large diameter TKP unless there is hypotony or severe anterior segment disease.
  - Some maneuvers can be performed open sky before suturing TKP, i.e., checking the infusion line, removing AC intraocular lens (IOL), etc. Be wary of potential complications during this stage and keep this time to a minimum to reduce the risk of expulsive bleeding.
  - The TKP is sutured in place with 8–0 or 10-0 nylon suture.
  - Perform all the necessary work required for the case, e.g., core vitrectomy, PVD induction, and laser. As visualization of the fundus after placing the corneal graft can be difficult due to edema and folds of the corneal button, it might be best to perform AFX with the TKP still in before placing the corneal graft.
  - Finally, gas/air exchange or silicone oil (SO)/air exchange can be performed at this stage. Generally, it is best to avoid SO use in aphakic eyes with corneal grafts.

- Suture the new corneal graft in place with 10–0 nylon suture. The size of the graft is usually similar to the size of the TKP used.
- If the eye requires an IOL, we elect to do that as a secondary procedure after 3 months provided the situation is stable (stable retina, optimum IOP control, and some visual potential).

5 Case Scenario

1. A 30-year-old patient was referred because of a right scarred cornea, traumatic cataract, and two small IOFBs from a war injury (Fig. 1) (a). Surgery comprised corneal trephination of 7.5 mm extracapsular cataract extraction, 8.2 mm sutured Landers trunkless TKP, 23 g pars plana vitrectomy, and posterior capsulotomy then IOFB extraction (b). The wide-field view allowed vitreous base shaving (c and d). One sclerotomy was enlarged to allow the 20-g instruments into the eye. The first foreign body using a backflush cannula. The other foreign body was removed by suction through a 20-g vitreous cutter. ILM peeling was undertaken to reduce the risk of postoperative ERM (e). A large PMMA IOL was implanted in the bag. The donor cornea button of 7.75 mm diameter was sutured with 10–0 interrupted sutures after removal of TKP, followed by air-fluid exchange (f).
2. An 89-year-old man underwent phacoemulsification with a corneal suture and developed a corneal abscess and acute endophthalmitis postoperatively. We undertook combined PPV and corneal graft surgery with the use of Landers TKP (Video 2).

Key Points
- Despite a hazy corneal view, PPV can be completed in many cases with standard widefield endoillumination and viewing systems.
- In the presence of severe opaque cornea, successful management requires collaboration between cornea and retina specialists, and the utilization of advanced techniques such as TKP or surgical endoscopy.
- TKP provides an excellent view of the posterior segment for vitreoretinal surgery.
- Careful surgical technique is needed when using TKP matching the sizes of the TKP, the corneal trephine and the corneal graft.

References

1. Saragas S, Krah D, Miller D. Improved visualisation through cataracts using intravitreal illumination. Ann Ophthalmol. 1984;16:311–3.
2. McCannel CA. Improved intraoperative fundus visualisation in corneal oedema: the viscoat trick. Retina. 2012;32:189–90.
3. Li, et al. Modified deep anterior lamellar dissection for corneal opacity during vitrectomy: case reports. BMC Ophthalmol. 2020;20:317.

4. Garcia-Valenzuela E, Blair NP, Shapiro MJ, et al. Outcome of vitreoretinal surgery and penetrating keratoplasty using temporary keratoprosthesis. Retina. 1999;19:424–9.
5. Park H, Fayyad F, Landers M III. An improved temporary. keratoprosthesis. Retina Today. 2014:42–4.
6. Skevas C, Bigdon E, Steinhorst A, Katz T, Schindler P, Kromer R, Spitzer MS. A novel temporary keratoprosthesis technique for vitreoretinal surgery. Int J Ophthalmol. 2021;14(11):1791–5.

Cataract Surgery and Vitreoretinal Surgery

Abdelrahman M. Elhusseiny, Mohammad Z. Siddiqui, and Riley Sanders

1 Introduction

- This chapter discusses the surgical considerations for cataract surgery during or after pars plana vitrectomy (PPV).
- We strongly encourage aspiring retina surgeons to continue to perform and master cataract surgery. Phacoemulsification provides the operator with a fantastic skill set. In our view, a good cataract surgeon makes a great retina surgeon!

2 Lens Feathering Due to Vitrectomy Surgery

- A clear crystalline lens can develop feathering opacity of the posterior subcapsular fibers at the time of PPV or in the early postoperative period. This happens more commonly during prolonged vitrectomy cases and with the use of vitreous tamponade including air, gas, or silicone oil (SO) (Fig. 1). Lens feathering is

Supplementary Information The online version contains supplementary material available at https://doi.org/10.1007/978-3-031-47827-7_34.

A. M. Elhusseiny
Ophthalmology, University of Arkansas for Medical Sciences, Little Rock, AR, USA
e-mail: ElhusseinyAbdelrahma@uams.edu

M. Z. Siddiqui
Jones Eye Institute, University of Arkansas for Medical Sciences, Little Rock, AR, USA

R. Sanders (✉)
Ophthalmology/Retina, University of Arkansas for Medical Sciences, Little Rock, AR, USA

A. B. Sallam et al. (eds.), *Practical Manual of Vitreoretinal Surgery*, https://doi.org/10.1007/978-3-031-47827-7_34

451

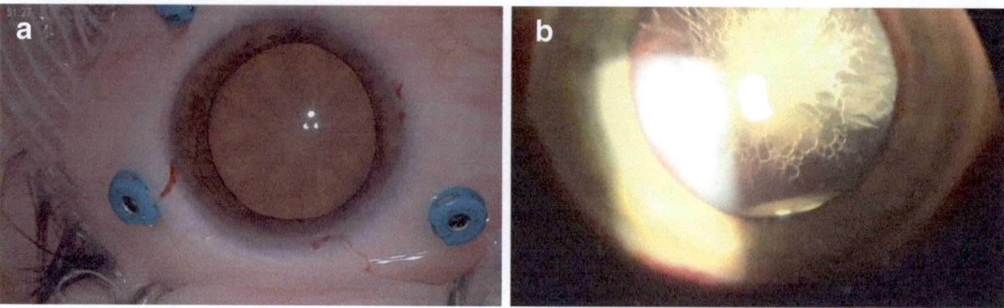

Fig. 1 Posterior lens feathering of a clear crystalline lens in a 40-year-old patient during diabetic vitrectomy necessitating lens removal to complete surgery (**a**). Postoperative lens feathering in a 33-year-old patient with traumatic vitreous hemorrhage and retinal detachment operated with pars plana vitrectomy + C3F8 gas (**b**)

thought to happen due to either hydration of the lens fibers or altered metabolism from the contact of the vitreous tamponade with the back of the lens [1, 2].

- Some cases of lens feathering can self-resolve with postoperative prone positioning to keep the tamponade away from the lens. It can also progress to permanent cataracts.
- If lens feathering happens near the end of the vitrectomy surgery, it is best to leave the lens alone and finish the operation. However, should intraoperative visualization become an issue, e.g., feathering hinders laser application or continuing delamination of diabetic membranes, you will need to remove the crystalline lens.

3 Cataract Development after Pars Plana Vitrectomy Surgery

- The most frequent complication of pars plana vitrectomy (PPV) is cataract formation, particularly nuclear sclerotic cataracts [3]. In the Vitrectomy for Macular Hole Study, 100% of phakic eyes had cataract progression by 2 years following PPV. In a large national registry data-based study from the UK that involved more than 2000 eyes with PPV performed for different indications, the risk of cataract surgery following PPV was in the range of 40% and the 1-, 2-, 3-, and 5-year cataract surgery rates were 50, 70, 75, and 85%, respectively [4].
- Although the exact mechanism of cataract formation or progression after PPV is unclear, several theories have been proposed, including increased oxygen tension after PPV with oxidative damage of crystalline lens proteins.
- Factors that increase the risk of cataract progression after PPV include older age and the use of tamponade, particularly long-acting gas, and complex extended PPV surgery [4].
- Factors that are protective against post-vitrectomy cataracts include young age, preservation of the anterior hyaloid, and being diabetic [5].

- Lens touch in phakic eye occurs in approximately 4% of patients and is more frequent during the learning curve and in eyes requiring complex proliferative vitreoretinopathy (PVR) or diabetic delamination surgery or shallow orbit (Video 1). Postoperative cataract may develop quicker in these eyes, and there is an increased risk of posterior capsule rupture (PCR) (10%) [6].

4 Simultaneous Cataract PPV Surgery

- Because cataracts will eventually develop in patients over the age of 50 after PPV, there are two surgical approaches when performing PPV: either performing combined phacoemulsification and PPV or performing a lens-sparing vitrectomy and then performing phacoemulsification at a different setting when needed [7].
- Advantages of combined surgery include easier and more complete removal of the peripheral vitreous mitigating the risk of touching the back surface of the crystalline lens. The combined approach may allow for earlier patient visual rehabilitation and is more cost-effective than a staged procedure.
- On the other hand, a combined cataract PPV approach results in loss of accommodation in young patients under the age of 40 years. It also increases the surgical time and carries the risk of intraoperative corneal edema and narrow pupil, which may make PPV technically more challenging. In addition, prolonged surgery may increase the risk of postoperative anterior chamber reaction, fibrinous exudate formation, and posterior synechiae. Using gas tamponade also increases the risk of anterior decentration of the intraocular lens (IOL) up to pupillary capture. Also, IOL calculation is challenging in a patient with a macula off retinal detachment or significant vitreous opacities and is usually based on measurements taken from the other eye.

5 Staged (Sequential) PPV Cataract Surgery

- A staged procedure avoids the disadvantages of simultaneous cataract PPV surgery.
- However, cataract surgery after PPV may also be challenging for cataract surgeons. Lack of vitreous support may result in anterior chamber fluctuation that may be severe in lens-iris diaphragm retropulsion syndrome (LIDRS). Furthermore, direct zonular or crystalline lens damage (lens touch) may occur during PPV, thereby increasing the risk of zonular dialysis in subsequent cataract surgery by 2-fold [4]. There is also added cost of another surgery, and there may be delayed visual rehabilitation.

6 Our Approach

- We prefer to keep PPV surgery simple and only remove the crystalline lens if there is significant lens opacity that will interfere with visualization during surgery.
- Nevertheless, we may perform combined phacoemulsification with PPV in two other scenarios:
  - Anterior PVR and cyclitic membrane that requires anterior access and dissection.
  - Vitreous hemorrhage with a significant dusting of the anterior hyaloid behind the lens capsule.
- These two situations are difficult to manage in phakic eyes without removing the lens. It is much easier if this is dealt with from the outset before inadvertent lens trauma and posterior capsular injury.

7 Surgical Considerations for Phacoemulsification Surgery in Combined Cataract Pars Plana Vitrectomy

7.1 Preoperatively

- The presence and the density of cataracts must be carefully assessed before surgery, and a decision made as to whether combined surgery or only PPV is to be performed accordingly.
- For IOL power calculation, similar to other cataract cases, it is essential to consider the refraction of the other eye, particularly in high myopic patients, to avoid postoperative intolerable anisometropia of more than two diopters. Caution is also needed when calculating IOL power in eyes with a coexisting macula off retinal detachment, as the axial length will be false. In this case, calculations are usually based on the axial length of the fellow eye.
- There is evidence of systematic slight myopic shift induced in phacovitrectomy eyes. However, newer formula such as the Kane formula, has been found to have the highest percentage of eyes within 0.25 diopters of postoperative spherical equivalence in eyes that have undergone phacovitrectomy [3, 4]. Additionally, modern formulas such Barrett UII, Hill-RBF, and Kane have been more accurate than older formulas in silicone-filled eyes [8, 9]. In combined cataract and epiretinal membrane (ERM) PPV surgery, it is possible that the myopic shift is due to that available A scan technology utilizes the anterior ERM peak and not the retinal pigment epithelium (RPE) peak in its calculations. Careful interrogation of the A scans to choose the correct posterior RPE peak, can mitigate this error [10].
- In SO-filled eyes, the axial length measurement by ultrasound biometry will be falsely long because silicone oil attenuates the speed of the ultrasound. In these

cases, a compensating factor could be used, which depends on the silicone oil viscosity [11]. This will not be an issue for optical biometry if the vitreous media is set to "silicone oil."

- It is best to have IOL calculations for any phakic patient undergoing PPV, particularly in eyes where PPV surgery is expected to be prolonged, and the lens can become cloudy during surgery.
- We routinely use hydrophobic acrylic lenses. Hydrophobic acrylic IOLs are preferred over silicone lenses with less risk of posterior capsule opacification. Silicone IOLs can also interfere with the fundus view during vitrectomy. If the posterior capsule is opened, there is a higher chance of droplets of residual infusion fluid remaining on the posterior surface of the IOL without coalescing during the fluid air exchange step. Furthermore, if silicone oil is used, the risk of oil droplets adhering to the surface of the silicone IOLs, preventing visualization of the fundus, is many folds higher as compared to acrylic IOLs. Optically advanced IOLs (i.e., multifocal IOLs) should also be avoided or used with extreme caution due to the high risk of IOL tilt and decentration in vitrectomized eyes. Multifocal IOL may also impair crisp fundus visualization during future PPV surgery [12].

7.2   Intraoperatively (Video 2)

- Place the vitrectomy trocars at the outset of the surgery before making the phacoemulsification wounds while the eye is still firm. Trocar placement after cataract extraction is more difficult as the globe is softer and scleral pressure may cause corneal wound leakage, even when the wound is sutured.
- When performing combined surgery, we opt for a slightly smaller capsulorhexis, about 5 mm, to better secure the IOL and decrease the possible decentration in combined surgery, particularly when using gas or SO tamponade. Unless the cataract is soft in a young patient, it is best to perform in-the-bag phacoemulsification utilizing the surgeon's preferred technique, away from the corneal endothelium.
- After complete cataract extraction, we prefer to implant the IOL before PPV. Hydrophobic acrylic IOL with anterior haptic angulation is preferred, and silicone IOLs should be avoided. We remove the ophthalmic viscoelastic device (OVD) from the anterior chamber before starting PPV and after IOL placement.
- If the pupil becomes smaller during cataract surgery, we find intracameral epinephrine 0.025%/lidocaine 0.75% (epi-Shugarcaine) very helpful in dilating the pupil. In this instance, we also recommend leaving the OVD until after the PPV to avoid further pupil miosis. While removing the OVD by irrigation/aspiration after finishing the PPV, it is important to do this while the vitreous cavity is filled with balanced salt solution (BSS) or perfluorocarbon liquid (PFCL) not air, and to switch off the posterior segment infusion to avoid shallowing of the anterior chamber from backpressure.

- We defer wound hydration till after the PPV to avoid corneal edema that may hinder the retinal view during PPV. We do not usually suture the corneal wound; a well-constructed corneal incision should not leak during pars plana infusion. However, if the wound is short, or if the anterior chamber continues to be shallow during PPV, we will not hesitate to suture the intracorneal path of the wound is using an interrupted 10/0 nylon or Vicryl suture. Some surgeons may prefer to place a corneal suture in all cases. This suture may be removed at the closing of surgery when the wound is hydrated.
- Finally, if air or gas tamponade is used, we favor placing a bubble of air in the anterior chamber to balance the pressure on the IOL from the gas in the vitreous cavity and decrease the risk of IOL decentration (Fig. 3) [13].

7.3   Chandelier-Assisted Cataract Surgery in the Setting of Vitreous Hemorrhage

- Cataract surgery in the setting of dense vitreous hemorrhage is challenging because of the absence of the red reflex. Staining the anterior capsule with trypan blue helps perform the capsulorrhexis somewhat, but the visualization problem remains during the subsequent steps of lens removal. Retroillumination using a chandelier is helpful in these cases to visualize the lens structures [14] (Video 3). Holding an endoilluminator light pipe is also an option that spares the added expense of a chandelier light. The light is only held during the capsulorrhexis and cortical removal. Nuclear removal is usually accomplished via phaco chop, which does not rely on visualization of the red reflex. The direction of the light can be reintroduced after the nuclear removal and directed more anteriorly to

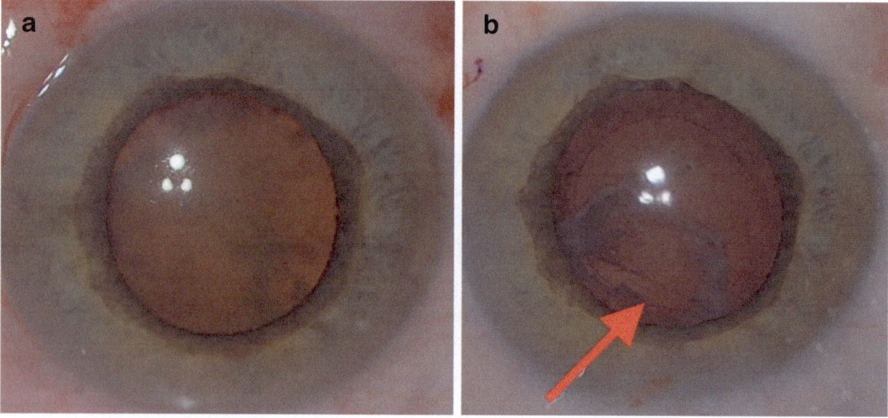

Fig. 2 Crystalline lens touch post-vitrectomy. Patient with significant posterior subcapsular cataract after vitrectomy (**a**). After lens removal, a linear capsular opening (arrow) could be seen along the path of the vitrectomy probe, with a surrounding posterior capsular plaque (**b**)

Fig. 3 Decentered posterior chamber intraocular lens with pupillary capture of the optic after combined phacovitrectomy with the use of gas tamponade

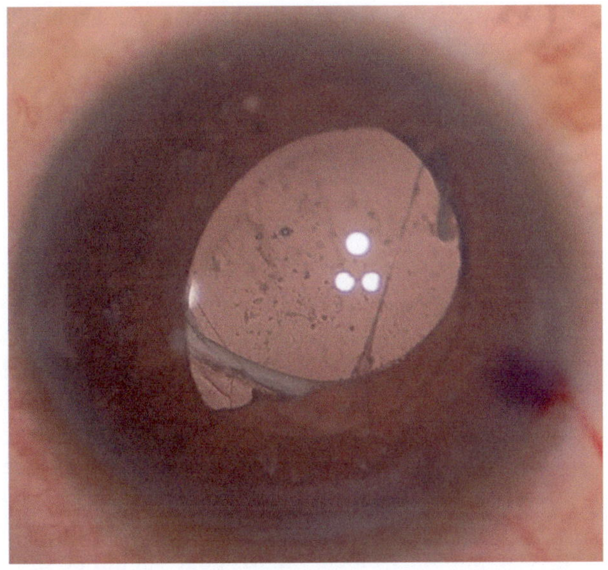

help visualize the lens cortex while it is aspirated. The surgeon must be mindful of the light pipe position while using this technique; it needs only to enter slightly inside the trocar port to avoid inadvertent lens or retina touch.

8   Surgical Considerations for Post-Vitrectomy Cataract Surgery

8.1   *Preoperatively*

- Before deciding to proceed with cataract extraction, surgeons should review the ocular history and evaluate the density of the cataract to determine if the diminution of vision is because of the cataract only or the preexisting retinal condition. This is very important for patient counseling.
- Careful slit lamp and fundus examination are necessary to identify any zonular instability, frank phacodonesis, or occult posterior capsular rupture before surgery including linear marks on the posterior surface of the lens or fibrotic patches (Fig. 2a). Rapid progression of cataracts shortly after PPV and the presence of persistent uveitis in the anterior chamber may be an indicator of posterior capsular injury (Fig. 2b).
- A poorly dilated pupil is common in diabetics, uveitic patients, and patients with floppy iris syndrome. Performing phacoemulsification in a small pupil is challenging, making capsulorrhexis and cataract extraction technically more difficult. In addition, it increases the risk of iris and posterior capsular injuries. Surgeons should be prepared to use iris hooks or ring expansion rings as needed.

- It is important to determine if there is a coexisting fundus pathology that needs to be addressed during the same setting after cataract extraction, such as SO removal or ERM peeling. In case of coexisting cystoid macular edema (CME), intravitreal steroids can be injected before or at the time of cataract extraction.

8.2 *Intraoperatively*

- Posterior capsular rupture and dropped lens fragment should be anticipated in cases of preexisting capsular injury from prior vitrectomy. These cases are best handled by a surgeon who can perform both cataract and retina surgery or by an anterior segment surgeon in collaboration with a retina specialist.
- Because the anterior chamber depth may be exaggerated in vitrectomized eyes with the lack of vitreous support, it is best to place appropriate length corneal incisions. A long corneal tunnel may result in placing the instruments more vertically, distorting the cornea and making the surgery more difficult. In the case of reverse pupillary block, the iris edge should be lifted off the anterior capsule to allow fluid equilibrium between the anterior and posterior chambers.
- Capsulorrhexis may be more challenging because of the exaggerated anterior chamber depth. One sign of occult zonular dialysis is difficulty initiating the capsulorhexis tear with a backward movement of the lens due to a lack of zonular counterpressure or lens movement during the progress of the capsulorhexis.
- Hydrodissection is better avoided if there is concern from preoperative examination about possible posterior lens trauma/touch. Instead, hydrodelineation and viscodissection are performed, and nuclear removal proceeds via a non-rotational technique.
- Excessive movement of the lens iris diaphragm with fluctuation in the anterior chamber depth is common in vitrectomized eyes, which increases the risk of intraoperative aqueous misdirection syndrome, pupillary constriction, and postoperative inflammation. Maintaining fluid equilibrium and a stable anterior chamber is necessary to avoid these complications. Surgical instruments should be handled gently and not be removed suddenly during the surgery. Hydration of the corneal incision before final OVD aspiration reduces the risk of anterior chamber collapse.
- Chopping techniques might be best suited for these cases because of exaggerated anterior chamber depth.
- The surgeon should be prepared for the possibility of using a capsular tension ring or segment in case of significant zonular compromise. We found a higher rate of zonular dialysis (not PCR) in post-vitrectomy cataract surgery in a large cataract surgery series [4]. The rate of PCR is high in eyes with previous lens touch during PPV [6].
- Intravitreal injections, for example, for treating coexisting CME, are best placed before removing OVD with the eye being firm to avoid inadvertent retinal injury.

8.3 *Cataract Surgery in Silicone Oil-Filled Eyes*

- For these cases, we usually remove the cataract first then proceed with SO removal.
- We insert all trocars before starting the cataract surgery similar to how we manage cases with combined cataract vitrectomy surgery.
- Sometimes, emulsified silicone floats in the anterior chamber obscuring the visualization. Through the corneal incisions, emulsified silicone in the anterior chamber can be removed with irrigation-aspiration, the phacoemulsification tip or excahnged with OVD depending on the stage of the surgery.
- After cataract extraction, we create a posterior capsulorrhexis to use for removing the SO. A SO extractor using a 20-g cannula is inserted through the main corneal incision draining SO through the posterior capsulorhexis. This technique is very efficient, particularly for removing high-viscosity SO, and lends itself well to small gauge vitrectomy, avoiding the need for a large sclerotomy to remove the SO.
- After removing the SO from the vitreous cavity, the retina is examined with the endoillumination to see if any additional surgical step is needed, such as ERM peeling or laser.
- At the end, a one-piece acrylic IOL is inserted in the capsular bag and the case is closed.
- An alternative technique is to finish the cataract surgery, place the IOL in the capsular bag, and then remove the SO through a superior 23-g or 20-g sclerotomy.

Key Points
- In the absence of significant cataract, we perform combined surgery only in anterior PVR or in the case of vitreous hemorrhage with a significant dusting of the anterior hyaloid.
- In the combined approach, a slightly smaller capsulorhexis is recommended to secure the IOL and reduce the risk of its decentration, especially if gas tamponade is to be used.
- Retinal condition may limit visual outcomes of cataract extraction post-PPV, and patient counseling is essential.
- There is an increased risk of zonular dialysis in post-vitrectomy cataract surgery compared to routine cataract surgery by twofold (1.3% vs. 0.6%).

References

1. Harlan JB Jr, Lee ET, Jensen PS, de Juan E Jr. Effect of humidity on posterior lens opacification during fluid-air exchange. Arch Ophthalmol. 1999;117:802–4.
2. Matsui E, Matsushima H, Mukai K, Senoo T. Mechanism of gas cataract is mainly related with oxidation. Invest Ophthalmol Vis Sci. 2008;49:2281.

3. Jackson TL, Donachie PHJ, Sparrow JM, Johnston RL. United Kingdom National Ophthalmology Database Study of vitreoretinal surgery: report 1; case mix, complications, and cataract. Eye (Basingstoke). 2013;27:27.
4. Soliman MK, Hardin JS, Jawed F, et al. A database study of visual outcomes and intraoperative complications of Postvitrectomy cataract surgery. Ophthalmology. 2018;125:1683.
5. Faramawi MF, Delhey LM, Chancellor JR, Sallam AB. The Influence of Diabetes Status on the Rate of Cataract Surgery Following Pars Plana Vitrectomy. Ophthalmology Retina. 2020;4(5):486–93.
6. Elhousseini Z, Lee E, Williamson TH. Incidence of lens touch during pars plana vitrectomy and outcomes from subsequent cataract surgery. Retina. 2016;36(4):825–9.
7. Elhusseiny AM, Soliman MK, Shakarchi AF, Fouad YA, Yang YC, Sallam AB. Visual outcomes and complications of combined vs sequential cataract surgery and pars plana vitrectomy: multicenter database study Journal of Cataract and Refractive Surgery. 2023;49(2):142–47.
8. Hipólito-Fernandes D, Elisa Luís M, Maleita D, et al. Intraocular lens power calculation formulas accuracy in combined phacovitrectomy: An 8-formulas comparison study. Int J Retina Vitreous. 2021;7:1–8.
9. Lwowski C, Miraka K, Müller M, et al. IOL calculation using eight formulas in silicone oil filled eyes undergoing silicone oil removal and phacoemulsification after retinal detachment. Am J Ophthalmol. 2022;0:166.
10. Wilson Heriot. Postoperative refractive outcomes in eyes undergoing combined phacovitrectomy surgery for Epiretinal Membrane. Pressentation in European Vitreoeretinal Society Meeting, August 2023, Turkey.
11. Murray DC, Durrani OM, Good P, et al. Biometry of the silicone oil-filled eye: II. Eye (Lond). 2002;16:727–30.
12. Tan X, Liu Z, Chen X, et al. Characteristics and risk factors of intraocular lens tilt and Decentration of phacoemulsification after pars plana vitrectomy. Transl Vis Sci Technol. 2021;10:10.
13. Tye A, Klufas MA, McCannel CA, McCannel TA. Intracameral air in phacovitrectomy for maintaining intraocular lens position. Retina. 2017;37(6):1207–8.
14. Bilgin O, Kayikcioglu. Chandelier retroillumination-assisted cataract surgery during vitrectomy Eye. 2016;30(8):1123–5.

Appendix: Rates and Numbers

Joseph H. Toma and Hudson de Carvalho Nakamura

Anatomy

- *Equator of the eye:*

  - From outside: 9–12 mm from the limbus and 2–4 mm anterior to the vortex veins exit.
  - From inside: the site of vortex veins ampulla, just anterior to the second bifurcation of the retinal blood vessels.

- *Vitreous base:* extends 2 mm anterior and 2–3 mm posterior to the ora serrata.
- *Ora serrata:* 5.5 mm from the limbus nasally and 7 mm temporally.
- *Recti muscle insertion:* medial, inferior, lateral, and superior recti muscles are inserted 5.5 mm, 6.5 mm, 6.9 mm, and 7.7 mm from the limbus, respectively.
- *Thickness of the retina:* 2–4 mm at the posterior pole and 1–2 mm near the ora serrata.

Vitreoretinal Anesthesia

- *Local anesthesia:*

J. H. Toma
Ophthalmology, Faculty of Medicine-Ain Shams University, Cairo, Egypt
e-mail: OutputMedium="None">joseph.hany.toma@gmail.com

H. de Carvalho Nakamura
Department of Retina and Vitreous, The Hospital of The Eye Bank Foundation of Goias, Brazil, Goiânia, Goiás, Brazil
e-mail: hudson.nakamura@alumni.utoronto.ca

© The Editor(s) (if applicable) and The Author(s), under exclusive license to Springer Nature Switzerland AG 2024
A. B. Sallam et al. (eds.), *Practical Manual of Vitreoretinal Surgery*,
https://doi.org/10.1007/978-3-031-47827-7

- Retrobulbar block: 5 mL anesthetic injected inside the muscle cone after penetrating the orbital septum; the needle is redirected 30–45° superonasally and advanced into the intraconal space.
- Peribulbar block: 10 mL anesthetic injected outside the muscle cone; the needle is advanced parallel to the orbital floor all through.

Basic Vitrectomy

- *Trocars insertion*: 3.5 (in pseudophakic and aphakic eyes) to 4 mm (in phakic eyes) from the limbus.
- *Entry site retinal tears incidence*: <1% in small-gauge vitrectomy vs. 10% in 20-g with no trocars.

Vitreous Substitutes

	Air/gas	PFCL	SO	Water
Specific gravity (g/ml)	0.001	1.7–2	0.97	1
Viscosity (mPas)	0.018	24–48	1000–5000	1
Interfacial tension against water (mN/m)	72 (highest)	50	40 (lowest)	NA
Refractive index	1	1.3	1.4	1.33

	Air	SF6	C3F8
Expansion (times original size)	NA	2	4
Time to maximum expansion (hours)	NA	24-48	72-96
Non-expansile concentration	NA	0.18	0.14
Longevity	5–7 days	1–2 weeks	6–8 weeks
Volume used in pneumatic retinopexy	1.2 mL	0.6 mL	0.3 mL

Vitreous Hemorrhage

- Risk of retinal tear with acute symptomatic posterior vitreous detachment (PVD): 7%.
- Risk of retinal tear with acute symptomatic PVD + vitreous hemorrhage or pigments: 70%.

Retinal Breaks and Pneumatic Retinopexy

- *Primary rhegmatogenous retinal detachment (RRD) incidence:* 1 per 10,000.
- *Risk of RRD with symptomatic horseshoe tear:* 50%, with laser retinopexy it decreases to 5%.
- *New breaks may develop after laser retinopexy:* in 5–15%.
- *Risk of RRD with symptomatic operculated tear:* 16%.
- *Risk of RRD with atrophic retinal hole(s):* 1–2%.
- *Risk of RRD after YAG posterior capsulotomy* 0.5%.
- *Risk of RRD after phacoemulsification surgery:* 1 per 1000.
- *Risk of RRD after phacoemulsification surgery with posterior capsule rupture (PCR):* 3%.
- *Risk of RRD after phacoemulsification surgery in high myopes:* 3%.
- *Fellow eye RRD general risk:* 10–15% (1% of RRD cases presents with bilateral RRD).

  - if fellow eye has a complete PVD: 3%,
  - if fellow eye has attached hyaloid: 8%,
  - if fellow eye has attached hyaloid then PVD occurs: 24% RRD risk and 18% retinal breaks without RD risk.

- *Peneumatic retinopexy (PnR) gas injection volume:* 0.6 mL SF6 or 0.3 mL C3F8.
- *Laser retinopexy chorioretinal adhesions:* start after 1 day and become adequate after 1 week.
- *Cryopexy chorioretinal adhesions:* start after 2 day and become adequate after 12 days.

Pars plana vitrectomy (PPV) in Primary RRD.

- *Advisable Timing for surgery in acute RRD:* within 24 h if macula ON and within 3–7 if macula OFF.
- *No detectable breaks preoperatively in RRD:* 5%.
- *Single surgery success rate in RRD:* 91.7% in scleral buckle, 83.1% in PPV, 81% in PnR.
- *Retinal displacement* 16% in scleral buckle, 45% in PPV, 7% in PnR.
- *Retained subfoveal fluid* 35% in scleral buckle, 10–15% in PPV and PnR.

Scleral Buckle

- *Encirclement buckle examples:* 41 band (3.5 mm width) or a narrower 240 band (2.5 mm width).

- *Sutures placement:*

  - Anterior limb of the anchoring suture: 4 mm behind the insertion of the recti muscles.
  - Posterior limb is usually placed 1 mm behind the posterior edge of the band.

- *Segmental 5 mm scleral buckle examples:* 510 (flat), 505 (round), and 506 (oval).
- *Separation of suture bites in segmental buckle:* 1.5 mm × width of buckle, i.e., for a 5 mm buckle, we would separate the suture bites by 7.5 mm.

Giant Retinal Tear (GRT)

- *GRT:* ≥3 clock hours.
- *GRT detachment:* 1.5% of all RRD cases.
- *Single surgery success rate in GRT detachment:* 80%.

Proliferative Vitreoretinopathy (PVR)

- *PVR incidence:* 5.1–11.7% in general and 10% after scleral buckle vs. 15% in PPV.
- *Visual outcome after PVR surgery:* 11–25% only achieving VA ≥ 20/100.
- *Anatomical (retinal reattachment) success rate after PVR surgery:* 75%.

Retinoschisis

- *Incidence of degenerative retinoschisis; 2% in adults.*
- Schisis *RRD in degenerative retinoschisis:* 6%.
- *Progressive RRD in degenerative retinoschisis:* <1%.
- *Single surgery success rate in progressive retinoschisis detachment:* 70%.

Epiretinal Membrane (ERM)

- *Visual outcome after ERM peel:* 80% of patients have visual improvement of about 2–3 Snellen lines with significant early improvement of distortion, 40% have visual acuity of ≥20/40 after 3–6 months.
- *ERM recurrence post peel:* 10%, 5% requires reoperation.

Lamellar Macular Hole (LMH)

- *Prevalence of LMH in the general population ranges from 1.1 to 3.6%.*
- *Risk of LMH changing to full thickness macular hole (FTMH): 10% in 5 years.*
- *Visual outcome after LMH surgery is not as robust as in FTMH. Discordant outcomes have been reported ranging from no vision improvement to a 2–3 Snellen line gain.*
- *Risk of post-PPV surgery, LMH changing to FTMH in the degenrative type: 10%.*

Macular Hole Surgery

Annual incidence of idiopathic FTMH: 4–8.7 per 100,000.

- *Fellow eye MH:* 10% risk, higher up to 40% with VMT.
- *MH stages:*

Stage	Size	Spontaneous closure
1	Impending hole	50%
2	<400 microns and VMT	11%
3	>400 microns and VMT	3%
4	>400 microns and PVD	

- *PPV with ILM peel success rates:*

  - 90% in idiopathic MH with minimal linear diameter of 400–649 microns.
  - 76% with minimal linear diameter of >650 microns.
  - <50% in chronic holes more than 1 year.
  - 100% in axial length < 26 mm—91% in axial length 26–29.9 mm and 0% with axial length > 30 mm.

Optic Disc Pit

- *Optic disc pit incidence:* 1 in 10,000.
- *Optic disc pit maculopathy:* 25–75% of optic disc pit cases.
- *PPV in optic disc pit maculopathy success rate:* 60% improvement of at least 1 Snellen line VA.

Myopic Traction Maculopathy (MTM)

- *High myopia:* Spherical equivalent >6D and/or axial length > 26 mm.
- *MTM incidence in high myopes:* 9–34%.

Diabetic Delamination Surgery

- *Anti-VEGF injection before PPV for diabetic delamination:* 2–3 days before surgery (fibrous component increases after 10 days).
- *Diabetic delamination PPV success rate:* Visual success (≥ 3 Snellen lines gain) in 60% of eyes, and visual loss in 15%, and 15% of eyes required further PPV.
- *Postoperative vitreous cavity hemorrhage after diabetic PPV:* 50%–65% in early postoperative period (90% of these will resolve on their own in the first month).

Surgery for Sickle Cell Retinopathy

- *Anterior chamber wash in hyphema complicating sickle cell retinopathy:* intraocular pressure (IOP) > 24 mmHg for 24 h, or any IOP >30 mmHg.
- *Outcome of PPV in tractional retinal detachment complicating sickle cell retinopathy:* 80% final re-attachment rate.
- *Rate of iatrogenic retinal breaks during PPV in sickle cell retinopathy cases with retinal detachment:* 12–30%.

Suprachoroidal Hemorrhage (SCH)

- *Incidence of SCH in ophthalmic surgeries:* 0.06–1.9%.
- *Visual outcomes in SCH:* 60% of patients with phacoemulsification-related SCH attained a vision of >20/200.

Submacular Hemorrhage

- *Natural course of submacular hemorrhage:* loss of approximately ≥3 lines of vision and poor vision of <20/200 in most cases.
- *Pneumatic displacement and PPV offer similar outcomes for submacular hemorrhage.*

Uveal Effusion Syndrome (UES)

- *Very rare, 1 in 10 million.*
- *Axial length in UES:* type 1 -- > nanophthalmic eye (axial length < 19 mm) and type 2 -- > normal axial length (average 21 mm).
- UES resolves with one scleral surgery: 85%.

Glaucoma and Vitreoretinal Surgery

- PPV, even without the use of tamponade, may increase the risk of subsequent primary open-angle glaucoma compared to the general population by nearly 10x (9% vs 1%).
- *Rate of chronic elevated IOP with silicon oil tamponade*: 10% of eyes after 36 months.

Posterior Segment Complications of Cataract Surgery

- *Ocular perforation with local anesthesia*: Retrobulbar anesthesia 1 in 10,000 and peribulbar anesthesia 1 in 16,000.
- *Visual outcomes after ocular perforation management*: >50% of eyes achieved acuity ≥20/80 while 25% between 20/120 and 20/200.

Vitreoretinal Surgery in Uveitis

- Yield of vitreous culture in bacterial endophthalmitis: 50%.
- Yield of vitreous culture in fungal endophthalmitis: 50%.
- Yield of viral PCR from vitreous or aqueous: >90%.
- Yield of Toxoplasma PCR: 65%.
- Yield of Lymphoma flow/immunohistochemistry: 65%.

Endophthalmitis

- *Postoperative endophthalmitis incidence:*
    - Cataract surgery: 0.04%. Increased incidence by 1.5-fold if patient is diabetic, 3-fold if cataract surgery is combined with PPV or in eyes that had previous PPV, and 7-fold if PCR occured.
    - PPV: 0.05–0.157%
    - Intravitreal Injection: 0.017–0.025%.
    - Keratoprosthesis: 5% and can present late and without pain.
    - Posttraumatic endophthalmitis: 3% and higher (30%) with intraocular foreign body, wounds contaminated with organic lens matter and lens capsule disruption.

- *Dose of intravitreal injections in endophthalmitis:*

  - Antibiotics: Vancomycin 1–2 mg in 0.1 mL and Ceftazidime 2.25 mg in 0.1 mL.
  - Corticosteroids: Dexamethasone 0.4 mg in 0.1 mL.

Pediatric Vitreoretinal Surgery

- *Sclerotomies site in newborns* till 6 months of age: 1.5 mm from limbus.
- *Anatomical success rates in retinopathy of prematurity (ROP) surgery*: 90% for stage 4A, 45% for stage 4B, and 14% for stage 5.
- *Coats disease prognosis*: poor visual outcome (20/200 or worse) in 53% with stage 2, 74% with stage 3, and 100% of stages 4 and 5 and 16% of eyes with Coats disease are enucleated because of blind and painful eye.

Retinal and Choroidal Tumors

- *Choroidal nevus prevalence:* 8% of general population.
- *The 5-year malignant transformation risk of choroidal nevus:* 1% if no risk factors present, 11% with 1 factor, 22% with 2 factors, 34% with 3 factors, 51% with 4 factors, and 55% with 5 factors.
- *Choroidal melanoma incidence:* 0.2 to 8.6 per million.
- *Retinoblastoma incidence*: 1 in every 14,000–20,000.

Cataract Extraction During or After PPV

- *Cataract surgery rate after PPV*: 50% in 1 year and 85% in 5 years.
- *Crystalline lens touch during PPV*: 4% and 10% of those have PCR during subsequent cataract surgery.
- *Pseudophakic cystoid macular edema rates (CME) rates:*

  - Uncomplicated phacoemulsification surgery: 1%.
  - Diabetic patients, no retinopathy: 2%.
  - NPDR: 3–8%.
  - PDR: 10%.
  - Complicated phacoemulsification with PCR: 3%.
  - Prior uveitis, retinal vein occlusion, retinal detachment repair, and epiretinal membrane: 3–6%.
  - Fellow eye CME among those with first-eye CME: 11%.

Index

© The Editor(s) (if applicable) and The Author(s), under exclusive license to   469
Springer Nature Switzerland AG 2024
A. B. Sallam et al. (eds.), *Practical Manual of Vitreoretinal Surgery*,
https://doi.org/10.1007/978-3-031-47827-7

Correction to: Scleral Buckle Surgery

Ahmed Roshdy Alagorie, Ahmed B. Sallam, and Sherif A. Dabour

Correction to:
Chapter 9 in: A. B. Sallam et al. (eds.),
Practical Manual of Vitreoretinal Surgery,
https://doi.org/10.1007/978-3-031-47827-7_9

The original version of Chapter 9 was inadvertently published with the below errors:

1. The reference to "blue arrow" has been corrected to "green arrow" for the caption of Fig. 5 on page 118.
2. The value 721,813 has been reformatted to 721/813 on page 126.

The updated version of this chapter can be found at https://doi.org/10.1007/978-3-031-47827-7_9

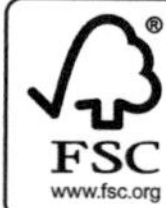

MIX
Papier aus verantwortungsvollen Quellen
Paper from responsible sources
FSC® C105338

If you have any concerns about our products,
you can contact us on
ProductSafety@springernature.com

In case Publisher is established outside the EU,
the EU authorized representative is:
Springer Nature Customer Service Center GmbH
Europaplatz 3, 69115 Heidelberg, Germany

Printed by Libri Plureos GmbH
in Hamburg, Germany